THE SENSITIVE NERVOUS SYSTEM

ACKNOWLEDGEMENTS

First, I wish to acknowledge those who have researched any aspect of neurodynamics.

I wish to thank the behind the scenes noigroup team for their constant support and help: Peter Barrett, Carolyn Berryman, Melissa Cadzow, Megan Dalton, Rob Dick, Dinah Edwards, Siri Kennedy, Frank Navacchi, Lynne Potts, Michael Shacklock, Helen Slater and Peter Vroom.

Thanks to Jim Matheson for his chapter on neurodynamics and research.

Thanks to Michel Coppieters for his advice and discussion on research issues.

To the artwork team, thanks to: Areti Boyaci for the line drawings, Cecilia Gunnarsson for the cover artwork, Catherine Gasmier for photography and Kirsten Britcher for layout and design.

Thanks to Sonia Russo and Juliet Gore for proof reading.

Thanks to Ted Huber and Colin Feneley for the drinks and neurally orientated discussions.

To Jan Heath and the librarians at the University of South Australia, thanks: You run the most cheerful and helpful library on the planet.

But I am keeping most of my thanks for Juliet who was really the one who got it done.

David Butler

September 2000, Adelaide.

THE SENSITIVE NERVOUS SYSTEM

DAVID S BUTLER, B PHTY, GDAMT, M APP SC, PT
With a contribution by James Matheson, MS, PT, CSCS
Artwork by Areti Boyaci

Noigroup Publications, Adelaide, Australia, 2000
PO Box 41 Unley DC 5061 Australia.

NOTE TO READERS

Although I would prefer to write in gender neutral language in this book, I was unable to do so. For clarity of explanations, ease of reading and because I am male and my model for this book is female, I have used the masculine gender pronoun to refer to the therapist and the feminine to refer to the patient.

Published by Noigroup Publications for NOI Australasia, Pty Ltd.

Printed and bound in Australia by Griffin Press.

Layout Design by Kirsten Britcher.

Noigroup Publications,
NOI Australasia Pty Ltd, PO Box 41 Unley DC, 5061 Australia.
www.noigroup.com
Ph/fax +61 (0)8 8271 8147

Butler, David S.
The Sensitive Nervous System
First reprint 2001
Includes index

ISBN 0 646 40251 X

National Library of Australia
A catalogue record for this book is available from the National Library of Australia.

State Library of South Australia
A catalogue record for this book is available from the State Library of South Australia.

CONTENTS

PREFACE

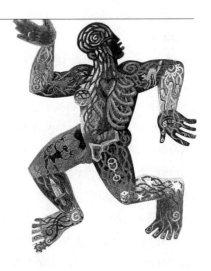

PREFACE

"There is a crack, a crack in everything; that's how the light gets in".

Leonard Cohen (1992)

In 1990, my publisher had to wrench "Mobilisation of the Nervous System" away from me. I knew it wasn't complete and I knew the pressures and forces for change in manual therapy practice were growing and uniting. I was beginning to realise the potential difficulties of encouraging examination of another mobile tissue without an adequately sophisticated clinical framework to handle it.

"Mobilisation of the Nervous System" is very much on a structural and mechanical level. A multi-tissue approach to management was proposed with the nervous system added to muscle joint and fascia as a mobile tissue to examine. Altered slump tests and straight leg raises were explained in terms of neurobiomechanics, innervated connective tissues and blood flow to nerves. A management strategy aimed at restoring physical health of the nervous system was proposed. "The Sensitive Nervous System" updates and revolutionises this framework. Pain states can be dissected much further than ever before. In particular, manual therapists are urged to begin to consider the targets of their therapy on a synaptic and molecular level and to evaluate on a framework of understanding biological, societal and psychological inputs to nervous system processing. "The Sensitive Nervous System" is written for anyone who uses movement as part of therapy.

We know so much more now about the nervous system; its plasticity, complexity and ability to represent our bodies, environments and survival needs within itself. However, this must occur within a structure which continually glides and slides and stretches and angulates as it adapts to the movements it orchestrates. In this book, "The Sensitive Nervous System" I wish to present the story of "neurodynamics" - the physical and related physiological abilities of the nervous system, again. This time, I will set it in a framework of as much broader scientific evidence as possible using neurobiology, available clinical research, and in particular, uncorrupted clinical reasoning science which allows due attention to experience and clinical creativity. Evidence means little if we cannot get it to the clinic.

David Butler

Adelaide, September 2000.

CHAPTER 1

INTRODUCTION –
PAINTING ON A BIGGER CANVAS

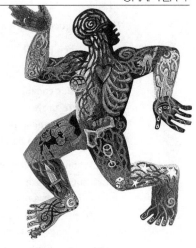

INTRODUCTION

Sometimes, to be able to truly and objectively look at what we do, it is necessary to view it from a different vantage point - to see things from above and to see ourselves as part of a bigger picture. History is one way to do this. In figure 1.1 I have shown my perspective on the origins, development and what appears to be the beginning of a merging of the major systems of western orthodox manual therapy. This representation will hopefully create discussion and argument, but its main purpose it to provide readers with a new vantage point from which to view the movement based therapies, to contemplate the future and to create the "big picture" framework for the material in this book.

SOME HISTORY

Manual therapy has been around for centuries. The dominant movement based orthodox therapy approaches of today arose from the integration of "bone setting" techniques by medical and non-medical practitioners, the work of Mennell and Cyriax, the integration of some chiropractic and osteopathic techniques and the skills and perceptions of individual clinicians.

Joint manipulation was first taught to physiotherapy students in 1916 at St. Thomas' Hospital in London, first by Mennell and then later by Cyriax. Chiropractic and osteopathy have a slightly longer history, over 100 years in the case of chiropractic and a little shorter in the case of osteopathy. The first osteopathy school opened in Missouri in 1892 and chiropractic began formal education at about the same time (Schiotz and Cyriax 1975). The first edition of the osteopath Stoddard's classic text, often used in manual therapy, appeared in 1962. From Mennell/Cyriax and osteopathy, and individual insight and expertise, arose the Norwegian based approach of Kaltenborn/Evjenth. This biomechanical, joint based approach spread through much of Europe and to North America, where it was carried on by Lamb and Paris among others, adding muscle assessment and management skills along the way. The Maitland/Grieve system arose a few years later. This concept was Australian/English originally before spreading to many parts of the world such as California, Switzerland and South Africa. This too was a joint based approach derived from Cyriax and others, but also Maitland's unique clinical approach. Maitland's signs and symptoms approach was neatly balanced by Grieve's methodical attention to pathology. Some years later, the McKenzie approach also spawned off Cyriax and others and McKenzie's careful clinical observations. This approach initially focused on clinical classifications of disc damage with a "hands off" management system which was novel at the time.

Exercise therapy has always been a part of manual therapy, although passive manual therapies came to dominate through the nineteen seventies and nineteen eighties and are only now being challenged to some degree. In much of Europe and elsewhere there were and still are varieties of non-specific exercise therapies in the form of gymnastics, aerobics, yoga and fitness programmes. In more recent years, specific exercise therapies were developed. The medical exercise group in Norway, and the Janda and Lewit concepts are examples. In later years, this specificity in exercise prescription was carried on by Sahrmann, McConnell, Jull and Hodges among others.

For much of the past 50 years, there have been manual therapy concepts that have dealt with the rehabilitation of the severely neurologically injured, such as patients with strokes, head

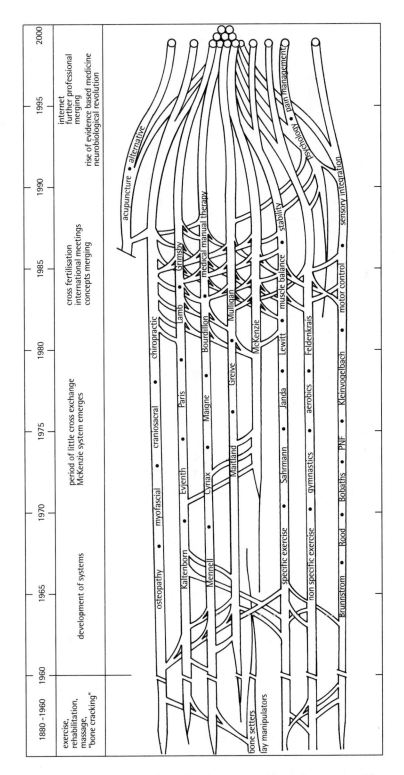

1.1   A broad historical overview of the origins, development and future of western manual therapy concepts

injuries and neurological diseases. These concepts such as Bobath and Proprioceptive Neuromuscular Facilitation (PNF), have existed and grown almost completely separate to the more orthopaedically biased manual therapies. In retrospect this is both remarkable and tragic; both groups need something of the skills of the other. Our patients are ultimately all neurological, although at different extremes of the injury spectrum and we are all eventually going to meet at the brain.

By the mid 60s (Fig. 1.1), once systems became established, a period of little cross exchange and isolationism ensued. This was perhaps assisted in part by the fact that the Norwegian and Australian systems were at either end of the earth. Groups may even have been suspicious of each other, and early IFOMT (International Federation of Orthopedic Manual Therapists) meetings were reportedly testy. The first meeting was in 1973, and the organisation was well established by the1984 Vancouver and 1988 Cambridge meetings. During this time significant cross fertilisation and international standardisation began. This cross fertilisation period was assisted by greater international travel, a growing awareness of the limitations of individual concepts and more international meetings. Although a significant sharing of ideas occurred through the 80s, the groups still kept their differences and identities, as much for political purposes as anything. However it appears that in the 1990s, many of the approaches appear to be coming together and integrating. The forces of evidence based medicine, greater stakeholder power residing with those who pay, and a greater awareness of neurobiology and commonality in approaches have allowed and cajoled this.

Further merging occurred through the 1990s and still appears to be happening. The internet of course is the essential glue which is bringing diverse systems, concepts and people together. For example, we are now interested in and have immediate access to global studies and other countries' recommendations for the management of low back pain. An aware Australian therapist is likely to be interested in an epidemiological study which may be performed in a Norwegian village. There are many similarities in seminars given by progressive, evidence based and aware members of the McKenzie and Kaltenborn groups for example. Also noticeable is the integration of therapies and concepts which were once thought to be out of the scope of manual therapy, for example, psychological techniques, counselling, exercise physiology and acupuncture. During the latter part of the 1990's a pain management movement in physiotherapy has arisen, especially in the United Kingdom. There appears to be the beginnings of a return to rehabilitation principles which were essentially active exercise based movements and which were used prior to the rise of the manual therapy systems. Maybe the names of the pioneering teachers to whom we owe so much are beginning to go.

KEY POINTS FROM THE HISTORY

There are a number of key points that emerge from contemplation of figure 1.1. First, we are young. Orthodox manual therapy is little more than 2 generations old. It is therefore still likely to be a changeable profession as it settles, finds its place in health systems and undergoes definition. Second, there have been changes and they have occurred rapidly. Each decade has involved a significant distinguishing period, from the development of systems in the 60s to the period of little exchange in the 70s, to the cross fertilisation period of the mid 80s and the recent merging and drawing together period. Major changes will probably occur with greater frequency in future years, especially as the rapidly changing world of neurobiology, evidence based medicine and stakeholders other than clinicians shape professional behaviour.

Third, the approaches tend to rely on particular tissues, usually muscle or joint. These skills must be merged into a wider rehabilitation system. Fourth, readers could look at the figure and contemplate their own professional roots. Some practitioners move from concept to concept collecting a bag of disparate techniques and ideas. This is great if it can be held together in a clinical reasoning framework. Perhaps for others, the new techniques and the personalities behind the concepts have provided serial relief from the burnout which so frequently stalks the people based professions.

Finally, we should also consider figure 1.1 from a patient's viewpoint. A patient could rightfully ask whether there should be so many ways to treat a spinal pain. How do they know who is best? Each profession or group presumably has something different to offer and surely they all can't be correct. Somehow we need to extract what is common and beneficial from the various groups.

HISTORICAL REFLECTIONS – NEURODYNAMICS

A "neurodynamics" or "neural tension" approach is not mentioned in figure 1.1. The main protagonists for examining the physical health of the nervous system (Elvey 1986; Maitland 1986; Butler 1991) have never presented it as a concept that stands alone. The preferred approach has been that the physical health of the nervous system issues are integrated into existing neurological/orthopaedic assessment bases using a best clinical reasoning approach.

Neurodynamic testing is not that new or "way out". The practice of straight leg raise, even the slump test have been described for many years (see chapter 11). The upper limb neurodynamic test for the ulnar nerve (chapter 12) was superbly described in Germany by Bragard (1929). Much of the current neurodynamic work can be traced to Cyriax and concepts of dural pain and the clinical anecdotal work of Maitland. It should be self evident that we have been encouraging the nervous system to move for many years with muscle, joint and myofascial techniques, without being fully aware of all the tissues we were moving and the biological processes we were affecting.

Maitland began exploring the use of the slump test in the late 1970s. In 1979, Elvey introduced the brachial plexus tension test, also known as the upper limb neurodynamic test (ULNT). The driving force was simply clinicians seeking answers to what they encountered daily in their clinics. There is an almost universal use of the straight leg raise, passive neck flexion and prone knee bend tests as assessment tools in orthopaedics and neurology. However new tests such as slump and ULNT and the concept of using the tests as part of treatment have stayed predominantly in the manual therapy arena, with considerable interest from neurological rehabilitation and sports medicine. Neurodynamics has spread to all the other approaches illustrated in figure 1.1 in some way including chiropractic, osteopathy and some of the neurological rehabilitation approaches. The important thing is that it has been integrated and absorbed. Neurodynamics should be another force for the merging of concepts.

Neurodynamics became very popular in the 1880s under the term "nerve stretching" (Cavafy 1881; Symington 1882; Marshall 1883). However the patient selection and strength of technique would make any clinician shudder and it was a blessing that it passed into obscurity at that time. Has the neurodynamics of the last 20 years been a passing fad then? After all, there are lots of fads in medicine and physiotherapy. An experiment is not needed to expose many of them, just some good existing basic sciences, logic and time to think. Examples in physiotherapy are faradic foot baths, grade 1 mobilisations and laser. All professions have fads. They persist for a few years, are grabbed at by all with great enthusiasm, and some diehard enthusiasts usually persist. Hopefully the beneficial aspects of what was once a fad can be held onto and integrated into a bigger and better therapy. I propose that neurodynamics, rather than being a fad destined to the fate of the faradic footbath, is here to stay and it signifies a milestone in the maturing of our profession as it links movement, tissues and the entire nervous system.

We do need better physical tests (Waddell 1998) and we need bigger and better ideas and concepts to manage spinal pain (Deyo and Phillips 1996; Cherkin 1998). My task now is to present skilled physical evaluation and management of the nervous system and place it in a framework of best available basic and clinical science.

REFERENCES CHAPTER 1

Bragard K (1929) Die nervendehnung als diagnostisches prinzip ergibt eine reihe neuer nervenphenomene. Münchener Medizinische Wochenschrift 76: 1999-2003.

Butler DS (1991) Mobilisation of the Nervous System, Churchill Livingstone, Melbourne.

Cavafy J (1881) A case of sciatic nerve-stretching in locomotor ataxy: with remarks on the operation. The British Medical Journal Dec 17: 973-974.

Cherkin DC (1998) Primary care research on low back pain. Spine 23: 1997-2002.

Deyo RA & Phillips WR (1996) Low back pain. A primary care challenge. Spine 21: 2826-2832.

Elvey RL (1979) Brachial plexus tension tests and the pathoanatomical origin of arm pain. In: Idczak R (ed.) Aspects of Manipulative Therapy, Manipulative Physiotherapists Association of Australia, Melbourne.

Elvey RL (1986) Treatment of arm pain associated with abnormal brachial plexus tension. The Australian Journal of Physiotherapy 32: 225-230.

Maitland GD (1986) Vertebral Manipulation, 6th edn. Butterworths, London.

Marshall J (1883) Nerve-stretching for the relief or cure of pain. The British Medical Journal Dec 15: 1173-1179.

Schiotz EH & Cyriax J (1975) Manipulation Past and Present, Heinemann, London.

Symington J (1882) The physics of nerve-stretching. The British Medical Journal May, 27: 770-771.

Waddell G (1998) The Back Pain Revolution, Churchill Livingstone, Edinburgh.

CHAPTER 2

A BIRD'S EYE VIEW
OF THE NERVOUS SYSTEM

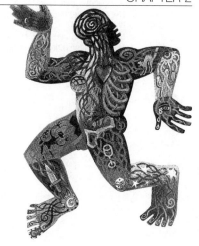

INTRODUCTION

THE ASSOCIATIVE, DISTRIBUTED, PLASTIC, REACTIVE AND REPRESENTATIONAL NERVOUS SYSTEM

THE COMPLEX SIGNALLING CAPABILITY OF THE CENTRAL NERVOUS SYSTEM

HARDWARE AND BIG NUMBERS
WETWARE
ION CHANNELS AND RECEPTORS
RESTING POTENTIAL, GENERATOR POTENTIAL AND THE SPIKE

PUTTING IT TOGETHER – THE NERVOUS SYSTEM AS A DISTRIBUTED SYSTEM

PARALLEL PROCESSING
BILATERAL PROCESSING
MOTOR CONTROL AREAS AS PART OF THE DISTRIBUTED PAIN EXPERIENCE
ACTIVE AND PASSIVE MOVEMENT

RECEPTIVE FIELDS AND HOMONCULI

CONCEPT OF RECEPTIVE FIELD
PLASTICITY IN THE CENTRAL NERVOUS SYSTEM
REPRESENTATIONS ARE DYNAMICALLY MAINTAINED
A VARIETY OF INPUTS CAN ALTER REPRESENTATIONS
THE MESSAGES OF PHANTOM LIMB PAIN
THE MECHANISMS BEHIND CORTICAL PLASTICITY

THE ULTIMATE REPRESENTATIONAL DEVICE

CLINICAL REPERCUSSIONS OF THE PLASTIC REPRESENTATIONAL NERVOUS SYSTEM

THE BIRD'S EYE VIEW AND THERAPY

MODELS TO ENGAGE PAIN AND SENSITIVITY

METAPHORS FOR THE NERVOUS SYSTEM

HOW DOES IT ACTUALLY WORK? – CONCLUSION

INTRODUCTION

There are many ways of viewing the nervous system. Most scientists take a tiny piece of it and spend their lives analysing it. The management strategies of many movement based clinicians often seem to focus at either end of the nervous system. In this chapter I wish to provide a functional bird's eye view of how the nervous system might work. There are no details, just a broad view. I hope that it helps to unite the numerous and disparate movement based professions. I also hope it begins to establish the new and better scientific construct for neurodynamics which Jim Matheson calls for in chapter 13. You can seek the neuroanatomy details elsewhere. The texts which I have found the most useful are the paperbacks, Barker and Barrassi (1999), Pritchard and Alloway (1999), and the texts, Kandel (1995), Zigmond et al. (1999), Bear (1996) and a neuroscience book written for therapists (Lundy-Ekman 1998).

I discuss pain a lot in this book, in particular pain related to movement. Pain is common to all branches of therapy, no matter which end of the nervous system your focus may be on. It has huge intra and extra-professional linking potential. And it provides direction. If you dissect out the components of pain, you will be taken to a basic sciences world ranging from gross anatomy to molecular biology, and to an understanding of the range and power of mixed societal, biological and psychological inputs to the pain experience. A big bird's eye view of pain may even engender a healthy re-look at professional definition (chapter 6).

But to conceptualise pain, I believe we all need an updated view of how the nervous system might work. Views about how it may work are changing rapidly. I have selected five descriptive terms to provide a viewpoint.

THE ASSOCIATIVE, DISTRIBUTED, PLASTIC, REACTIVE AND REPRESENTATIONAL NERVOUS SYSTEM

The nervous system has been traditionally presented as an input/ processing/output hierarchical structure. "In sensory and out motor" is how many of us were taught. This view is changing to one where the nervous system is an active constructor of activity, one that evolves and learns patterns of activity rather than computing it. As such, it is not a passive recipient of information, it can construct a pain experience (eg. Chapman et al. 1997; McCrone 1997).

Some modern descriptive nervous system terms would include associative, plastic, reactive, distributed and representational. It is associative in that the effects of any physical, psychological or environmental input will be determined by co-existing inputs and processing. By plastic, I mean individual neurones and neuronal networks are dynamically maintained and can change their function. It is reactive because it has the potential to consciously and subconsciously ascribe value to all inputs and react in a coordinated way via multiple systems such as the endocrine, motor and immune systems. The nervous system may well process inputs in terms of available response systems (Wall 1999a). The system is widely distributed. There is no one master pool of neurones for any one sensation or function. For example with noxious stimuli, brain areas such as the contralateral insular cortex, the cerebellar vermis, thalamus, the contralateral anterior cingulate and the premotor cortex will be active. These are all areas which have roles apart from pain perception (eg. Casey 1999). Consciousness, whatever that is, must also be a continuous feature of processing.

I think representational is the best overall descriptor. Through its transmitters, modulators and changing architectural hardware, the system has the ability to represent the anatomy and physiology of bodily parts and sensory, emotional and cognitive aspects of injuries and diseases in ways that allow maximal survival and comfort in society. The phantom limb phenomenon is a sharp reminder that it is not necessary to have a piece of anatomy for the nervous system to maintain a representation of that anatomy and its function.

Suddenly, physical examination and the neurodynamic tests such as the straight leg raise and the slump test can seem crude and far away. They don't have to be but we do need to link physical evaluation of the nervous system strategies with a modern view of nervous system function. A bird's eye view of the nervous system is necessary to better understand patients' movement patterns and responses to physical inputs. An ultimate goal is to quantify and qualify physical status in terms of the processing state of the nervous system. Importantly, big picture modern views of the nervous system strongly support bio-psycho-social management constructs. I have discussed some of the clinical consequences of the bird's eye view later in the chapter.

I want to try and build up a story of complexity and look at some of the critical parts of nervous system functioning which are relevant to movement based therapists.

THE COMPLEX SIGNALLING CAPABILITY OF THE NERVOUS SYSTEM

Hardware and wetware are rather jargonistic computer terms which were useful to explain how a computer worked. They can help with an understanding of the more complex nervous system as well. Let's look at the hardware first.

HARDWARE AND BIG NUMBERS

In the nervous system, a genetically determined blueprint of neural connection and pattern of activity (eg. reflexes) in those connections is present. Many of these connections are "ready to run" if used. Through life, enormous modification of this hardware occurs in response to various inputs.

The activities of one neurone resembles the entire central nervous system's behaviour. One neurone receives a variety of inputs at different places and times. The output of the neurone may be in the form of excitation through some pathways and inhibition through others. Its own chemical effects are signalled back to it. The neurone will maintain a chemical history of events that it has dealt with. This is just one neurone.

With electron microscopes, estimates of the hardware have been made. The adult brain contains in the order of 10^{11} neurones (about 100 billion) and these are interconnected by something in the order of 10^{14} synapses (Kandel et al. 1995; Swanson 1995). As Swanson notes, there is also a macrocircuitry about which little is known. There are about 10^3 "centres" or "nodes" connected by the order of 10^5 pathways. Neurones are outnumbered 10 to 1 by glial cells. Glial cells such as oligodendrocytes, Schwann cells and astrocytes provide structural and metabolic support for neurones and are also a source of immune signalling molecules.

Each neurone is studded with approximately 5000 spines on which other neurones connect (Fig. 2.1). Most of these connections will be part of feedback loops from neighbouring neurones. Only a small percentage will come directly from the associated sense organs. "Every neurone is plumbed into a sea of feedback" (McCrone 1997). This gives the nervous system a recursive structure that allows the system to repeat itself again and again. This will allow a continual check/recheck on its actions.

The numbers are hard to get a feel for and popular texts are useful to try to get the message over. Kotulak (1996), based on evidence from electron microscopy research, says that there are about 350 million connections in a pinhead size speck of brain tissue. But, the big numbers are just the start. It is the combination of connections possible which is awesome. Edelman (1992) reasoned that there were more possible combinations of connections than positively charged particles in the universe. There must be an extraordinary density of coding behind the connections and combinations, allowing patterns of activity which can all be replayed if needed or quickly adapted for future responses. Our ultimate behaviour is a result of this coding. There is surely enough space for the memories of a lifetime including all painful experiences, their contexts, the actual and possible responses at the time and future responses.

WETWARE

Hardware needs wetware to drive it. Various chemical substances form the wetware of the nervous system - the neurotransmitters and neuromodulators. The major groups are the inhibitory and excitatory amino acids, neuropeptides, acetylcholine and the amines such as serotonin and noradrenaline.

Intracellular communication doesn't only occur via synapses. Hormones such as adrenocorticotrophic hormone (ACTH), and immune molecules such as the interleukins, important in the stress response (chapter 4) offer long range signalling. Once the membrane of a neurone is disturbed, further signalling can occur via a cascade of cellular responses which activates second messenger systems within the neurone. The major neurotransmitters and neuromodulators are briefly discussed below.

AMINO ACIDS

The major inhibitory neurotransmitter is the amino acid GABA (gamma-aminobutyric acid). Anti-anxiety drugs such as the benzodiazepines target GABA receptors and try to mimic the effect of GABA. GABA is distributed right through the central nervous system. Glycine, another inhibitory neurotransmitter, is found in the spinal cord.

Glutamate is the key excitatory transmitter in the brain and the spinal cord. The cerebral cortex contains more glutamate than any other part of the body. Between 60 and 70% of all synapses in the brain are glutamate synapses (Nadler 2000). Glutamate will act on a number

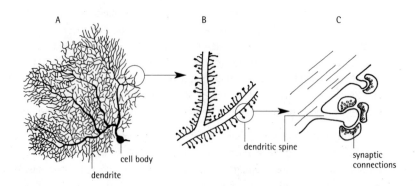

A   B   C

cell body
dendrite
dendritic spine
synaptic connections

2.1   A. Representation of a Purkinje neurone and its dense plexus of dendrites in the cerebellum
       B. Spinous processes from one branching dendrite.
       C. Synaptic connections onto a dendritic spine. Adapted from Pritchard and Alloway (1999).

of receptors including the NMDA receptor (N-methyl-D-aspartate) and AMPA (alpha-amino-3 hydroxy-methyl-4-isoxazole propionic acid) receptors. Best to stick to the shortened terms! The NMDA receptor seems to be important in memory acquisition and long term sensitivity changes. However excessive glutamate, like an excess of most of the neurotransmitters can be injurious to neurones (see chapter 4).

NEUROPEPTIDES

There are many different types of neuropeptides functioning as neurotransmitters and modulators. They include the hypothalamic peptides and the opioid peptides. The hypothalamic peptides include oxytocin and vasopressin (antidiuretic hormone). The opioid peptides such as enkephalin and endorphins are well known for their effect on pain perception. The peptides have effects on central and peripheral nerve activation. Substance P is the most studied of these. It is particularly associated with pain and touch sensations.

ACETYLCHOLINE

Acetylcholine has a major role in the peripheral nervous system at the neuromuscular junction. It is also a key neurotransmitter in the autonomic nervous system and in the CNS it is related to attention and autonomic regulation. Cholinergic synapses are the targets of surgical anaesthesia.

AMINES

The catecholamine (adrenaline, noradrenaline and dopamine) responsive neurones originate from a home base in the brainstem and then project right across the central nervous system. In the United States, noradrenaline is known as norepinephrine, and adrenaline is known as epinephrine. The catecholamines are essential for the normal functioning of the autonomic and endocrine circuits. When life gets a bit stressful or thrilling, up goes the noradrenaline and dopamine levels. Upregulation or dysfunction of the system leads to fear and behaviours seen in post traumatic stress disorders.

Serotonin (5-hydroxytryptamine) or 5HT is a very similar neurotransmitter to the catecholamines. Serotonergic neurones are widely distributed to all areas of the nervous system including descending projections to the spinal cord. Serotonin has general inhibitory effects as it suppresses sensory input. Low levels are associated with clinical depression.

The gases nitric oxide and carbon monoxide also act as neurotransmitters and neuromodulators. These act as hormones modulating local activity and are induced as part of chemical cascades occurring at central nervous system synapses.

FURTHER COMPLEXITY

To this point, I have discussed multiple neuronal populations interconnected by synapsing and modulated by a variety of wetware. Further complexity arises because the anatomy of the brain does not match up with the chemistry. There is no exclusive transmitter to one brain region although they tend to have a home base. Wetware effects are widespread. For example, figure 2.2 shows the wide distribution of noradrenergic neurones. Many neurones in the brain are very long and can extend right across the brain to make links. In addition, some neurones synthesise a neuropeptide and a classic neurotransmitter at the same time. Inputs related to thoughts, injuries and feelings drives the wetware to activate pathways.

To activate pathways, receptors and ion channels are required. Here is yet another contributor to the complexity of processing. Neuronal activity depends on ion channels opening or closing. Some neurotransmitters may influence a variety of receptors with short or long term effects. Some neurotransmitters (antagonists) close ion channels and thus inhibit function while others (agonists) will open them. Ion channels could be considered the molecular targets of manual therapy.

ION CHANNELS AND RECEPTORS

For the wetware to work and influence neurones, the hardware must contain ion channels. This is one of the most fundamental concepts in cell biology. Ion channels are passages constructed from protein subunits. They span the cell membrane. Ion channels are gated and can be either opened or closed (Fig. 2.3). Channels open in response to various stimuli and thus allow passage of ions. There are channels which will open to electrical current (voltage gated), various chemicals (ligand gated) and stretch or pressure (mechanically gated channels). Receptors are proteins usually associated with a ligand gated channel (Fig. 2.3). In the simplest case, when a neurotransmitter binds to the receptor, the channel will open in the case of an agonistic transmitter, or close in the case of an antagonistic neurotransmitter. While a neurotransmitter is usually specific for a particular receptor there are often subgroups of receptors.

Some receptors are not coupled directly to an ion channel but to an enzyme which then opens the channel via activation of a G protein. These are much more slowly acting receptors referred to as metabotrophic receptors. They allow the ion channel to stay open for longer (maybe minutes) and perhaps cause more long lasting changes in the neurone via gene activation and production of more or different ion channels. The mechanosensitive channels, often called stretch activated channels (Sachs 1986), exist mainly in the peripheral nervous system. There are also channels whose ionic conductance will vary with temperature. Along the cell membrane, there will always be some channels open and these will contribute to the resting membrane potential.

An ion is an atom minus or plus an electron. Hundreds of thousands of ions can flow through a channel each second. Membrane potentials and spikes rely on the exchange of four ions:

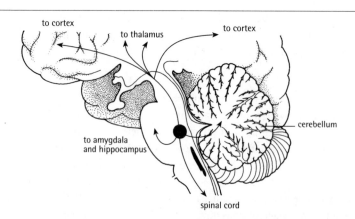

2.2   The widespread noradrenaline system. Adapted from Martin JH (1996) Neuroanatomy Text and Atlas, 2nd edn. Appleton & Lange, Stamford.

sodium (Na⁺), Potassium (K⁺), Chloride (Cl⁻) and Calcium (Ca²⁺). The membrane is oily, and can be penetrated only if the ion channels are open.

The term "messenger systems" is often applied to chemical signalling. The first messenger is the neurotransmitter delivering the message to the receptor. The second messenger in the receiving cell conveys the message to the cell nucleus and to other receptors in the cell and this could result in the opening of more ion channels, calcium liberation and gene activation. Examples of second messengers are cyclic adenosine monophosphate (cAMP) and arachidonic acid.

Reading chapters on ion channels in major modern texts such as Zigmond (1999) and Kandel (1995) or reviews (Waxman 2000) may send many of us into a tailspin. It is an extremely complex and changing area. There are a number of key points related to ion channels which movement based therapists should be aware of. These points will help to make sense of the next 2 chapters and provide a base for rational, biologically based therapies.

SEVEN KEY ION CHANNEL POINTS

1. Ion channels are a collection of proteins shaped to form a channel. This channel is bound in the membrane of the neurone (axolemma). These channels are synthesised on ribosomes around the nucleus, all to a genetic instruction. Channels are transported in the axoplasm (nerve cytoplasm) and they are then inserted into the axolemma.

2. They form a plug in the axolemma with a hole through it. The hole can open or close and if it is open then ions flow through, according to the electrochemical gradient. This will cause a depolarisation and then, secondary to other chemical events, the channel will usually shut.

3. There are many different kinds of channels expressed by genes. Some channels will open to specific modalities such as stretch or temperature changes. Other channels will open in response to changes in electrical potential or a neurotransmitter binding to it.

4. An ionotrophic (eg. ligand gated channel) will only open for a few milliseconds and thus allow equalisation of the electrical gradient. Another class of ion channels (G protein) will open for much longer, perhaps minutes and instigate changes in the next neurone including second messenger activation and gene expression.

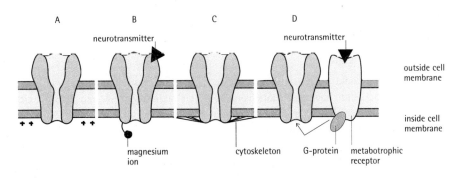

2.3   Four different kinds of open ion channels. A is an electrically gated channel, B is a ligand gated channel, including a magnesium plug. Neurotransmitters "dock" into the protein, opening or closing the gate. C is a mechanically gated channel. The cytoskeleton may pull the channel open. D is a metabotrophic channel or G protein gated channel. The receptor is separated from the ion channel and G protein activation is required to open the channel.

5. Ion channels are continually changing. There is a constant insertion and degradation of channels. The half-life of an ion channel such as the Na+ channel may only be a few days (Schmidt and Catterall 1986). This allows a self-regulatory process which defines synaptic function. For example, in a stressful situation the number of adrenosensitive channels could increase. It is likely that different forms of injury induces production of different forms of ion channels (eg. Perl 1999; Waxman et al. 1999).

6. Ion channels are not distributed evenly. There are more channels at the cell body, axon hillock, dendrites, terminals and the nodes of Ranvier (Waxman 1977; Waxman 2000). This allows saltatory conduction. An area such as the axon hillock is a possible site for insertion of additional channels if needed.

7. Ion channel number, kind and activity at any one time is a fair representation of the sensitivity needed for best survival in society as computed for that individual. There is thus a plasticity in ion channel expression. In injury states the pattern of channel expression and insertion can change dramatically and receptor numbers in areas such as the amygdala, hippocampus and dorsal root ganglia increase. In peripheral nerves, myelin normally resists channel insertion. However, after demyelination, the bared segment can acquire a high density of channels (Foster and Whalen 1980). This is thought to be the basis of abnormal impulse generating sites in peripheral neurones (Devor and Seltzer 1999) (chapter 3).

RESTING POTENTIAL, GENERATOR POTENTIAL AND THE SPIKE

Ions will not cross the oily axolemma while the neurone is in the resting state. The resting membrane potential of a neurone is the difference between the electrical potential on the inside of the cell and the electrical potential on the outside. By this convention the membrane potential is negative and somewhere between -60 and -70 millivolts. Any signalling (the generator potential) will result from a change in this resting potential. An influx of sodium ions (Na^+) and calcium ions (Ca^{2+}) depolarises the membrane. Then with the closure of the Na^+ channels and an efflux of potassium ions (K^+), the membrane will be repolarised by restoring the resting potential. There is a threshold where a critical level of depolarisation must be reached in order for the cell to respond with the opening of voltage gated channels and an all or none action potential or "spike" will follow (Fig. 2.4).

This sequence will be repeated if the stimulus evoked generator current is still present, for example, if a peripheral nerve is still irritated or the particular thought continues. Because of the all or none spike, frequency of action potential rather than magnitude of firing is the coding used by the nervous system.

THRESHOLD FOR FIRING

Threshold is the relationship between incoming and outgoing currents. There is no obvious benefit to have continual spiking. With the Na^+ inflow, the K^+ ions flow out creating a balance which dampens down the depolarisation process unless overpowered by the generator current, ie. the stimulus. The threshold for firing (Fig. 2.4) is not a set current, it is a relationship between the two currents and it will always be variable depending on the health status of the nervous system and the needs of the person. It comes down to the number of ion channels open. It could be likened to the difference between a car motor just "ticking over" or one which is "revving and about to go". This and similar metaphors could be very useful to pass onto patients.

Injured nerves develop the ability to repeatedly fire. A persistent stimulus and thus generator potential bring the membrane repeatedly back to a spike. Sensory neurones, especially injured ones, exhibit a spontaneous oscillation of the membrane potential, the peaks of which may reach threshold and cause repetitive firing (Amir et al. 1999). Some injured nerves may sit just under the threshold for firing and thus require only minor stimuli to make them spike and persistently discharge (Devor and Seltzer 1999). Because of the various kinds of ion channels, this stimulus could be variable, for example, slight heat, noradrenaline or a mechanical distortion.

We know a lot about all the parts of the nervous system - things like the spike, the pathways and the chemicals. How it is all put together is still a mystery. How do billions of action potentials combine to form a perception? Here are a few thoughts.

PUTTING IT TOGETHER – THE NERVOUS SYSTEM AS A DISTRIBUTED SYSTEM

I had always thought that when I had memories of my grandmother, there would be a sort of "grandmother node" in my brain that lit up and sparkled as I thought about her. I had it wrong of course. Pain was thought of in the same way for decades with the thalamus singled out as the major pain node. Brain imaging studies have dispelled that along with the grandmother node. While the thalamus is an important centre, there are many neurones and groups of neurones including those in the limbic system and cortex that are involved in the pain experience. In certain pain states, activation of some thalamic nuclei decreases (Iadorola et al. 1995). Sensory processing is distributed around the nervous system in a way which is markedly unique in every person and probably for every pain. The processing of psychological and sensory inputs are similar events which are all converted into interacting action potentials. The term "neuromatrix" has been introduced by Melzack (1996) to describe "the entire network whose spatial distribution and synaptic links are initially determined genetically and later sculpted by sensory inputs". Perhaps more than sculpted, the brain demands and learns about the body and environment and sculpts itself.

Classical theories of a singular brain cluster of cells in relation to pain have been swept away with the advent of modern brain scanning. But we should have known this years ago. There are many examples where destruction of brain or spinal cord tissues will not completely

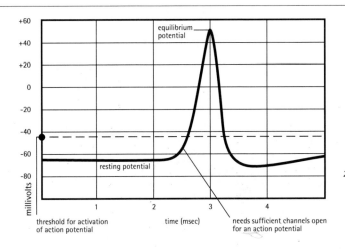

2.4 The spike and its components. Note that the resting membrane potential and the threshold for firing have a variable relationship.

abolish the pain experience (White and Sweet 1969; Lahuerta et al. 1994). Long held concepts from Head's day (Head and Holmes 1911) that, apart from meninges and blood vessels the brain was insensitive, have contributed to concepts that the brain has had little to do with pain. The new science of brain imaging and the associated colourful brain imaging pictures has put it out there in front of us and is making us reflect. Techniques such as positron emission tomography (PET) and functional magnetic resonance imaging (fMRI) among others allow a measure of synaptic activity. See Ingvarana and Hsieh (1999) and Casey and Bushnell (2000) for further information.

With experimental noxious stimuli, various brain areas show activity. For example, a typical PET analysis (eg. Casey 1999) shows that painful input causes significant activity in the contralateral insular cortex, the cerebellum, the contralateral thalamus, primary and secondary somatosensory cortex, anterior cingulate cortex, putamen, prefrontal cortex and the premotor cortex (Fig. 2.5). See Coghill (1999) and Ingvar and Hsieh (1999) for a review. All these areas have functions other than pain perceptions. These functions include motor, sensory, association and emotional functions. It does raise the idea of special pain areas again, but while the thalamus, hypothalamus and anterior cingulate cortex are usually active pain evoked areas, the fact that they have many other functions, and that activation is not the same in all individuals (Davis 2000) should point away from set nodal responses to pain.

There are repeated reports that the somatosensory cortex is involved in the pain experience, but is not crucial to the pain experience, as damage or removal of the somatosensory cortex has only a partial impact on an individual's pain experience (Coghill 1999). This is a feature of parallel processing.

PARALLEL PROCESSING

When you have a painful experience, you get the whole package at once. It doesn't happen serially such that a tissue stimulates a C fibre which activates spinal cord tracts, then the thalamus, limbic system, cortex, amygdala etc. It all happens together and any one processing component can probably initiate it. In phantom limb pain there may be no peripheral initiating input. You cannot have injury without immediate psychological and social input. For example, when you are cut, part of the inputs the processor has to contend with could include

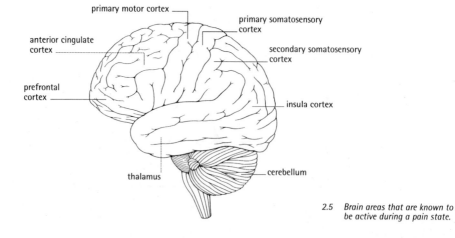

2.5   *Brain areas that are known to be active during a pain state.*

"stupid me, I have cut myself, the blood is making a mess". If you take a chocolate cake out of the oven, and before you get to the table you realise you are being burnt, you don't drop your beautiful cake, you process the whole deal and get the cake to the table, then lick your fingers. Human behaviour relies on the concurrent processing of a variety of inputs, context and concurrent apportioning to the response and homeostatic systems.

Parallel processing is a feature of a distributed system. Serial processing follows a more hierarchical line system (Fig. 2.6). Tactile processing appears to have more serial components (Pons et al. 1987; Pons et al. 1992; Mima et al. 1998) although with considerable feedback mechanisms. The more complex pain phenomenon is processed in a parallel fashion. This means that there must be neural architecture including reciprocal feedback loops to support parallel processing. This exists. For example, there are multiple routes for the processing of information from the thalamus to the cortex and vice-versa. Thalamic plasticity depends on feedback connections from the cortex (Kaas 1999; Krupa et al. 1999). For a review of pathways, see Craig (1999).

Serial processing can be risky as disruption to a part will have severe consequences for the whole processing. Plus, it creates a greater distance for an impulse to travel (Fig. 2.6). Its advantage is that processing can occur without much competition. However with injury to a part, the distributed system will survive as other parts are sufficient to process the pain experience. This is why heroic neurosurgery for chronic pain will usually fail (White and Sweet 1969), as will any therapy which aims at just one part of the experience. Distributed processing probably explains part of the individual variations seen in brain scanning experiments. Why would person A process his/her pain state the same as person B anyway? The terms primary and secondary as in the somatosensory cortex are suggestive of serial processing but even here the processing is parallel (Ploner et al. 1999).

It is this processing in parallel that allows the integration of various cognitions and emotions into the overall experience. Inputs related to a straight leg raise will arise from multiple tissues, activated memory banks, time of day, level of pain evoked, therapist/patient interactional events and current emotional status. It must be processed in parallel. Pain processing is not only parallel, it occurs on both sides of the brain.

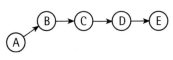

serial processing

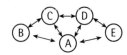

distributed (parallel) processing

2.6   Parallel and serial processing. With serial processing an injury at one part will prevent transfer of information from A to E. With parallel (distributed) processing, a similar lesion would have a minimal impact. Adapted from Coghill (1999).

BILATERAL PROCESSING

The image of decussation of the sensory pathways at the pyramids and the resultant rule that the sensations of one side are dealt with by the contralateral cortex has held for years. It's not quite true.

Some neurones in the somatosensory cortex will react to stimulation from both sides of the body. These neurones therefore have bilateral receptive fields. This occurs particularly for midline structures such as the trunk and mouth. The process is sometimes called midline fusion theory (Manzoni et al. 1989). However the feet and especially the hands have recently been shown to activate neurones with bilateral receptive fields, ie. one neurone will respond to input from both sides. An extension of the midline fusion theory is that where body parts work together, such as the hands and the mouth/tongue/oral cavity, there will be more relevant neurones in the brain with bilateral receptive fields. The feet are used reciprocally and therefore are represented by a smaller number of neurones with bilateral receptive fields (Iwamura 2000).

Numerous scanning studies have shown bilateral brain activation from ipsilateral nociceptive input. Bilateral activation of the thalamus has been shown for example (Casey et al. 1996; Derbyshire et al. 1997; Iadorola et al. 1998; Paulson et al. 1998).

Bilateral spread of pain is a feature of chronic pain states which clinicians and patients have found difficult to accept or explain. It doesn't fit with models of decussation at the pyramids. In a recent review of commonly used nerve constriction models, Pither noted (1999) that a sensitivity in the other limb will also occur, probably due to CNS upregulation. Bilateral spread of pain is common in some chronic pain states which are in initiated by an ipsilateral stimulus. complex regional pain syndromes and nerve root disorders are examples. I think many patients may not report bilateral spread of pain for fear that their health provider will think they are malingering. Different use of the other side may be one explanation, but the presence and activation of nociceptive neurones with bilateral representations is a better explanation. Hopefully these people will begin to be better understood by health carers.

MOTOR CONTROL AREAS AS PART OF THE DISTRIBUTED PAIN EXPERIENCE

One of the more surprising findings of the last decade of brain imaging was that areas of the brain which were always considered to be the domains of motor control showed activity during pain state investigations. This includes areas such as the motor and premotor cortices and subcortical sites such as the cerebellum, basal ganglia and putamen. Coupled with this is the fact there are about a million fibres in the corticospinal tract, compared to a few thousand in the spinothalamic tract (Blinkov and Glezer 1968). Motor control and its relationship with pain management is clearly a topic for further study. As Coghill (1999) reports, subjects for brain scanning experiments have to remain still and silent to minimise movement artifacts. Thus the normal motor responses of avoidance and articulation are suppressed and a motor control process is engaged. Note that the premotor cortex, cerebellum and basal ganglia are concerned with motor planning, not necessarily movement. The cerebellum and basal ganglia receive input from almost all areas of the cerebral cortex. The basal ganglia have been proposed as structures supporting attentional mechanisms in the prefrontal region, facilitating motor program recall and movement based thoughts (Brown and Marsden 1998). It is likely that the anterior cingulate cortex plays a role in motor control in addition and related to its role in attention. A recent functional MRI study (Lotze et al. 1999) showed that motor imagery and motor performance possess similar neural substrates in the cortex and cerebellum.

Wall (1999a) proposes that the brain analyses sensory input in terms of what it might be able to do about it. Bilaterally distributed processing in the existing neuronal architecture would allow this. The proposal gives new meaning to the analysis of motor function. It also encourages novel management strategies. If motor activation is a contributor to pain processing, then can the motor areas be disengaged from the pain experience? After all, disengaging the anterior cingulate by distraction will alter pain perception. Motor inputs, either novel, new, trick, meaningful or otherwise which can be accepted by the nervous system as nonpainful or non stressful may have a role in retraining the brain processing which constructs the pain experience. An upper limb neurodynamic test may be painful. Perform it in another order, different context and place and with additional meaning and it may be accepted by the CNS without contributing to a painful experience. Once accepted, the repeat performance should be easier.

ACTIVE AND PASSIVE MOVEMENT

There have been some brain mapping studies performed comparing active and passive movement. The first brain imaging study suggested that brain activation was similar in active and passive movements (Weiller et al. 1996), though more recent studies have shown significant differences in active and passive finger movements (Mima et al. 1999). Passive movements activate the contralateral primary and secondary somatosensory cortex whereas other areas including the basal ganglia, cerebellum and the premotor cortex are engaged in active movements. These experiments use passive movements via machinery. I expect that the cognitive and emotional aspects of having another human perform movements would activate other brain areas and the activation would be dependent on subject/therapist interaction. These studies have yet to be done.

RECEPTIVE FIELDS AND HOMONCULI

CONCEPT OF RECEPTIVE FIELD

Since Sherrington's time (1906), a receptive field (RF) has been considered the region of sensory surface which must be stimulated to obtain a response in any given neurone or group of neurones. The simplest RF belongs to a peripheral sensory neurone, with the field being a tiny piece of skin, about 100 mm^2 in the case of a C fibre (Schmidt et al. 1997). Due to convergence, a number of primary afferent neurones connect to one second order neurone, thus one second order neurone now looks after the combined fields of a number of primary afferent neurones (Fig. 2.7). This does not mean a loss of clarity for the second order neurone as inhibitory and excitatory influences come into play. For example, the process of lateral inhibition allows the inhibition of submaximally activated primary afferent neurones and thus allows a good spatial contrast. A third order neurone will carry the receptive fields of the first and second neurones, although now there is far greater number of possible inhibitory and excitatory influences in action. Thus the receptive fields of a single neurone become larger, more complex and more dynamic with each stage of information processing, yet at the same time maintaining an ability to know the fine details of what the first neurone can report on. An "input filtering" process is in operation (Jenkins et al. 1990) and is part of what must be perturbed when receptive field changes occur. This complexity extends to the interlaminar layers of the cortex. Thus at each level of processing, neurones receive convergent information from the previous level and diverge to another level, receiving feedback on their actions, but ultimately forming larger and more complex receptive fields (Buonomano and Merzenich 1998). However it's not just an increasing complexity all the way up to the cortex. There are ten times more fibres projecting from the cortex to the thalamus than vice versa. Changes at one level are not necessarily passed on to the next and this gating could occur at any level of the nervous system.

SOMATOTOPY

Somatotopy is a feature of receptive field arrangement. The body is represented in the nervous system in an orderly arrangement which preserves the relationships of the body parts. The rule is that adjacent body parts are represented in adjacent sites of the nervous system. This design anatomically facilitates plasticity and may allow neighbouring parts to take over function in the case of injury. Somatotopy occurs throughout the entire nervous system, including peripheral nerve (Hallin 1990), spinal cord (Fig. 2.8) (Swett and Woolf 1985) and in many parts of higher brain centres. The best known example of somatotopy is in the primary somatosensory cortex (S1), known as the sensory homonculus (Penfield and Boldrey 1937). This "brain map" is finely delineated, even down to individual joints of individual fingers (Fig. 2.9).

This famous homonculus is not alone. At least 11 other homonculi have been discovered in S1. Some will respond to deep stimulation and others to skin stimulation (McComas 1999). There

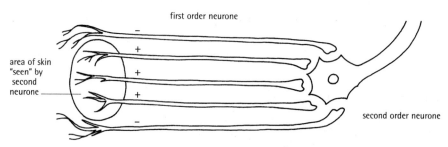

2.7   *Concept of receptive fields. The outer two neurones prove a lateral inhibition so that the second order neurone has a clear "view" of the target tissues.*

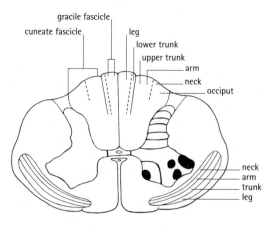

2.8   *Somatotopic organisation in the tracts in the spinal cord. Adapted from Martin JH (1996) Neuroanatomy Text and Atlas, 2nd edn. Appleton & Lange, Stamford.*

are other homonculi elsewhere in the motor cortex, lateral thalamus and cerebellum (Rijntjes et al. 1999) and scanning experiments continue to find more. Movements are represented through various homoncular arrangements in the motor cortex (Nudo et al. 1992; Nudo et al. 1996). Movement of particular parts, eg. index finger versus thumb, will activate different parts of the motor cortex (Lotze et al. 2000).

It is not only the body surfaces which have a representation in the cortex. The visual system has a topographic representation (retinopy) and so does the auditory system (tonotopy). However the key thing is that these representations are not fixed, and are quite plastic.

PLASTICITY IN THE CENTRAL NERVOUS SYSTEM

After birth, our neurones will not replicate, although Gould et al. (1999) recently showed that we may get a daily dose of a small number of fresh neurones. There is however a remarkable degree of adaptation, neuronal connectivity and dieback as the central nervous system is sculpted partly in response to external input and in part to what it learns about variations in homeostatic function.

Neuroplasticity means a change in function of a neurone and group of neurones. This includes receptive field changes. There are obviously huge advantages for an animal to have modifiable synapses and neurones right through life. It was believed a decade ago, that when the trying period of adolescence passed and teenagers grew a mature cortex to sit on the more primitive midbrain, not much more happened. This is not true, the representations are dynamic

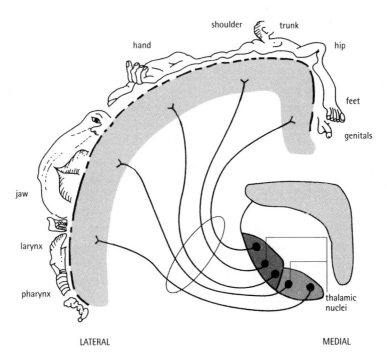

2.9   The primary somatosensory homunculus.
Adapted from Pritchard and Alloway (1999).

throughout life. The brain mapping projects alluded to earlier promise to have as much influence on changing health care as the human genome project. For one thing, expectations of possible outcomes should be higher.

The major focus of the neuroplasticity research has been in the primary somatosensory cortex of the monkey hand. It is two dimensional, extremely precise down to individual digits and is exposed on the brain surface (Kaas 2000).

REPRESENTATIONS ARE DYNAMICALLY MAINTAINED

The somatotopic representations such as the sensory homonculus are not fixed. Although relatively stable across time and individuals, the representations reflect not only the anatomy and function of the part but also the history of stimuli to the part. The representations can be easily altered by various changes in peripheral input and thus their contribution to parallel processing alters (eg. Merzenich et al. 1984; Byl et al. 1997; Buonomano and Merzenich 1998; Kaas 2000). A whiplash injury with resultant brain stem shakeup (Duckett and Duckett 1993) cannot be advantageous to processing.

Representational change can be useful, such as the empowered and enriched cortical representation of a Braille user's index finger (Pascual-Leone and Torres 1993), or destructive, in the case of cortical changes in phantom limb pain (Flor et al. 1995) or focal dystonia (Byl et al. 1997). Representational change not only occurs in the somatosensory cortex. It occurs at subcortical level, for example in the thalamus and cerebellum (Florence et al. 1993; Buonomano and Merzenich 1998; Dostrovsky 1999; Kaas et al. 1999). It also occurs in the spinal cord (eg. Doubell et al. 1999), and at the terminals of neurones, the membrane can alter to represent its share of the nervous system's construction of reality (eg. Carlton and Coggeshall 1999).

Amputation of the finger or nerve ligation will mean that a segment of cortex will lose its input and be "silenced", at least initially. However this presumably "unused" piece of cortex will begin to adopt the properties of the surrounding neurones, or put another way, the surrounding neural structures will "invade" the unused or now susceptible area of nervous system. In addition, with the amputation of the hand, the digits of the intact hand will now get a larger cortical representation (Elbert et al. 1997). A similar process occurs in the visual system when input is removed from the matching part of the retina (Darian-Smith and Gilbert 1995).

Review the homonculus in figure 2.9 again. The body is obviously not an exact representation. First, the areas requiring greater sensation for function are larger. Second, the body is broken up. In particular the face is near the hand and the foot representation sits next to the genitals. A phenomenon occurs in people with a phantom limb sensation after upper limb amputation where they can map the phantom digits on their face (Fig. 2.10). This can be quite specific, and it has been reported within 24 hours of amputation (Doetsch 1997). So it appears that the facial representational area which is presumably quite active and powerful "takes over" the hand area and is able to in part represent the hand. The overall processing output perception is that the area touched must be hand.

Cortical plasticity is brought to life by Ramachandran in his book and various publications (1992; 1995; 1998). Ramachandran and Blakesee (1998) also share a case study where a patient reports the sensation of orgasm in their phantom foot. Presumably a similar process is happening here given the cortical representation of the foot close to the genitals. Map changes have been found in the auditory cortex in tinnitis sufferers, hence tinnitus has been suggested as an auditory phantom phenomena (Muhlnickel et al. 1998).

A VARIETY OF INPUTS CAN ALTER REPRESENTATIONS

Overuse, lack of use, minor injuries, and associated cognitions will also alter representations. Amputation simply serves as a dramatic example.

There are some remarkable examples of representational changes. In a person who has been blind since birth and who has communicated through Braille, the index finger representation in the brain is greater than the other fingers (Pascual-Leone and Torres 1993). Also, in subjects who have been blind since birth, using Braille activates the visual cortex, showing a marked and powerful brain mutability (Sadato et al. 1996). Compared to non-musicians, violinists, cellists and guitarists have a greater cortical activation from fingertip stimulation (Elbert et al. 1995) (Fig. 2.11).

Syndactyly is a rare condition where a person is born with two or more webbed fingers. The brains of two people with syndactyly were mapped in a study by Mogliner et al. (1993). A compressed cortical representation of the two fingers was noted, meaning that stimulation anywhere on either of the webbed fingers activated the same representation in the brain. However one week after surgery, the map in one of the patients approached normality and separate fingers could be perceived. Similarly in primates, surgical fusion of two digits in primates will result in a merging of their cortical zones in the somatosensory cortex (Allard et al. 1991).

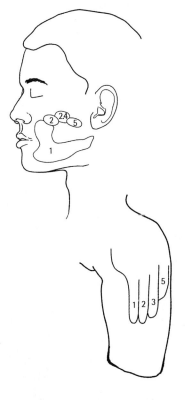

2.10 *Phantom sensations and trigger zones. This patient's left arm had been amputated 10 years prior to testing. A map of digits 1-5 can be seen on the face and upper arm. Sensory input to these zones activates old hand territory in the brain. When these points are touched, the sensations are as though it was the missing hand that was touched. From: Ramachandran, VS and Blakeslee S (1998) Phantoms in the Brain, William Morrow and Co. New York, with permission.*

As suggested by the musicians and Braille users, attention to stimuli appears to be a necessary prerequisite for cortical changes to occur. Attending to the stimuli and thus activating neuromodulatory circuits in associative brain areas such as the anterior cingulate cortex creates powerful changes in the cortical representations. For an overview of the importance of attention in altering circuits, see Recanzone (2000).

The motor cortex also shows representational changes. The representation of the dominant hand in monkeys is larger and more spatially complex than the non-dominant hand (Nudo et al. 1992). The motor cortical representation of a movement will improve with training as has been shown in wrist and finger exercises in monkeys (Nudo et al. 1996) and humans (Karni et al. 1995). Whether a well established homoncular pattern makes it more resistant to change is not known. However it may lead to a decrease in performance at another task (Nudo et al. 1996; Recanzone 2000).

THE MESSAGES OF PHANTOM LIMB PAIN

Phantom limb pains are usually regarded as medical odd baskets, although no one could doubt or fail to feel for patients suffering what must be among the most frustrating of all pains. Phantom limb sensations occur in over 80% of traumatic amputations such as surgery, and in up to 80% of those the phantom is a painful one (Sherman and Sherman 1983; Jensen et al. 1985).

Phantoms are becoming more and more understandable. In the case of a below knee amputation, there is obviously no anatomy below the knee any more. However there is a foot and lower leg representation, although perturbed, still held in the various homonculi. The external reality of the leg is gone but a powerful and sometimes destructive internal reality continues. Phantom pains are more likely and often worse if the amputated limb has been painful (Jensen et al. 1985; Weiss and Lindell 1996). Phantom pains are also very similar to the pre-amputation pains (Katz and Melzack 1990). There is no use operating on the somatosensory cortex or thalamus for phantom limb pain because it will fail (White and Sweet 1969). As Melzack (1996) comments, the brain generates the experiences, sensory experiences only modulate it. We should also note that stress such as frustration will make many phantom limb pains worse (Arena et al. 1990).

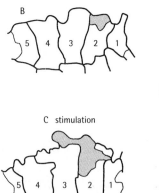
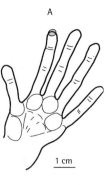

2.11 The size of receptive fields in the primary somatosensory cortex will alter with behaviour modification.
A. An owl monkey was repeatedly trained to stimulate the tip of the second digit.
In B, the area of the somatosensory cortex (area 3b) normally responsive to digit stimulation is shown, the stippled area represents the fingertip.
C. After repeated stimulation over three months, the portion of the area 3b now representing the digit has expanded. From: Jenkins, WM, Merzenich MM, Ochs MT et al. (1990) Functional reorganisation of primary somatosensory cortex in adult owl monkeys after behaviourally controlled stimulation. Journal of Neurophysiology 63: 82-104, (with permission).

People suffering phantom limb pains have had their brains mapped. The findings are likely to have great relevance to manual therapists. The greater the magnitude of phantom limb pain, the greater the amount of sensory cortical reorganisation (Flor et al. 1995). Birbaumer et al. (1997) could show that cortical reorganisation was eliminated instantly in half the phantom limb pain sufferers, by an injection of local anaesthetic at the brachial plexus. This was an instant reduction of pain and and elimination of cortical reorganisation. In the other half, cortical reorganisation and the pain was unchanged. Note also, these studies showed that where there is no phantom, no cortical reorganisation occurs. The findings suggest that in some patients, more peripheral components exist, in others the mechanism is more central.

As the work of Birbaumer et al. (1997) suggests, plastic changes are not fixed either, they continually change - a form of "plasticity of plasticity" (Knecht et al. 1998). The suggestion is that when somatosensory representations are "smudged", altered processing could lead to spread of pain as well as causing various motor perturbations. That chronic low back pain also involves some reorganisation of the somatosensory cortex (Flor et al. 1997) should be of interest to manual therapists. It seems likely that chronic pain anywhere may be linked to plastic changes in the nervous system. However, the very notion of plasticity should lift hopes and expectations in dealing with chronic pain.

THE MECHANISMS BEHIND CORTICAL PLASTICITY

The cortical plasticity mechanisms are essentially unknown but it is likely that several biological processes will be involved. The rapid reorganisation can be attributed to a reprocessing including a rebalancing of excitatory and inhibitory inputs (Kaas 1999). This must include an unmasking and recruitment of previously silent synapses.

Long term changes must involve the process of long term potentiation (LTP). This is a repetitious-use evoked increase in the strength of synaptic transmission which lasts for more than a few minutes. Most study has been on hippocampal cells where a few seconds of intense activity will cause synaptic strength increases for hours. There are obvious links to memory acquisition. The reverse, a process of long term depression, occurs also, otherwise synaptic strengths would just keep increasing. Extended low frequency stimulation appears to decrease synaptic strength.

A high frequency train of input will make the next cell more excitable, lasting at least several days if:

• More than one cell is activated (cooperativity).

• Contributing fibres and postsynaptic cells must be activated at the same time (associativity).

• Potentiation must be specific to only the activated pathway (specificity). See Kandel et al. (1995) for a review.

Glutamate and the NMDA receptor appears essential to LTP as cortical map changes can prevented by blocking NMDA receptors (Kano et al. 1991; Garraghty and Muja 1996). Modulation of NMDA activity occurs from many of the neuromodulators, such as nitric oxide (Kara and Friedlander 1998) noradrenaline, acetylcholine, dopamine and serotonin (Kilgard and Merzenich 1998; Kirkwood et al. 1999). This means that many brain centres are involved in map restructuring and memory acquisition. The NMDA receptor changes are discussed in chapter 4 in the section on dorsal horn cell changes. Other related processes may occur. The dendritic spines of neurones which will house the majority of synaptic contacts are continually being modified. In addition, dendritic spines are somewhat mobile which perhaps physically helps to create synaptic links (Fischer et al. 1998).

THE ULTIMATE REPRESENTATIONAL DEVICE

In summary, the nervous system is the ultimate representational device. The entire nervous system, from receptors in the neuronal terminals to the distributed, bilateral and dynamic processing brain has the infrastructure and ability to represent anatomy, physiology, function, disease, past use, current activity, perhaps future presumed use. The basic forces behind the representations are probably survival first and then survival in comfort. The complexity is such that having the anatomical part may not be necessary. Processing can still be accomplished, though perturbed, if a brain part is missing or malfunctioning.

In a way, anatomy and physiology as subjects by themselves are somewhat rendered obsolete, unless their representation in another system in the same body can also be taken into account. There are a number of clinical repercussions of this viewpoint.

CLINICAL REPERCUSSIONS OF THE PLASTIC REPRESENTATIONAL NERVOUS SYSTEM

THE BIRD'S EYE VIEW AND THERAPY

All of this may be interesting reading, but what are the implications for management from this perhaps new perspective? And what does a manual therapist do about the central nervous system, when for many (including myself), our initial education finished at the atlanto-occipital joint?

A SHIFT IN THINKING IS NECESSARY

For professions whose operational premise is pain and pathological movement states, a slight but powerful shift in management focus seems necessary. The nervous system could be seen more as an organ which constructs and exerts a complex and dynamic threshold control over input, sometimes "listening" to that input and sometimes not. A desirable shift, depending on the pain state, would be to place more emphasis on components of the threshold control. For example, this may involve "priming" the system prior to any active or passive physical inputs, it might involve considering a "hands off" approach and timing of a "hands on" approach. It raises the importance of a healing, helping environment that includes education, understanding, empathy and skilled use of the placebo.

Perhaps, on the basis of current research and understanding, if it were possible to perform an amputation of someone's lumbar spine for chronic low back pain, in many cases, there would be a phantom back pain.

WHAT WE ENCOUNTER CLINICALLY IS AN EXPRESSION OF THAT DISTRIBUTED REPRESENTATIONAL PROCESSING

All that we encounter in the clinic - the patient's thoughts, motor patterns, responses to any inputs are expressions of the processing. That sounds simple perhaps, but it must have repercussions on rational clinical behaviour. Any input is processed in terms of coexisting and competing inputs. These can be grouped into psychological, biological and societal inputs. Thus the modern nervous system concepts strongly support what many now call the bio-psycho-social approach to disturbed sensorimotor states.

Allied to this is support for the interdisciplinary approach. Various professions with an understanding of, and tools to identify and manage the processes contributing to a patient's pain and disability may be required. Or in less severe states, one profession may have the necessary tools.

Where interdisciplinary management is used, all contributing members need to speak the same language otherwise another set of conflicting neural representations will emerge. The distributed processing in itself should make us aware that an alteration of part of that distributed processing could have wide-ranging effects on the whole. For example resolution of a workplace issue could affect memory, quality of movement, and tissue healing. Equally, skilled management of a physical dysfunction in tissues could have many beneficial "side effects".

NORMAL MOVEMENT AS SOON AS POSSIBLE SEEMS IDEAL FOR THE REPRESENTATIONS

Rest is a great analgesic, but there are side effects. It is now well known that rest is usually harmful for most spinal conditions and early movement associated with anxiety reduction is far better for recovery and mortality (eg. Malmivaara et al. 1995; Indahl et al. 1998). The anatomical structures which are likely to benefit from this are not only injured muscles, joints and nerves, but also nervous system tissues and representations. "Smudging" of representations in the sensory and motor cortices and elsewhere are best avoided by return to normal activities. The brain is the ultimate "use it or lose it" machine. It seems clear that functionally meaningful and goal directed inputs will be better accepted by the brain processing. Movements that are feared, avoided and context dependent will have to be presented to the brain in different ways, for example in different environments, or the movement "broken down" or paced (see chapter 14). Clearly, the more functional the movement and the more it links to desired activity and achievable goals, the better.

STILL UNDEFINED MANAGEMENT STRATEGIES

There is likely to be hitherto novel management strategies based on neuroplasticity and distributed processing. There are current suggestions that therapy could be based more on representation restoration (eg. Nudo et al. 1996; Byl and Melnick 1997; Candia et al. 1999). This includes introducing useful motor, sensory and cognitive input and retraining the brain so that input which it once instantly identified as a contributor to a pain experience does not necessarily have to always be so. It also includes repeated input to try and re-establish lost representations.

The large mindful movements such as those encouraged in Tai Chi and yoga could be considered in a more scientific light. I also think expectations can be lifted, especially in the elderly. You may well encourage a person to move better by telling them "use it or lose it" stories pertaining to both brain and tissues.

There are many questions here- What about retraining neighbouring representations, or use of the contralateral side. What can we do with mirrors (Ramachandran and Rogers-Ramachandran 1996) to provide input in brains deprived of normal input? What of creative inputs and activities to not only add to movement repertoires available to the brain but to add to distraction, mastery and sense of accomplishment? The neurodynamic concepts can help here.

In this framework there are also likely to be useful developments in peripherally based management inputs. This could be improved skills in managing sensitive joints, a piece of mechanosensitive nervous system or a muscle which is not performing adequately.

Somehow, your interaction with the patient is processed with the pain experience. Perhaps in some chronic pain states, visiting you may even be a cue for the perception (or reduction) of pain! The real skill in manual therapy in my view, comes down to facilitating the best possible patient interaction to allow your evidence based inputs, be they exercise, education, manipulation or all three, every chance of working.

NEURODYNAMICS AND MODERN NERVOUS SYSTEM CONCEPTS

A simple, crude but effective way to link the brain concepts to manual therapy is to consider that a straight leg raise test is also a straight leg raise of the various homonculi in the brain. If the initial vision is one of the leg being lifted in the sensory homonculus, then that's fine. A straight leg raise which accesses the injury either by physical means (eg. tethered nerve root) and/or psychological (eg. provides a reminder of a limitation) will all be processed in a distributed manner. The activation may have links to other brain areas which are related to anticipation, attention, selection, learning and various memory banks. The leg representations may be "smudged" with resultant altered pain area perceptions and motor responses. In a particular patient, the SLR based inputs could be processed by an amygdala studded with noradrenaline receptors, a hippocampus with cell death and an easily activated limbic/hypothalamic input related to fear because that person knows it is really going to hurt.

Manual therapists should aim to identify the state of processing of the nervous system which the SLR and ULNT presumes to test.

MODELS TO ENGAGE PAIN AND SENSITIVITY

Frameworks for clinically engaging the nervous system are necessary. A general clinical reasoning framework is proposed in this book, but an additional coexisting framework to engage sensitivity would also assist.

Traditional models go from the tissues up and into the brain. This is often called the "bottom up" approach. It is simple, widely accepted by patients and it fits with body concepts that sensations go "into" the body. The "bottom up" model has its uses and fits with the concept that the representations are in part, input driven. The problem is that there is no place for concurrent cognitions and emotions, leading to therapies dominated by "the bottom". This approach can be useful in acute pains but it will be only part of the ideal management process for chronic pains, indeed any pain state.

There is a simple piece of evidence, shown many times and easily observable in ourselves, that signalling events into the CNS do not have a fixed response in so-called normals, and in those who are injured. A tickle sometimes tickles yet at other times it does not. What hurts one hour or one day may not hurt the next hour or the next day. Responses depend on the value the CNS gives the input. Value processing is extremely complex. A "top down" model, that is from the brain downwards enables us to engage this. This approach is closer to the view of the brain as a constructor of reality and it allows us to consider the central nervous system as providing threshold control assisted by reciprocal links with the endocrine, autonomic and immune systems.

This "top down" approach is clearly very useful. However what actually makes up "the top" needs defining. There are layers of processing right through the brain and the cortex. If the top was the cortex, then it is obvious that a lot can happen between the "bottom" and the "top". Even in the absence of injury to neural structures between the top and bottom, processing related to the brainstem, spinal cord and dorsal root ganglion areas and interaction with homeostatic and response systems needs inclusion.

Circular models can help. With circular models there is no start and no finish, a pain process can be initiated anywhere along the process and it will have repercussions around the circle. These have been in use for some years, best articulated for physiotherapy by Louis Gifford (1998). See figure 2.12. A circular model allows a greater sense of feedback, reciprocality and awareness of variation and change within the nervous system. It allows something of a balance between the health of the tissues and the nervous system. In the next few chapters I will discuss the integration of tissue and nervous system pathobiology into a meaningful clinical approach.

METAPHORS FOR THE NERVOUS SYSTEM

Sometimes for our own appreciation of the brain and to share brain stories with patients, metaphors and descriptive text can be helpful. These are some of the metaphors and rejected metaphors which have helped me.

THE CREAMY WRINKLED SOFT OBJECT

Sometimes books aimed at the general public such as Greenfield (1997), Kotulak (1996) and Carter (1998) can be helpful. Greenfield (1997) reminds us that the brain is a "creamy, coloured, wrinkled object of around 1kg in weight with the consistency of a soft boiled egg".

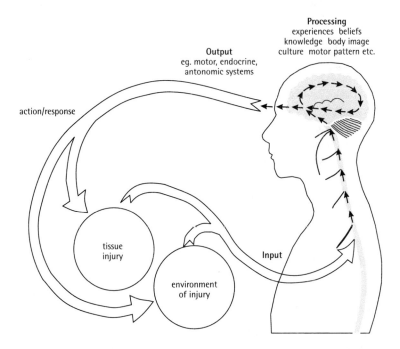

2.12 A circular model represents the interacting components of sensitivity. Adapted from Gifford LS (1998) Pain, the tissues and the nervous system. Physiotherapy 84: 27-33.

Brains are hard, grey and very motionless in anatomy laboratories. We may have forgotten the creamy coloured soft thing, yet it may be the first step to engaging the brain as a plastic object.

The brain is the greediest bodily organ in terms of fuel consumption. It will burn about 10 times as much oxygen and glucose as the other body systems at rest. Although only 2 and half percent of body weight it will take about 20 percent of energy consumption. And as we know if it runs out of oxygen, neurones will die very rapidly. It helps to establish how alive the brain is. Take the greediness a step further - the central nervous system is always searching and seeking and trying to reward itself. This takes a lot of energy.

YOUR BRAIN IS TURNED ON ALL THE TIME

The statement that "your brain is turned on all the time" (McCrone 1997) can be helpful. It is not something which is activated only when there is input. Cells in the brain are always active which gives the brain a background tone, allowing some sort of maintained but defocused representation of that person's entire memory bank. While many inputs and combinations of inputs are not turned on all the time, the brain is. A shift from input driven to an active constructor of experiences is a better way to consider it.

THE HUNGRY GREEDY SPONGE

The brain continually seeks information. It wants to be "fed" and is a greedy structure. This relates to the "use it or lose it" metaphor mentioned next. Perhaps like an addiction, it craves and seeks feedback for what it has constructed. In simple terms for patients, it might be the awareness that they have not had their shoulder above their head for some time. Your brain is waiting and wants that activity, but it won't wait forever. The various representations to handle the movement are there but need activating. When you dust the roller blades off or get the skates or skis out, it does take a little time to get back in the smooth and rolling action again.

With some patients, I have used a garden metaphor. The brain is like a garden. It needs to be watered and likes a bit of fertiliser (movement) now and then. However make sure all parts of the garden are watered, otherwise the well fertilised and watered parts will take over. So look at that computer activity. It's all hands and wrists. Time to give the shoulders and elbows a "feed". I must admit to readers here, that some people look at me rather oddly but others run right with the metaphor.

"USE IT OR LOSE IT"

This phrase is often used, quite correctly, aimed at limb flexibility and muscle strength. "Use it or lose it" applies to the central nervous system as well, in a mechanical sense (chapter 5) and also in a representational sense. Feeding representations via movement is a rather new concept, but when you consider the poor quality of movement of chronic pain patients and their limited movement responses to input, it makes you realise how important variety and quality of movement is for the brain.

Perhaps some of the research into what keeps an older mind agile helps. According to Albert and Moss (1996), education level, some strenuous activity, good lung function and the feeling that what you do in life makes a difference are determinants of retention of older person's mental agility. The Seattle Longitudinal Study (Schaie 1996) showed that seven factors stood out among people who kept their intellectual prowess as they aged. These were a lack of chronic diseases, active engagement in reading, clubs, travel, professional education and cultural events, a willing to change, a smart spouse, an ability to rapidly grasp new ideas and satisfaction with achievements.

"BALANCE THE BRAIN"

Practice at a task will provoke a change in cortical representation. Whether this is beneficial for the person depends on the task. The inference is that in movement, deficient, chronic pain states, a repeated limp or maladaptive movement habit will strengthen synaptic weights in various homonculi related to that movement. This may be one reason why movement patterns can be difficult to change, but also one which encourages a variety of novel, useful creative inputs as therapy.

This metaphor is supported by research such as the Braille user's larger index finger representation in the somatosensory cortex, discussed earlier. If one part gets a stronger representation then what happens to weakened and less well represented parts? There are suggestions that they degrade (Nudo et al. 1996; Recanzone 2000). An elite sports person is rarely skilled to the same level at another sport or at other components of the same sport. The golfer who performs his swing in reverse as part of practice may well be balancing the representations in the brain.

A sports person should revel in the concept and process of strengthening and balancing synapses as well as muscles. General stretch, strengthening and balance protocols will have a beneficial brain representational component as well as aiding tissues, cardiovascular and immune systems.

BRAIN OUTPUT IS LIKE A BAKED CAKE

There are many ingredients which can go into a cake, they can be mixed in different orders and ways, but it all comes out as a single product at the end. Psychological input and physical input mix and merge and the perception of pain and the resultant behaviour are the products. In the baked cake, the ingredients, ie. emotions, thoughts, beliefs and inputs from sensitive tissues cannot be separated (Nicholas et al. 2000).

IT'S NOT LIKE A TELEPHONE SYSTEM

It was often taught that the nervous system was like a telephone system with all inputs going to a central exchange. This was replaced by a computer metaphor. If the phone line was cut, then no messages could get through. This metaphor was unfortunately applied to the nervous system, which is why operations were commonly performed cutting nerves and tracts to stop pain. It didn't work. In the peripheral nervous system, cutting a nerve is not like cutting a phone line. There will be activity in other parts of the nervous system and the distal end of the cut nerve will undergo changes. The cut nerve is still part of the processing.

IT'S NOT LIKE A COMPUTER EITHER

The computer metaphor was useful to express the complexity in the system, but it is rapidly losing its power and holding back conceptual development. The main difference is that in a computer, the connections are fixed, yet in the nervous system the connections are plastic and continually changing and reassembling. Transient alterations in neuronal connections must be occurring with every thought.

The computer cannot completely represent a neurone, let alone a brain. Perhaps nervous system function is more like the internet than the computer?

HOW DOES IT ACTUALLY WORK? – CONCLUSION

There is no single answer to how the nervous system works. It seems that we are rapidly gaining knowledge about its component parts but how it all fits together and functions is still lacking. How do billions of action potentials combine to form perceptions? I believe that the headings of representational, plastic, reactive, and distributed are a way of giving relevance to brain function and allowing the concepts to be introduced into manual therapy. I believe they will also encourage change in manual therapy practice.

There are two quotes which caught my eye.

From Wall (1995), "...brain activity is a spatiotemporal activity that is never repeated, a combined action of existing architecture and neurotransmitters with reciprocal connections and effects that are long lasting".

When I first become aware of plasticity and the extent and speed of representational changes it seemed remarkable. However, if there is an existing view that the brain is alive and hungry and changing continually with every thought and physiological alteration, then the representational changes are not that awesome.

The second quote is a much-used one from Sherrington, from a lecture he gave in the 1930s: "It is as if the milky way entered upon some cosmic dance. Swiftly the brain becomes an enchanted loom where millions of flashing shuttles weave a dissolving pattern, through never an abiding one; a shifting harmony of subpatterns".

REFERENCES CHAPTER 2

Albert M & Moss M (1996) Neuropsychology of aging: Findings in humans and monkeys. In: Schneider E, Rowe J, Johnson T et al. (eds.) Handbook of the Biology of Aging, Academic Press, San Diego.

Allard T, Clark SA & Jenkins WM (1991) Reorganisation of somatosensory area 3b representations in adult owl monkeys after digital syndactyly. Journal of Neurophysiology 66: 1048-1058.

Amir M, Michaelis M & Devor M (1999) Membrane potential oscillations in dorsal root ganglion neurons: role in normal electrogenesis and neuropathic pain. Journal of Neuroscience 19: 8589-8596.

Arena JG, Sherman RA, Bruno GM, et al. (1990) The relationship between situational stress and phantom limb pain: cross-lagged correctional data from six month pain logs. Journal of Psychosomatic Research 34: 71-79.

Barker RA & Barasi S (1999) Neuroscience at a Glance, Blackwell, Oxford.

Bear MF, Connors BW & Paradiso MA (1996) Neuroscience. Exploring the Brain, Williams & Wilkins, Baltimore.

Birbaumer N, Lutzenberger W, Montoya P, et al. (1997) Effects of regional anaesthesia on phantom limb pain are mirrored in changes in cortical reorganisation. Journal of Neuroscience 17: 5503-5508.

Blinkov SM & Glezer II (1968) The Human Brain in Figures and Tables, Plenum Press, New York.

Brown P & Marsden CD (1998) What do basal ganglia do? Lancet 351: 1801-1804.

Buonomano DV & Merzenich MM (1998) Cortical plasticity: from synapses to maps. Annual Review of Neuroscience 21: 149-186.

Byl NN & Melnick M (1997) The neural consequences of repetition: clinical implications of a learning hypothesis. Journal of Hand Therapy 10: 160-174.

Byl NN, Merzenich MM, Cheung S, et al. (1997) A primate model for studying focal dystonia and repetitive strain injury: Effects on the primary somatosensory cortex. Physical Therapy 77: 269-284.

Candia V, Elbert T, Altenmuller E, et al. (1999) Constraint-induced movement therapy for focal dystonia in musicians. Lancet 353: 42.

Carlton SM & Coggeshall RE (1999) Inflammation-induced changes in peripheral glutamate receptor populations. Brain Research 820: 63-70.

Carter R (1998) Mapping the Mind, Weidenfeld and Nicholson, London.

Casey KL (1999) Forebrain mechanisms of nociception and pain. Proceedings of the National Academy of Science 96: 7668-7674.

Casey KL & Bushnell MC (2000) Pain imaging. Pain: Clinical Updates 8: 1-4.

Casey KL, Minoshima S, Morrow TJ, et al. (1996) Comparison of human cerebral activation pattern during cutaneous warmth, heat pain and deep cold pain. Journal of Neurophysiology 76: 571-581.

Chapman RC, Oka S & Jacobson RC (1997) Phasic pupil dilation response to noxious stimulation in humans. In: Jensen TS, Turner JA & Wiesenfeld Z (eds.) Proceedings of the 8th World Congress on Pain, IASP Press, Seattle.

Coghill RC (1999) Brain mechanisms supporting the pain experience: a distributed processing system. In: Max M (ed.) Pain 1999 - An Updated Review, IASP Press, Seattle.

Craig AD (1999) Functional anatomy of supraspinal pain processing with reference to the central pain syndrome. In: Max M (ed.) Pain 1999 - An Updated Review, IASP Press, Seattle.

Darian-Smith C & Gilbert CD (1995) Topographic reorganization in the striate cortex of the adult cat and monkey is cortically mediated. Journal of Neuroscience 15: 1631-1647.

Davis KD (2000) The neural circuitry of pain as explored with functional MRI. Neurological Research 22: 313-317.

Derbyshire SWG, Jones AK, Devani P, et al. (1997) Pain processing during three levels of noxious stimulation produces differential patterns of central activity. Pain 73: 431-445.

Devor M & Seltzer Z (1999) Pathophysiology of damaged nerves in relation to chronic pain. In: Wall PD & Melzack R (eds.) Textbook of Pain, 4th edn. Churchill Livingstone, Edinburgh.

Doetsch GS (1997) Progressive changes in cutaneous trigger zones for sensation referred to a phantom hand: a case report and review with implications for cortical reorganisation. Somatosensory & Motor Research 14: 6-16.

Dostrovsky JO (1999) Immediate and long-term plasticity in human somatosensory thalamus and its involvement in phantom limbs. Pain Supplement 6: S37-S43.

Doubell TP, Mannion RJ & Woolf CJ (1999) The dorsal horn: state dependent sensory processing, plasticity and the generation of pain. In: Wall PD & Melzack R (eds.) Textbook of Pain, 4th edn. Churchill Livingstone, Edinburgh.

Duckett S & Duckett S (1993) The neuropathology of the minor head injury syndrome. In: Mandel S, Thayer Sataloff R & Schapiro SR (eds.) Minor Head Trauma, Springer Verlag, New York.

Edelman G (1992) Brilliant Air, Bright Fire, Penquin, London.

Elbert T, Sterr A, Flor H, et al. (1997) Input-increase and input-decrease types of cortical reorganisation after upper extremity amputation in humans. Experimental Brain Research 117: 161-164.

Elbert TC, Pantev C, Wienbruch C, et al. (1995) Increased cortical representation of the fingers of the left hand in string players. Science 270: 305-307.

Fischer M, Kaech S, Knutti D, et al. (1998) Rapid actin based plasticity in dendritic spines. Neuron 20: 847-854.

Flor H, Braun C, Elbert T, et al. (1997) Extensive reorganisation of primary somatosensory cortex in chronic back pain patients. Neuroscience Letters 244: 5-8.

Flor H, Elbert T, Knecht C, et al. (1995) Phantom limb pain as a perceptual correlate of cortical reorganisation following arm amputation. Nature 375: 482-484.

Florence SL, Garraghty PE, Carlson M, et al. (1993) Sprouting of peripheral nerve axons in the spinal cord of monkeys. Brain Research 601: 343-348.

Foster RE & Whalen CC (1980) Reorganisation of the axonal membrane of demyelinated nerve fibres. Science 210: 661-663.

Garraghty PE & Muja N (1996) NMDA receptors and plasticity in adult primate somatosensory cortex. Journal of Comparative Neurology 367: 319-326.

Gifford LS (1998) Pain, the tissues and the nervous system. Physiotherapy 84: 27-33.

Gould E, Reeves AJ, Graziano MSA, et al. (1999) Neurogenesis in the neocortex of adult primates. Science 286: 548-550.

Greenfield S (1997) The Human Brain. A Guided Tour, Weidenfeld & Nicolson, London.

Hallin RG (1990) Microneurography in relation to internal topography: Somatotopic organisation of median nerve fascicles in humans. Journal of Neurology, Neurosurgery and Psychiatry 53: 736-740.

Head H & Holmes G (1911) Sensory disturbances from cerebral lesions. Brain 34: 102-254.

Iadorola MJ, Berman KF, Zeffiro TA, et al. (1998) Neural activation during acute capsaicin-evoked pain and allodynia assessed with positron emission tomography. Brain 121: 931-947.

Iadorola MJ, Max MB, Berman KF, et al. (1995) Unilateral decrease in thalamic activity observed with positron emission tomography in patients with chronic neuropathic pain. Pain 63: 55-64.

Indahl A, Haldorsen EH & al. e (1998) Five year follow-up study of a controlled clinical trial using light mobilization and an informative approach to back pain. Spine 23: 2625-2630.

Ingvar M & Hsieh J-C (1999) The image of pain. In: Wall PD & Melzack R (eds.) Textbook of Pain, 4th edn. Churchill Livingstone, Edinburgh.

Iwamura Y (2000) Bilateral receptive fields neurons and callosal connections in the somatosensory cortex. Philosophical Transcripts of the Royal Society of London 355: 267-273.

Jenkins WM, Merzenich MM, Ochs MT, et al. (1990) Functional reorganisation of primary somatosensory cortex in adult owl monkeys after behaviourally controlled tactile stimulation. Journal of Neurophysiology 63: 82-104.

Jensen TS, Krebs B, J. N, et al. (1985) Immediate and long term phantom limb pain in amputees: incidence, clinical characteristics and relationship to pre-amputation pain. Pain 21: 267-268.

Kaas JH (1999) Is most of the neural plasticity in the thalamus cortical? Proceedings of the National Academy of Science USA 96: 7622-7623.

Kaas JH (2000) The reorganisation of sensory and motor maps after injury in adult mammals. In: Gazzaniga MS (ed.) The New Cognitive Neurosciences, 2nd edn. MIT Press, Cambridge.

Kaas JH, Florence SL & Jain N (1999) Subcortical contributions to massive cortical reorganizations. Neuron 22: 657-660.

Kandel ER, Schwartz JH & Jessell TM (1995) Essentials of Neural Science and Behaviour, Appleton & Lange, Norwalk.

Kano M, Lino K & Kano M (1991) Functional reorganisation of adult cat somatosensory cortex is dependent on NMDA receptors. Neuroreport 2: 77-80.

Kara P & Friedlander MJ (1998) Dynamic modulation of cerebral cortex synaptic function by nitric oxide. Progress in Brain Research 118: 183-198.

Karni AG, Meyer P, Jezzard MM, et al. (1995) Functional MRI evidence for adult motor cortex plasticity during motor skill learning. Nature 377: 155-188.

Katz J & Melzack R (1990) Pain 'memories' in phantom limbs: review and clinical observations. Pain 43: 319-336.

Kilgard MP & Merzenich M (1998) Cortical map reorganisation enabled by nucleus basalis activity. Science 279: 1714-1718.

Kirkwood A, Rozas C, Kirkwood J, et al. (1999) Modulation of long-term synaptic depression in visual cortex by acetylcholine and norepinephrine. Journal of Neuroscience 19: 1599-1609.

Knecht S, Henningsen H, Hohling C, et al. (1998) Plasticity of plasticity? Changes in the pattern of perceptual correlates of reorganisation after amputation. Brain 121: 717-724.

Kotulak R (1996) Inside the Brain, Andrews McMeel, Kansas City.

Krupa DJ, Ghazanfar AA & Nicolelis MAL (1999) Immediate thalamic sensory plasticity depends on corticothalamic feedback. Proceedings of the National Academy of Science USA 96: 8200-82005.

Lahuerta J, Bowsher D, Lipton S, et al. (1994) Percutaneous cervical cordotomy: a review of 181 operations on 146 patients with a study on the location of "pain fibres" in the C2 spinal cord segment of 29 cases. Journal of Neurosurgery 80: 975-985.

Lotze M, Erb M, Flor H, et al. (2000) fMRI evaluation of somatotopic representation in human primary motor cortex. Neuroimage 5 Pt 1: 473-481.

Lotze M, Montoya P, Erb M, et al. (1999) Activation of cortical and cerebellar motor areas during executed and imagined hand movements: an fMRI study. Journal of Cognitive Neuroscience 11:491-501.

Lundy-Ekman L (1998) Neuroscience. Fundamentals for Rehabilitation, WB Saunders, Philadelphia.

Malmivaara A, Hakkinen U & Aro T, et al (1995) The treatment of acute low back pain - bed-rest, exercises, or ordinary activity? The New England Journal of Medicine 332: 351-355.

Manzoni T, Barbaresi P, Conti F, et al. (1989) The callosal connections of the primary somatosensory cortex and the neural bases of midline fusion. Experimental Brain Research 76: 251-266.

McComas A (1999) The world of touch - from evoked potentials to conscious perception. The Canadian Journal of Neurological Sciences 26: 7-17.

McCrone J (1997) Wild minds. New Scientist 156: 26-30.

Melzack R (1996) Gate control theory: on the evolution of pain. Pain Forum 5: 128-138.

Merzenich MM, Nelson RJ, Stryker MP, et al. (1984) Somatosensory cortical map changes following digital amputation in adult monkeys. The Journal of Comparative Neurology 224: 591-605.

Mima T, Nagamine T, Nakamura K, et al. (1998) Attention modulates both primary and secondary somatosensory cortical activities in humans: a magnetoencephalographic study. Journal of Neurophysiology 80: 2215-2221.

Mima T, Sadato N, Yazawa S, et al. (1999) Brain structures related to active and passive finger movements in man. Brain 122: 1989-1997.

Mogliner A, Grossman JAI, Ribrary U, et al. (1993) Somatosensory cortical plasticity in adult humans revealed by magneto-encephalography. Proceedings of the National Academy of Sciences USA 90: 3593-3597.

Muhlnickel W, Elbert T, Taub E, et al. (1998) Reorganisation of the auditory cortex in tinnitus. Proceedings of the National Academy of Science USA 95: 10340-10343.

Nadler JV (2000) Excitatory amino acids. In: Fink G (ed.) Encyclopedia of Stress, Academic Press, San Diego.

Nicholas M, Molloy A, Tonkin L, et al. (2000) Manage your Pain, ABC Books, Sydney.

Nudo RJ, Jenkins WM, Merzenich MM, et al. (1992) Neurophysiological correlates of hand preference in primary motor cortex of adult squirrel monkeys. Journal of Neuroscience 12: 2918-2947.

Nudo RJ, Milliken GW & Jenkins WM (1996) Use-dependent alterations of movement representations of primary motor cortex of adult squirrel monkeys. Journal of Neuroscience 16: 785-807.

Pascual-Leone A & Torres F (1993) Plasticity of the sensorimotor cortex representation of the reading finger of Braille readers. Brain 116: 39-52.

Paulson PE, Minoshima S, Morrow TJ, et al. (1998) Gender differences in pain perception and patterns of cerebral activation during noxious heat stimulation in humans. Pain 76: 223-229.

Penfield W & Boldrey E (1937) Somatic, motor and sensory representation in the cerebral cortex of man as studied by electrical stimulation. Brain 60: 389-448.

Perl ER (1999) Causalgia, pathological pain, and adrenergic receptors. Proceedings of the National Academy of Science USA 96: 9664-7667.

Pither GM, Ritchie J & Henry JL (1999) Nerve constriction in the rat: model of neuropathic, surgical and central pain. Pain 83: 37-46.

Ploner M, Schmitz F, Freund HJ, et al. (1999) Parallel activation of primary and secondary somatosensory cortices in human pain processing. Journal of Neurophysiology 81: 3100-3104.

Pons TP, Garraghty PE, Friedman DP, et al. (1987) Physiological evidence for serial processing in somatosensory cortex. Science 237: 417-420.

Pons TP, Garraghty PE & Mishkin M (1992) Serial and parallel processing of tactual information in somatosensory cortex of rhesus monkeys. Journal of Neurophysiology 68: 518-527.

Pritchard TC & Alloway KD (1999) Medical Neuroscience, Fence Creek Publishing, Madison.

Ramachandran VS & Blakeslee S (1998) Phantoms in the Brain, William Morrow, New York.

Ramachandran VS & Rogers-Ramachandran D (1996) Synaesthesia in phantom limbs induced with mirrors. Proceedings of the Royal Society of London B. 236: 377-386.

Ramachandran VS, Rogers-Ramachandran D & Cobb S (1995) Touching the phantom limb. Nature 377: 489-490.

Ramachandran VS, Stewart M & Rogers-Ramachandran DC (1992) Perceptual correlates of massive cortical reorganisation. Neuroreport 3: 583-586.

Recanzone GH (2000) Cerebral cortical plasticity. In: Gazzaniga MS (ed.) The New Cognitive Neurosciences, 2nd edn. MIT Press, Cambridge.

Rijntjes M, Buechel C, Kiebel S, et al. (1999) Multiple somatotopic representations in the human cerebellum. Neuroreport 10: 3653-3658.

Sachs F (1986) Biophysics of mechanoreception. Membrane Biochemistry 6: 173-192.

Sadato N, Pascual-Leone A, Grafman J, et al. (1996) Activation of primary visual cortex by Braille reading in blind subjects. Nature 380: 526-528.

Schaie KW (1996) Intellectual Development in Adulthood: The Seattle Longitudinal Study, Cambridge University Press, Cambridge.

Schmidt JW & Catterall WA (1986) Biosynthesis and processing of the alpha subunit of the voltage-sensitive sodium channel in rat brain neurons. Cell 46: 437-445.

Schmidt R, Schmelz M, Ringkamp M, et al. (1997) Innervation territories of mechanically activated C nociceptor units in human skin. Journal of Neurophysiology 78: 2641-2648.

Sherman RA & Sherman CJ (1983) Prevalence and characteristics of chronic phantom limb pain among American veterans. American Journal of Physical Medicine 62: 227-238.

Sherrington C (1906) The Integrative Action of the Nervous System, Yale University Press, New Haven.

Swanson LW (1995) Mapping the human brain: past, present and future. Trends in Neuroscience 18: 471-474.

Swett JE & Woolf CJ (1985) Somatopic organisation of primary afferent terminals in the superficial dorsal horn of the rat spinal cord. Journal of Comparative Neurology 231: 66-71.

Wall PD (1995) Independent mechanisms converge on pain. Nature and Medicine 1: 740-741.

Wall PD (1999) Introduction to the fourth edition. In: Wall PD & Melzack R (eds.) Textbook of Pain, Churchill Livingstone, Edinburgh.

Wall PD (1999a) Pain. The Science of Suffering, Weidenfeld & Nicholson, London.

Waxman SG (1977) Conduction in myelinated, unmyelinated and demyelinated fibers. Archives of Neurology 34: 585-590.

Waxman SG (2000) The neuron as a dynamic electrogenic machine: modulation of sodium-channel expression as a basis for functional plasticity in neurons. Philosophical Transcripts of the Royal Society of London 355: 199-213.

Waxman SG, Dib-Hajj S, Cummins TR, et al. (1999) Sodium channels and pain. Proceedings of the National Academy of Science USA 96: 7635-7639.

Weiller C, Jüptner M, Fellows S, et al. (1996) Brain representation of active and passive movements. Neuroimage 4: 105-110.

Weiss SA & Lindell B (1996) Phantom limb pain and etiology of amputation in unilateral lower extremity amputees. Journal of Pain and Symptom Management 11: 3-17.

White JC & Sweet WH (1969) Pain and the Neurosurgeon, Charles C. Thomas, Springfield IL.

Zigmond MJ, Bloom FE, Landis SC, et al. eds. (1999) Fundamental Neuroscience, Academic Press, San Diego.

CHAPTER 3

PAIN MECHANISMS AND
PERIPHERAL SENSITIVITY

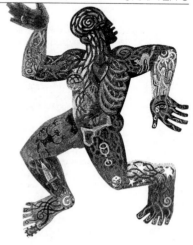

INTRODUCTION

PATHOBIOLOGICAL MECHANISMS IN INJURED AND DISEASED TISSUES

LIMITATIONS OF THE TISSUE INJURY MODEL

PATHOBIOLOGICAL MECHANISMS IN PAIN PERCEPTION

CURRENT CATEGORISATION
WHY FOCUS ON PAIN?
THE PAIN MECHANISMS

PAIN FROM TISSUES – NOCICEPTIVE PAIN

THE APPARATUS AND STIMULI FOR NOCICEPTIVE PAIN
NOCICEPTIVE PAIN AND INFLAMMATION
NOCICEPTIVE PAIN WITH MINIMAL INFLAMMATION
A SUGGESTED PATTERN OF NOCICEPTIVE PAIN
SOME THOUGHTS FOR CLINICIANS

PERIPHERAL NEUROGENIC PAIN

MODERN CONCEPTS
ABNORMAL IMPULSE GENERATING SITES (AIGS)
PROPOSED SYMPTOM PATTERN FOR PERIPHERAL NEUROGENIC PAIN
SOME THOUGHTS FOR CLINICIANS

PERIPHERAL INPUT TO THE CNS

CHAPTER SUMMARY

REFERENCES CHAPTER 3

INTRODUCTION

We can all ask patients to rotate their necks, perform muscle tests, and with a little practice, we can perform skilled neurodynamic tests. But what do the findings mean and how do the tests relate to management? A potentially powerful and recently available tool to add to existing clinical tools is the combination of clinical reasoning skills and knowledge of pathobiological mechanisms. Hence, instead of only thinking of the anatomical source of a problem, attention should be given to the pathobiological processes or mechanisms that are likely to be dominating the clinical picture.

For example, if a woman who does not normally suffer back pain said that her lumbar spine was a bit stiff and generally sore after a long drive in a car, it would be difficult to say what structure(s) such as discs, muscles, joints, ligaments and fascia could be responsible. You could guess, as clinicians and pain sufferers have always done. However, with some current neurobiological knowledge you could make a reasoned judgment about the mechanisms causing the pain and other symptoms. In this case, it's likely to be an ischaemic/inflammatory nociceptive pain mechanism, perhaps involving many tissues. The mechanism could be treated, for example, by spinal extension movements to restore the pH in tissues, by telling her it will be fine and that breaking up the drive will lessen the chance of pain. Perhaps a check and adjustment of the seat and maybe healthier and fitter tissues from exercises are all that is warranted. In this case of simple backache, your treatment strategy has involved knowledge of mechanisms of nociceptive pain rather than an actual tissue. This does not say that consideration of tissues is not important. A key part of this book is that clinical decision making strategies should include knowledge of pathobiological processes related to the tissues and pathobiological processes related to the perception of pain. We can do so much better than operational diagnoses such as "recurrent back strain".

PATHOBIOLOGICAL MECHANISMS IN INJURED AND DISEASED TISSUES

Pathobiological processes related to damaged and diseased tissues are well known to clinicians and provide the basis of current manual therapy. All injured tissues will go through a stage of inflammation, then cell proliferation followed by tissue remodelling. Different tissues take variable times to heal. For example skin often heals within days, while the less vascularised ligamentous tissues can take months before they reach their full healing potential. As noted by Gifford (1998), tissues heal by repair not regeneration and are unlikely to ever be the same again. Different disease processes will affect the rate and extent of tissue healing. Other healing variables will include age, previous injuries, management and stress. In some cases the tissues will be sensitive, in others not. A person's central nervous system has the ability to make nerve terminals more sensitive if the person decides consciously or subconsciously that there is a need to have sensitive tissues. Perhaps one reason arthritic joints are painful in some but not others is that a CNS processing decision has been made that the arthritic area needs protection. Some recommended texts on tissue healing include van Wingerden (1995), Leadbetter et al. (1990) and Woo and Buckwalter (1988).

LIMITATIONS OF THE TISSUE INJURY MODEL

Despite variability in healing rates, there is generally an even and predictable process of healing. On initial observation then, manual therapy and orthopaedic-based professions should be protocol driven and stress-free professions. They are clearly not. The tissue model, while extremely helpful does not explain many things. For example it cannot explain phantom limb pain; why pain often persists post healing; why a similar injury in one person heals much faster than in others; why between 10 and 14% of the population of industrialised western societies have an ongoing pain state (Magni et al. 1993; Verhaak et al. 1998). Nor does it explain why compressed nerve roots can be identified at autopsy, where in life there was no complaint of pain. The pain reports which nearly all patients bring in for our attention do not necessarily match the injury or the pathology. Many authors have written eloquently on this topic, none better than Patrick Wall (1996; 1999). It is for these reasons, that in management, attention to the pain processes as well as the processes in tissues may be beneficial.

In figure 3.1 some examples of the pain state/tissue injury mismatch are shown. Three common post injury overall pain scenarios are graphed with the injury and healing of tissues over time. In P1, the overall pain level relates to the time of injury and when healing is adequate, the overall pain level drifts back to nil. Perhaps this represents a typical ankle sprain. In P2, the pain starts before the time of injury, worsens with injury and then fluctuates and is always there. This could be an osteoarthritic hip. In P3, the pain begins shortly after the injury and then despite tissue healing, the pain levels remain severe. Some whiplash injuries are like this. There may be other variations, for example, there may be no pain at all or it may cycle. The point is that the pain state does not necessarily relate to the injury and disease over time, or if it does relate, there is variability over time. This why it is necessary to take some time to consider the pathobiological processes which are occurring to cause the pain.

The pain/tissue healing mismatch has been expressed in another way in figure 3.2. This has been adapted from an editorial by Haldeman (1990), entitled "Failure of the Pathology Model to Predict Back Pain". In 3.2A, the medical model is depicted. This means that pathology should equal pain. This is fine especially where pathology can be exhibited. It fits where someone has symptoms of diabetes and the pathology can be shown in a urine sample or in the case of rheumatoid arthritis, the pathology can be demonstrated via a blood test. Some nerve root problems fit nicely if relevant level compression can be shown on scanning. In 3.2B, the presumed effect of intervention is shown. An intervention such as a drug, surgery, list of exercises, or a manipulation, should stop the progress of the pathological changes and the person should return to a state of reasonable health. All this is well and good except in most back pains, whiplash, overuse syndromes, abdominal pains and headaches there is little

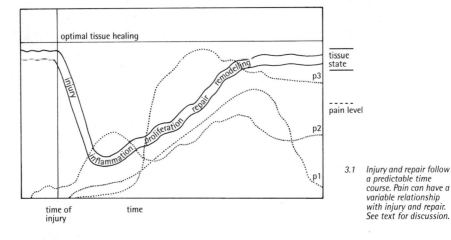

3.1   Injury and repair follow a predictable time course. Pain can have a variable relationship with injury and repair. See text for discussion.

evidence of pathological change. Thus, currently, the model fails for many people. What many clinicians encounter is shown in figure 3.2C. Here, patients have lots of symptoms, but the symptoms do not match pathological findings and in many cases, physical findings. This would be a typical pattern for many patients suffering low back pains and whiplash injuries. Presumably over a long period of time, with much soul searching and billions of dollars of research funds, the pathobiological mechanisms will be unearthed. However, we should be able to look at figure 3.2C these days with some hope. A better understanding of peripheral and central sensitivity is at least beginning to provide some explanations for some of these pains. So too, is an understanding of neurodynamics.

Let's spend some time contemplating figure 3.2D. Here, the patient (or more likely an ordinary citizen) has lots of pathological changes, but has little or no pain. There are many examples here where pathological findings and injury fail to match with pain and disability (eg. Boden et al. 1990; Jensen et al. 1994; Peterson et al. 2000). The most notable of these is that significant disc bulging and degeneration does not necessarily hurt or cause disability. There are three precious lessons which all clinicians should take from these figures. Firstly, there should be a lift in expectations and optimism for patients as outcomes do not necessarily have to be held back by knowledge of pathological findings. Secondly, the real meaning of pathological findings must be explained to patients, for example that disc degeneration is often a normal aging change and not necessarily an injury. Thirdly, it should be clear from figures 3.2C and 3.2D that clinical decision making models need to take a closer look at the processes of pain as well as the health of tissues.

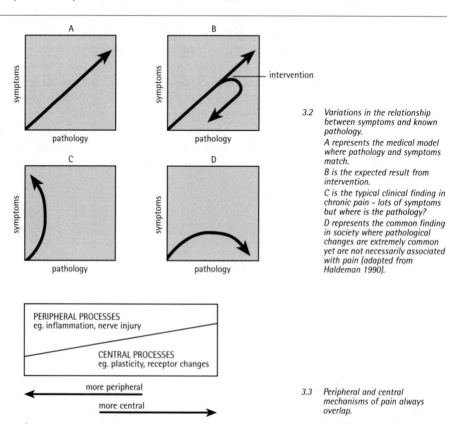

3.2 Variations in the relationship between symptoms and known pathology.
A represents the medical model where pathology and symptoms match.
B is the expected result from intervention.
C is the typical clinical finding in chronic pain - lots of symptoms but where is the pathology?
D represents the common finding in society where pathological changes are extremely common yet are not necessarily associated with pain (adapted from Haldeman 1990).

3.3 Peripheral and central mechanisms of pain always overlap.

PATHOBIOLOGICAL MECHANISMS IN PAIN PERCEPTION

The pain mechanisms concept has been within the pain sciences world for many years. However, it has taken clinicians (myself included) who were brought up on line labelled specificity theory (ie. tissue based problems signalled directly to a particular brain site) and biomechanical joint based manual therapy models, some time to realise its meaning and its power. In its simplest form a pathobiological pain process could involve predominantly peripheral mechanisms (eg. processes involved in an acute sprained ankle pain during the first 10 minutes after the sprain) or predominantly central processing (eg. phantom limb pain). See figure 3.3. This is at once extremely simplistic and clearly there could be overlap even in these extreme examples. The pathobiological process in the ankle sprain could also involve considerable central processing if the patient thought the ankle could be broken or if she began to think of the athletic event she planned to participate in that weekend. The phantom limb may have some peripheral components perhaps from tissue changes at the end of the stump. A comprehensive model of all pain states must include peripheral and central factors.

Closely related to the peripheral and central pain mechanisms are the terms **primary and secondary hyperalgesia**. Primary hyperalgesia is increased sensitivity to input at the site of injury. It is due to processes in damaged tissues. Secondary hyperalgesia is sensitivity in the uninjured tissues around the original injury (Lewis 1942). This is most likely to arise from central mechanisms. See Raja et al. (1999) for a review. Raja at al. state the important tenet "....the peripheral signal for pain does not reside exclusively with nociceptors. Under pathological circumstances, other receptor types, which are normally associated with the sensation of touch, acquire the capacity to evoke pain".

This simple categorisation of the relationship of peripheral and central biological processes is the first step in adopting pain mechanisms. Later in this chapter the peripheral mechanisms are divided into nociceptive and neurogenic. In chapter 4, central pain mechanisms associated with secondary hyperalgesia are introduced and pain mechanisms associated with the sympathetic, endocrine and immune system are discussed. The word "division" can be instant trouble because these mechanisms all occur in a continuum. All pain states probably involve all mechanisms, however in some, a dominance of one mechanism may become obvious. Pain mechanisms are not diseases or specific injuries. They simply represent a process or biological state.

CURRENT CATEGORISATION

Pain states are currently categorised by time (eg. acute/chronic), causative forces (eg. whiplash, repetitive strain injury, mouse user's wrist) or body part (eg. lateral elbow pain, headache). This labelling presents some difficulties because it does not predict outcome, give guidance to treatment, allow a search for risk factors, nor identify subcategories which may be responsive to certain therapies. In particular, the terms acute and chronic are very polarised. For some years there have been calls for bigger and better classification categories (eg. Deyo 1993; Cherkin 1998; Woolf et al. 1998). The suggestions by Woolf (1998) mirror an underlying theme from the International Association for the Study of Pain and the leading pain text, Wall and Melzack (1999), that pain can be categorised in terms of its mechanisms or processes, thus essentially its biochemistry.

Clinicians have always attempted to categorise their patients' presentations to lessen the clinical chaos and to try and best fit a set of signs and symptoms to a treatment. For example, classifications in common use in manual therapy include stages of disc injury, mechanical and inflammatory pain and patterns of movement. The proposal here is that the pain experience can be divided up and some attempt can be made to clinically categorise the pain experiences into operant mechanisms on the basis of known pathophysiology, clinical patterns and logic. For further details and a proposal of how this will fit into a bigger reasoning model, see chapters 6 and 7.

WHY FOCUS ON PAIN?

A frequent criticism of approaches which on first impression may appear to have a pain dominance is that the patient focuses on the pain and thus negative behavioural effects follow. It can be a precarious clinical balance here. On one side, pain is the "thing" that the patient brings in to have explained, ameliorated or managed and you need to know something about it to make decisions about its processes and its sources. The patient will want to tell you all about it; the more chronic the pain, the more time patients will want. On the other side, for the sake of therapy, "the pain" as a centre of discussion, even the word "pain" should recede in order to make the management process more focused on goals, function and realistic optimism. It could be said that a greater pain focus is necessary initially for diagnosis and for developing an interaction with the patient, but "the pain" as a point of reference increasingly loses its importance in subsequent management.

Dissection of the pain experience, however, is a rich source of information and understanding for both patients and clinicians alike. This is something which is analysed during the subjective and physical examination.

There is a logical reason from the wider perspective to take this pain revolution into your practice. Pain is seen as the doorway, the gateway to big picture pathobiology. To take it on means links to sometimes new and diverse fields of information such as psychology, endocrinology, counselling, psychoneuroimmunology, gross anatomy and molecular biology. It is also the most powerful linking force between various professions who are likely to engage in multidisciplinary management of chronic pain states.

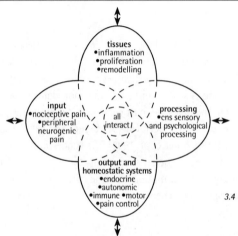

3.4   The pathobiological mechanisms involved in pain states including tissue mechanisms and pain mechanisms. The arrows represent varying contributions by mechanisms.

THE PAIN MECHANISMS

It is proposed that pathobiological mechanisms, in addition to the tissue mechanisms can be broken up into pain mechanisms related to input into the nervous system, mechanisms related to processing in the nervous system and mechanisms related to output of the nervous and other systems (Butler 1994; Gifford and Butler 1997; Gifford 1997; Butler 1998; Gifford 1998). Overlap of mechanisms is the key feature because the boundaries are often fuzzy. There will be differing contributions of mechanisms to the injury state over time, person and injury. All pathobiological mechanisms involved in the injury state need to be represented. See figure 3.4. The remainder of this chapter focuses on peripheral mechanisms.

PAIN FROM TISSUES - NOCICEPTIVE PAIN

Nociceptive pain means pain from tissues at the end of a neurone. It is in a sense a nerve pain, as all pain is neurogenic, but in this case the nerve endings are excited by mechanical or chemical processes originating from tissues in which the nerve endings embed themselves. It is often referred to as "nerve end" pain. Note that nociceptive pain could be caused by any tissue such as muscle, joint, cornea, urethra, fascia, pleura etc. The pain may behave according to the anatomical placement of the tissues, the functional demands on the tissue, its innervation density and its vascularity. Of course there will always be facilitatory/inhibitory CNS currents in operation. Although there is a pathobiological category for tissue mechanisms in clinical reasoning strategies, the reason that a category also exists for pain from tissues is that the pain and the health status of the tissues do not necessarily match. For recent reviews on the basic science of nociceptive pain see Westlund (1999), Levine and Reichling (1999), Raja (1999) and Dickenson (1996).

THE APPARATUS AND STIMULI FOR NOCICEPTIVE PAIN

For a tissue to hurt, it must be innervated by the nerve endings of A delta and/or the unmyelinated C fibres. Many C fibres are polymodal, meaning they will respond to chemical, thermal and mechanical stimulation. In some pain states, A beta fibre activation can cause pain, but this requires changes in the central nervous system as discussed in the next chapter.

The process of converting a force or a chemical into action potentials is not fully understood, but it must come back to ion channels (chapter 2). Recall that ion channels are either open or closed. If open, positive ions will flow into the cell, negative ions will flow out and a net flow of positive ions will excite the membrane and a spike will occur. Recall also from chapter 2, that there are many different kinds of ion channels and thus a specific key to the channel (a chemical, a certain current, mechanical force) is necessary to open the channels.

Normally, nerve endings have high firing thresholds - there is no use them firing off unless they really need to. In fact some of them have a rather boring life and will never fire. These are called silent nociceptors (Schaible and Schmidt 1988; Schmidt et al. 1994). They are widespread in the body, except perhaps in muscle (Mense 1996), but will fire in the presence of inflammation. It is estimated that one third of all nociceptors are silent (Schmidt 1996). It is remarkable that they could remain stable without use for a lifetime.

The stimuli which can cause nociceptive pain are illustrated in figure 3.5. They can be broadly divided into mechanical, thermal and chemical. The chemical stimuli are numerous and interactive and are best considered under the term "inflammatory soup" (Handwerker and Reeh 1991).

NOCICEPTIVE PAIN AND INFLAMMATION

Inflammation is an old and primitive method of defense. In invertebrates it is the only measure of defence. The swelling itself does not have a therapeutic value. However it allows the delivery and distribution of a variety of cells such as macrophages which are all there in the name of health and repair of the damaged tissues. Understanding inflammation is a critical aspect of understanding both chronic and acute pains.

With injury, pro-inflammatory mediators such as prostaglandins, serotonin, protons, bradykinin, leukotrienes, amines, nerve growth factor and cytokines are liberated from damaged tissues (Dray 1995; Levine and Reichling 1999; Raja et al. 1999). These are quite potent and specific, activating only nociceptive receptors at the nerve terminals and leaving other terminals alone (Reeh and Kress 1995), suggesting a specific "taste". Silent nociceptors will fire in the presence of inflammatory chemicals. Kinins (eg. bradykinin) may have a particular non-receptor action in inflammation, stimulating mast cells to release pro-inflammatory chemicals such as histamine and serotonin in addition to direct bradykinin receptor activation (Calixto et al. 2000). Overall, inflammation lowers the threshold of firing and increases the rate of firing. Mechanical forces that were not painful previously become painful. Sensitisation (learning) will occur following exposure to noxious stimulation (eg. Fitzgerald and Lynn 1997). This is all part of primary hyperalgesia.

In addition to the sensitisation caused by the inflammatory soup, intracellular second messenger systems are activated, often through G protein gated channels. This results in greater membrane permeability and excitability and perhaps gene transcription modification and thus more ion channel production and insertion into the terminals (Dray 1995). For example, sensory axons express more glutamate receptors during inflammation (Carlton and Coggeshall 1999).

Chronic inflammation is probably different to acute inflammation. The body may become depleted of inflammatory mediators, but in chronic inflammation, the receptive properties of sensory neurones may change. Nerve growth factor levels and receptor changes play a prominent role in this (Koltzenburg 1999; Shu and Mendell 1999).

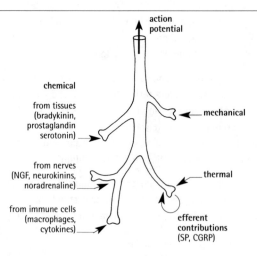

3.5   The various stimuli which will activate peripheral nerve endings. SP = substance P, CGRP = calcitonin gene related peptide, NGF = nerve growth factor (adapted from Dickenson 1996).

While the pro-inflammatory contributors to the inflammatory soup arise from blood and the damaged tissues, the nervous system will also contribute. A closer look at the glandular C fibres is warranted.

THE GLANDULAR C FIBRES AND INFLAMMATION

The way C fibres work demands our attention. There are more than double the number of C fibres compared to A fibres (Hulsebosch and Coggeshall 1981), four times as many according to Ochoa and Mair (1969). C fibres are unmyelinated and impulses travel at about 1% of the speed of A fibres. While they may not serve to signal the sharp pricking pains characteristic of A delta fibre stimulation, they will signal slower, less response demanding pains - sunburn sensations for example (Ochoa and Torebjork 1983; Raja et al. 1999). However, they also have an efferent, trophic function and could well be considered as glands of the peripheral nervous system (eg. Sann and Pierau 1998). C fibres contain neurotransmitters and neuromodulators such as excitatory amino acids, substance P (SP) and Calcitonin Gene Related Peptide (CGRP). These chemicals can be released into the dorsal horn but they can also be released into the target tissues. SP and CGRP are vasoactive peptides. They will make the cells of capillaries flatter, thus the capillaries become larger and leakier, causing plasma extravasation and thus swelling. The process is called neurogenic inflammation. This is a sterile and usually useful inflammatory process. Overall, it encourages healing (Kruger 1996) and beneficial immune system responses including the migration of leucocytes to the injury site (Nilsson et al. 1985). The process could evoke or increase vasodilation and pain as SP will make mast cells degranulate, releasing histamine or serotonin (Hagermark et al. 1978; Ebertz et al. 1987) and encouraging pro-inflammatory immune activity. It all makes the inflammatory soup a very sensitising soup for nerve endings.

The stimulus for the release of peptides into the target tissues is an antidromic impulse, which is an impulse that travels from proximal to distal in a C fibre (ie. the "wrong way"). An impulse which travels from distal to proximal in a C fibre is referred to as an orthodromic impulse (Fig. 3.6). This makes a neurone rather busy. The mechanisms for how it happens are not known, but the antidromic impulses somehow "fit" between the orthodromic impulses. Antidromic impulses can arise from injury along the nerve, the nerve terminals, or the dorsal root ganglion (Chahl and Ladd 1976; Wall and Devor 1983; Daemen et al. 1998). Perhaps oscillating membrane potentials (Amir et al. 1999), short of spike, may maintain inflammation via antidromic mechanisms. In addition, antidromic impulses can also arise from the spinal cord, where they are known as dorsal root reflexes (Sluka et al. 1995) (Fig. 3.6). Although C fibres are a focus here, antidromic impulses also occur in A delta fibres (Kolston and Lisney 1993). Spinal cord evoked antidromic impulses are of interest suggesting that central inhibitory influences may mediate peripheral inflammation.

The cranial nerves are also peripheral nerves. Peptides are also released via the trigeminal nerves. This may result in vasodilation and plasma extravasation in the dura and the pia mater, contributing to headaches (Moskowitz 1984; Moskowitz 1993) and probably reactions from tests which pull on the meninges such as the slump test (chapter 10). Neurogenic inflammation may have a role in many diseases such as gastrointestinal, ocular and respiratory disorders (Maggi and Meli 1988).

SYMPATHETIC NERVOUS SYSTEM AND INFLAMMATION

It seems only natural that such a widely distributed responsive system such as the sympathetic nervous system (SNS) will somehow respond at the site of the injury. Responses in sympathetic neurones and circuits are obvious after injury - ranging from varying degrees of stress, anxiety, fear, sweating, heart rate changes and interactions with the immune and endocrine systems. But there is also an interesting response at the injury site.

Catecholamines (adrenaline, noradrenaline) will not usually cause pain, otherwise every activity and thought would cause pain. It is only when a nerve is injured or there is a tissue inflammatory process that sympathetic activity can cause pain (Janig 1996). Catecholamines can maintain pain or enhance nociception in inflamed tissues. It appears that they enhance the activities of the pro-inflammatory chemicals, nerve growth factor, prostaglandin production and bradykinin (Levine and Reichling 1999). The aggregate evidence for this is that chemical or surgical sympathectomy can abolish pain and hyperalgesia associated with inflammation (eg. Loh and Nathan 1978; Campbell et al. 1992). Where patients had the benefit of such treatment, an injection of adrenaline could often rekindle the pain (Davis et al. 1991). The link here to modern manual therapy should be clear - any way of easing stress and making tissues healthier could have an effect on inflammation and healing and the efficacy of active and passive movement therapies.

NOCICEPTIVE PAIN WITH MINIMAL INFLAMMATION

LOWERED TISSUE pH - ISCHAEMIC NOCICEPTIVE PAIN

A pain state occurs where there appears to be little inflammation. This pain mechanism is more ischaemic in origin. This is a common and clinically detectable pain state. With persistent postural demands, lack of movement, perhaps stretch or tension in muscles, fluids are forced out of tissues and a painful ischaemia related to acidic tissues may occur. Acidic pH is associated with an increase in hydrogen ions and protons and it will cause pain in normal tissues (Steen and Reeh 1993; Dray 1995; Steen et al. 1995). There is a specific acid sensing ion channel which is activated by hydrogen ions (Bevan and Yeats 1991; Waldmann et al. 1997). Low pH is also a feature of inflamed tissues and there appears to be a synergistic effect of protons and inflammatory mediators (Steen et al. 1996).

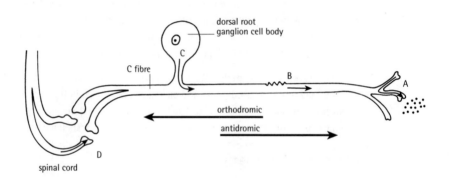

3.6   *Known sites of antidromic impulse generation from a C fibre. A. nerve terminals, B. damage mid axon, C. dorsal root ganglion, D. spinal cord*

There are powerful messages here to get people moving, to pause and change postures during sustained activity and to make sure the simple backache is diagnosed and managed as such. Management should also be easy, based on education about acidic tissues and the importance of active movement.

MECHANICAL PAIN

Much pain occurs in the absence of inflammation. If you slap your face there is an instant sharp stinging pain which must occur without inflammation and be a result of the fast A delta signalling. Even if you stub your toe there is an instant pain which occurs before there is time for inflammation. Much of this pain must be mechanically induced pain, presumably via opening of mechanosensitive ion channels. Much mechanical pain must be part of normal physiological pain although, if nerve endings are caught in scar, a mechanically dominant pain could be envisaged.

With persistent acidosis and mechanical pain, a slowly progressing inflammatory contribution to the pain state would be expected as would slow changes in CNS threshold levels.

A SUGGESTED PATTERN OF NOCICEPTIVE PAIN

In this chapter, patterns to help identify various peripherally dominant pain mechanisms are proposed. Nociceptive pain is likely to be more associated with acute injury, with damaged and healing tissues and postural pain. It will also be part of the pain mechanisms from weakened and deconditioned tissues of patients in chronic pain states. The key pattern to notice here is that stimulus intensity and sensation are reasonably related. The threshold for pain is lowered thus light touch instead of heavy pressure hurts, and any painful stimulation is magnified, thus a pinch is extremely painful. This is hyperalgesia, in this case primary hyperalgesia and it is a common feature of inflammation and injury. Note that sometimes sensitivity may be dynamic requiring movement (stroking hyperalgesia) and at other times, sensitivity may be to palpation.

MORE INFLAMMATORY PATTERN

When a more inflammatory nociceptive pain mechanism is in operation, these clinical features may be noted:

• the cardinal signs of acute inflammation - redness, oedema and heat.

• association with acute pain and tissue damage.

• a close relationship between a stimulus and a pain response.

• a diurnal pattern in pain and stiffness may exist, ie. worse in the morning and overnight.

• there may be hints that the nervous system is unhealthy (eg. entrapment, disease) and contributing via neurogenic inflammation.

• neurogenic inflammation, represented by redness or swelling or symptoms in a neural zone.

• beneficial effects of anti-inflammatory medication (stops the prostaglandin contribution to the soup).

Examples of inflammatory nociceptive pains include acute sprains and strains, post-activity muscle pains and rheumatoid arthritis.

MORE ISCHAEMIC/ACIDIC PATTERN

The features which may suggest a more ischaemic/acidic pattern include:

• symptoms after prolonged or unusual postures.

• rapid ease of symptoms after a change of posture, usually a change in the opposing direction.

• symptoms towards the end of the day or after the accumulation of activity.

• a poor response to anti-inflammatory medication.

• sometimes no evidence of actual trauma.

Some examples of this pattern would include postural pains or the simple backache described by Waddell (1998).

SOME THOUGHTS FOR CLINICIANS

In many cases of nociceptive pain it may be easier to pick the process than it is the actual structure(s) at fault. For example, postural neck strain such as that from sitting at a desk and working on a computer for many hours, the kind which improves when the neck is moved, could be argued to be nociceptive pain and probably ischaemic from changes in tissue pH. A number of tissues including skin, muscle and joints could be involved. While it would be ideal to identify tissues at fault, in many cases it may not matter. Activity which unloads the tissues will stop the pain. Certain exercises may make tissues more healthy and more robust to similar postural forces. There are likely to be worthwhile ergonomic interventions.

Recent research, reviewed in the next chapter is showing the influence of thoughts and emotions on tissue pain and healing. Clinicians have always been aware that optimism and coping skills are great healers. Some of the mechanisms here could be related to sympathetically mediated neurotransmitters and modulators added to the inflammatory soup, immune cell involvement in inflammation and dorsal root reflexes. The role of the nervous system in inflammation is intriguing. It may contribute to inflammation, which, as discussed above could be initiated from damaged peripheral nerve or altered central nervous system controls. Therefore it should be worth checking the physical health (chapters 8,9,10,11) of the nervous system and the patient's psychological status (chapter 7) regarding the injury/disease state. Even at tissue terminals, known neurobiological processes call for a bio-psycho-social approach to pain states.

Nociceptive pains are a big part of simple backache. Once these patterns are understood then the more complex neuropathic pain patterns arising from damaged nerves and altered central nervous system processing can be appreciated.

PERIPHERAL NEUROGENIC PAIN

There is over a metre in length between the extremities and the spinal cord and along the way is the dorsal root ganglion (DRG), the "brain" of the peripheral nervous system. A lot of processing can occur between tissues and cord. We must resist the urge to consider peripheral nerves as mere cables linking tissues to the central nervous system. Peripheral nerves are long, living, and responsive tissue components of the entire nervous system. Even when nerves are cut, pain is not turned off, but paradoxically, sensitivity often increases. Unfortunately this information has come too late for many who were subjected to nerve ablation techniques in the 60s and 70s. Even with sympathectomy, intact afferent fibres may develop adrenaline sensitivity (Bossut et al. 1996). A summary of modern concepts related to peripheral neurogenic pain follows.

MODERN CONCEPTS

1. The stability of peripheral nerve function, from nerve terminals to the cortex is incredible. First, consider the encoding, conducting, relay and processing functions and secondly, the mechanical forces being placed upon the system by normal human movement (Butler 1991). An axon can be over a metre long, have differing sources of blood, bend all the time, rub on various tissues and yet is just one cell. You can read more about the remarkable physical abilities of the nervous system in chapter 5.

2. Axons are designed to be "highways" and transmit impulses rather than generate them. Impulse generation and the transduction process are features of the nerve terminals and perhaps the dorsal root ganglion cells. For persistent nerve pain, impulses need to be somehow modified along the pathway. These modified sites are known as abnormal impulse generating sites (AIGS). Knowledge of AIGS is a key to understanding peripheral neurogenic pain.

3. The subtlety and variety of peripheral nerve contributions to pain states are not appreciated (Sunderland 1978; Loeser 1985; Ochoa 1993; Devor and Seltzer 1999; Serra 1999). Much symptomatology could relate to what Sunderland (1978) referred to as "perversions of function", referring to nerve problems which may not necessarily involve failing conduction and thus rate a diagnostic category of neurapraxia or Sunderland category 1. Classifications of peripheral neuropathies need updating to include abnormal impulse generating sites.

4. The connective tissues of peripheral nerve are innervated and hence capable of causing pain (Hromada 1963; Bove and Light 1997; Sauer et al. 1999). Not much is known about nerve sheath pain, although there is a discussion in chapter 5. Presumably, the healthier the connective tissues of the sheath, then the healthier conduction will be.

5. Despite the existence of many textbooks on focal nerve entrapment, it is unlikely that a focal neuropathy such as nerve compression syndrome will exist on its own. Interactions with nociceptive pain (via neurogenic inflammation), further changes in peripheral nerve (eg. DRG upregulation) and contributions to stress response activation and central sensitisation are likely. A mechanisms approach to pain states is necessary to fully include these components of the pain state.

6. A new area of study is the role of the immune system in peripheral neurogenic pain. Pro-inflammatory cytokines such as interleukins 1 and 6 and tumour necrosis factor appear far more pain provocative than ever realised. Even undamaged peripheral nerve can become sensitive in the presence of these mediators (Sorkin et al. 1997; Watkins and Maier 2000).

ABNORMAL IMPULSE GENERATING SITES (AIGS)

There are a number of ways in which a peripheral nerve can become a pain generator. The most obvious is for symptoms to arise from the innervated connective tissues of the nerve. We don't know much about this pain, although a tentative suggestion is that the nerve probably acts in a similar fashion to any ligamentous pain (Asbury and Fields 1984). The close proximity of the epineurium, perineurium and endoneurium to nerve fibres suggests that they may have a more important role than just mechanical support. More complex pain generating sites must involve the long conducting fibres and AIGS development. However it is likely that chemicals released by the nervi nervorum such as CGRP and Prostaglandin E2 (Bove and Light 1995) and proinflammatory cytokines (Sorkin et al. 1997) may react with damaged nerve fibres.

When injured, a segment of peripheral nerve may develop the ability to repeatedly generate its own impulses. Spontaneous activity and mechanosensitivity are the main features of an AIGS, thus neurodynamic testing is likely to evoke symptoms. For a detailed and excellent review see Devor & Seltzer (1999).

INSIDE THE AIGS

Briefly, the axolemma is always in a state of remodelling. Ion channels (chapter 2) are continually being replaced, and up/downregulated either naturally or in response to life's stressors. The key element of ectopic discharge must be that ion channel number, kind and excitability must have altered. In addition, there must be available mechanical and/or chemical stimuli to activate the channels.

There are various injury processes occurring in peripheral nerve which allow variations in ion channel number and kind. Myelin physically suppresses the insertion of ion channels so that anywhere it is absent is an opportunity for ion channel insertion. Therefore demyelinated patches, neuromas, regenerating axon sprouts and cells in the DRG, all of which have no myelin are likely places for channel accumulation (eg. Wall and Gutnick 1974; Calvin et al. 1982; Baker and Bostok 1992; Amir and Devor 1993; Janig et al. 1996; Tal and Eliav 1996; Chen and Devor 1998; England et al. 1998; Liu et al. 2000) (Fig. 3.7). A similar process may happen in the spinal cord (Smith and McDonald 1980). Note also that the kinds of ion channel will vary and will represent the perceived needs of the individual. Ion channels only have a half-life of a few days and thus are continually being turned over and replaced. A well supported hypothesis discussed below is that alpha1 adrenoceptors are expressed in nociceptors when conditions are favourable, such as bare axolemma. An action potential is due to a number of stimuli. Open noradrenaline sensitive channels may hold the membrane potential close to activation and then a small number of open mechanosensitive channels is all that is needed to cause a spike. An AIGS will thus occur and fire antidromically and orthodromically (Howe et al. 1977; Raminsky 1978).

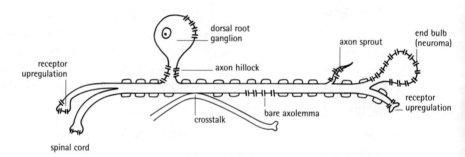

3.7   *Possible abnormal impulse generating sites represented in one neurone. Note bare axolemma, neuroma, nerve sprouts and that the DRG has no myelin. Note also cross excitation with a neighbouring neurone. II = ion channel.*

STIMULI WHICH FIRE AN AIGS

Various stimuli as illustrated in figure 3.8 have the capacity to activate an AIGS. A frequent stimulus will be mechanical forces opening mechanosensitive channels. Hence active movements, palpation of nerves and the neurodynamic tests may cause pain and/or dysaesthesias.

Temperature extremes of hot and cold may make the AIGS fire. Cooling excites C fibres and heating excites the A fibres (Matzner and Devor 1987), although more complex mechanisms exist (Craig 1999). Various metabolic and chemical stimuli can also excite the damaged and altered membrane. So can ischaemia, anoxia and blood gas changes (Devor and Seltzer 1999). The pro-inflammatory cytokine, tumor necrosis factor alpha has been shown to evoke C fibre ectopic firing in undamaged nerves (Sorkin et al. 1997; Junger and Sorkin 2000) and will stimulate production of other pro-inflammatory cytokines such as interleukin-1 (IL-1). These may prime the system for ectopic discharge (Bennett 1999). Pain, including referred pain from experimental neuritis from minor nerve damage can be initiated by cytokines (Eliav et al. 1999). Cytokines have also been linked to demyelination (Redford et al. 1995).

Zochodne et al. (1997) had the opportunity to see what was inside a mechanosensitive human sural nerve neuroma and compare it with a non-symptomatic contralateral nerve. Disorganised axon profiles were noted with axons containing SP and CGRP. The neuroma also contained large numbers of mast cells containing serotonin, which is a pro-inflammatory chemical in the periphery.

Spontaneous activity is a feature of an AIGS, especially if the dorsal root ganglion is injured. Clinically this may translate into a patient unable to give an example of an aggravating activity for a nerve root pain, or more likely the aggravating incident has been so minimal that it was not perceived.

ADRENALINE, NORADRENALINE AND NERVE PAIN

Adrenaline is the primary catecholamine released from the adrenal gland, noradrenaline is secreted by postganglionic sympathetic neurones. If adrenaline is injected around a stump neuroma or in the skin of a patient with postherpetic neuralgia, there will be an increase in spontaneous pain (Raja et al. 1998). An injection of noradrenaline into normal tissues does not hurt, hence it is likely that adrenaline receptors are connected to nociceptors in the case of

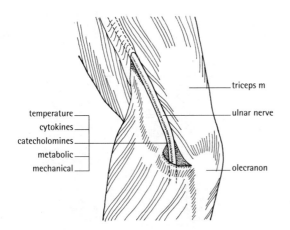

triceps m

ulnar nerve

temperature
cytokines
catecholomines
metabolic
mechanical

olecranon

3.8   The various stimuli which are known to activate an abnormal impulse generating site in a peripheral nerve.

neuromas. There are likely to be adrenoceptor density changes, expression of new adrenoceptors or existing receptors acquiring greater sensitivity (Perl 1999). The density of noradrenaline receptors in hyperalgesic skin of patients with reflex sympathetic dystrophy is increased compared to the normal skin of control subjects (Drummond et al. 1996).

Injured A and C fibres may become sensitive to sympathetic stimulation (Wall and Gutnick 1974; Habler et al. 1987; see review by Devor and Seltzer 1999). Post ganglionic sympathetic fibres are like leaky hoses and noradrenaline has easy access to neurones (Fig. 3.9). With nerve injury, even intact nociceptors and low threshold mechanoreceptors develop sensitivity to sympathetic stimulation (Sato and Perl 1991; Ali et al. 1999; Birder and Perl 1999), with peak excitatory effects 2-3 weeks after the injury (Sato and Perl 1991). Another process which may be clinically relevant is that sprouting of sympathetic fibres will occur in injured DRG and skin nerves (Chung et al. 1993; McLachlan et al. 1993; Small et al. 1996; for review see Ramer et al. 1999).

OTHER FEATURES OF AN AIGS

While an AIGS may be a source of local pain, it must be placed within a bigger clinical picture. An AIGS may affect dorsal horn cells, inevitably brain cells, the dorsal root ganglion, and it may contribute to neurogenic inflammation via antidromic impulse generation. An AIGS may contribute to another neuropathy along the nerve, known as "double crush" (see chapter 15).

When peripheral neurones are injured, neighbouring neurones also get excited. This is known as cross-excitation (Fig. 3.7). It may occur where myelin is lost and thus cells are in close contact, or after repetitive signalling which causes an increase in intracellular calcium that diffuses and excites neighbouring cells (Shinder and Devor 1994). Acute coupling vanishes very quickly but as a clinician, I am more interested to know that it returns in a few weeks in a more long lasting form. These cross-excitations may lead to a chain reaction as more neurones are recruited, resulting in shock like pain complaints, for example in trigeminal neuralgia (Rappaport and Devor 1994) and some nerve root injuries.

Extraterritorial pain after a nerve injury may well be due to central processes, although the contribution of the uninjured afferents to maintaining the CNS sensitivity has been suggested by some (Ro and Jacobs 1993; Tal and Bennett 1994; Sotgiu and Biella 1997).

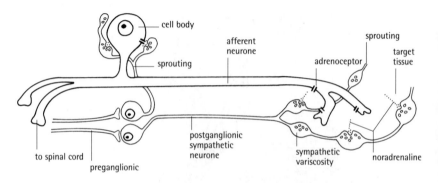

3.9   Afferent neurone/sympathetic coupling. More adrenoceptors are available in the DRG and target tissues. Sympathetic sprouting occurs in the DRG and in the target tissues. II = ion channel. Adapted from Janig et al. (1996).

Note also that AIGS occur in sensory nerves rather than motor nerves. There has been little investigation of the process in motor nerves although it would seem more appropriate for survival purposes for the afferent system to be more predisposed to sensitivity changes. We are just beginning to explore the role of genes and pain. While it is known that inherited forms of migraine and congenital insensitivity to pain involve gene mutations, there are sure to be other genetic links to pain (Mogil et al. 2000). It is also interesting that abnormal impulse generating sites seem to occur in certain species of rat suggesting a genetic predisposition to AIGS formation (Devor and Seltzer 1999).

Remember the discussion earlier in the chapter about pain not always relating to injury. This feature also occurs with nerve injuries. Histological studies of humans at autopsy have shown that 50% of cadavers have connective tissue and nerve fibre changes, particularly in vulnerable places such as the ulnar nerve at the elbow (Neary and Ochoa 1975). In life they never complained of pain. Various imaging techniques consistently reveal abnormally compressed nerve roots in 20-30% of adults who have no history of pain. The process of turning pathology into pain is a complex bio-psycho-social phenomenon of which peripheral neurogenic pain must be a part.

The dorsal root ganglion and nerve roots

The dorsal root ganglion is a rather special part of the peripheral nervous system. It is exquisitely mechanosensitive compared to nerve roots (Sugawara et al. 1996). It is also intrinsically rhythmogenic - firing orthodromically and antidromically, creating something of a background sensory field. Mechanical pressure placed upon uninjured nerve roots in awake patients undergoing low back surgery will not cause pain (Smyth and Wright 1958; Kuslich et al. 1991). At the most it will cause some paraesthesia. However, like the nerve terminals, the presence of inflammation makes the nerve root complex particularly sensitive. In addition to the inflammatory mediators discussed above, a further source of irritation are algogesic chemicals produced from the disc, in particular phospholipase A2, commonly known as PLA2 (Saal et al. 1990; Franson et al. 1992; Chen et al. 1997). Chronic exposure to PLA2 will cause nerve root demyelination (Chen et al. 1997) and thus more potential for ion channel density changes. Other known nerve irritants produced by cervical and lumbar discs include nitric oxide, cytokines, prostaglandins and metalloproteases (Kang et al. 1995; Kang et al. 1996). It may be the presence of these chemicals which cause neural irritation and radicular pain.

AIGS IN HUMANS

The effects of mechanical stimuli have also been measured in humans with known neuropathies, using microneurographic recordings from single nerve fibres (Vallbo et al. 1979). The study by Nordin et al. (1984) links the animal studies to clinical findings and indirectly to neurodynamic assessment. Nerve activity correlating to intensity and time course of symptoms was recorded in five patients. The first was in a patient with a Tinel's sign of ulnar nerve entrapment at the elbow. This patient had symptoms for two years and there were slight changes in motor nerve conduction. The second patient had residual minor ulnar based paraesthesia and weakness post brachial plexus decompression for a "thoracic outlet syndrome". Measurable nerve activity increased as he lifted his arm and experienced symptoms. The third patient had an L5-S1 radiculopathy from a herniated disc. Activity in the sural nerve could be reproduced by straining plus neck flexion. In the fourth patient, with radiculopathy and perineural fibrosis post surgery, nerve activity correlated with symptoms experienced during straight leg raising. The fifth patient had multiple sclerosis. The activity could be recorded in a median nerve fascicle during neck flexion (L'hermittes sign, chapter 8). This is also an indication of centrally induced antidromic impulse.

Spontaneously or mechanically evoked mid single axon impulses have been recorded in relation to Spurling's test (cervical extension, lateral flexion towards test side) (Ochoa et al. 1987) and in amputation neuromas (Nystrom and Hagbarth 1981). Subjective sensations of mechanically or spontaneously induced paraesthesia have been also been correlated with AIGS activity (Campero et al. 1998). These studies all support the likelihood of a neurodynamic test reproducing symptoms related to an AIGS.

AXOPLASM, CIRCULATION AND SCARRED NERVES

The discussion so far has been at the molecular end of the spectrum. An understanding of AIGS must be allied with the more macroscopic view of the peripheral nervous system such as vascularity, axoplasmic flow and the physical health of the connective tissue sheath. These issues have been discussed elsewhere (eg. Sunderland 1978; Lundborg 1988; Butler 1991; Rempel et al. 1999).

A discussion on AIGS must also be allied with the physical health of the nervous system (chapter 5). If the nervous system has lost some of its normal abilities to strain and glide, then it is logical that forces which may have normally been displaced can no longer be dispersed and thus more mechanical forces are placed on the AIGS. Lack of movement may also mean that dispersal of surrounding irritating chemicals cannot easily occur. The presence of scar tissue is often associated with mechanosensitive nerve roots. In reopened laminectomies, Kuslich (1991) always noted perineural fibrosis and suggested that scarring will compound nerve pain by fixing the nerve root in one position.

PROPOSED SYMPTOM PATTERN FOR PERIPHERAL NEUROGENIC PAIN

Symptoms could be related to hyperactivity or hypoactivity in peripheral nerves. Hyperactivity type symptoms from sensory axons relate to abnormal impulse generating sites and could be painful sensations, burning, feelings of coldness, crawling, tightness and prickling. Hypoactivity symptoms are more related to blocked conduction and could include sensory loss and weakness (Dyck 1993).

Below is a proposed pattern. It is not pathognomic, but it allows a clinical diagnosis of an operant mechanism. See chapters 6 and 7 for the use of patterns via clinical reasoning. Take care with its use. Some clinical presentations are clearly peripheral neurogenic. Others, because of the co-existence of peripheral and central sensitisation are much less clear.

AREA OF SYMPTOMS

Symptoms in the following distributions may suggest peripheral neurogenic pains.

• Pain or dysaesthesias in a neural zone such as a dermatomal or cutaneous innervation field (chapter 9). Some peripheral neuropathies are very well localised. Others may involve part of the field.

• Spot pain along a nerve. Palpation of the nerve may elicit symptoms.

• Pain along a nerve trunk (could be a line or strip).

QUALITY AND KIND OF SYMPTOMS

A wide spectrum of disorders exists, from a minor spot pain (perhaps a "trigger point") to a severe, debilitating nerve root disorder. Symptoms may include:

• appropriate motor involvement (chapter 9).

• "burning". This is a common complaint especially when cutaneous nerves are involved. The deeper nerves and nerves to muscles may cause a deep diffuse cramping sensation (Ochoa and Torebjork 1983).

• paraesthesia in a peripheral neural zone.

• noctural pain.

BEHAVIOUR

The behaviour of the symptoms can give many clues to the mechanism and sources. For example:

• Pain is usually evoked on movement of the nerve (eg. elevation of the arm) or changes in the surrounding tissues (eg. cervical zygapophyseal joints closing down onto cervical nerve roots). Mechanosensitivity could be in the form of a burst at the initiation of a stimulus, during the time of the stimulus, a burst on release of the stimulus, or it may leave an afterdischarge (Devor and Seltzer 1999) (Fig. 3.10). In general, the stimulus/response relationship will be present, although not as preserved as in nociceptive pain. For example, pulling on the nerve via a straight leg raise may hurt, ease the pressure, and the pain subsides. If the dorsal root ganglion is involved, the stimulus/response relationship may be less stable. There could even be spontaneous pain.

• There may be a link to stress states (eg. sympathetic nervous system coupling).

• There may be a link to inflammation (eg. neurogenic inflammation).

• Antalgic postures are quite common. Some examples are elevated shoulder girdles to take pressure off lower cervical nerve roots and ipsilateral lumbar lists which may take off some of the forces on sensitive lumbar nerve roots.

• The peripheral neurogenic mechanisms may evoke varied descriptive terms such as "strings pulling", "ants on me" and "electrical feelings". A new patient once described to me a sensation of "tight nerves". The more bizarre pain reports may make the central nervous system a target for consideration. However, it is obvious from animal and human research, that the capacity of an AIGS to contribute to apparently weird symptomatology should not be underestimated.

• It is worth noting that after injury, some AIGS remain silent for a few days before they become reactive.

SOME THOUGHTS FOR CLINICIANS

The AIGS concept may well force a reconsideration of certain diagnoses. Many trigger points may be small AIGS in cutaneous nerves struggling with their relationship to fascia and muscle and postural demands (see notalgia paraesthetica, chapter 15). Once well-defined disorders such as de Quervain's disease now appear to have a significant peripheral nerve component (Mackinnon and Dellon 1988). Any nerve, even tiny branches are capable of generating ectopic impulse production.

It would be beneficial to know the source(s) of the mechanisms, that is, the actual peripheral nerve structures causing the symptoms. This may be easy if there is a dermatomal or cutaneous field loss, or diminution of reflex which can point to involvement of a particular nerve or site along the nerve. This may be very simple in the clinical setting in neatly defined nerve compression syndromes. In others where there may be coexisting central sensitivity and multiple sites of nerve injury, the pattern is not as clear. Chapter 10 has further details about analysing neurodynamic findings.

Management can be targeted at the various stimuli (Fig. 3.8), meaning that the approach is aimed at biological targets as well as anatomical targets. Hence, a management aim will be to turn a firing nerve off. This may be achieved by altering sympathetic and immune inputs (eg. explain disorder, make goals, decrease fear) or encouraging better circulation (simple exercise), lessening mechanical forces (adapt postures, make nervous system more physically healthy), even altering the workplace if there is heat or cold sensitivity. Further details on management of specific peripheral neurogenic states such as carpal tunnel syndrome and nerve root disorders are discussed in chapter 14 and 15.

The importance of the barrage into the CNS from ectopia cannot be underestimated. While potentially a nasty local problem, the overall pain state may become much nastier in the presence of a maladaptively upregulated CNS (chapter 4). The CNS will respond of course to any afferent input, but while an AIGS keeps firing, the CNS is in a danger state for sensitisation, some of which may be long lasting. Because people have different levels of CNS threshold control and ascribe different meanings to painful input, some people may be more predisposed to CNS changes post AIGS barrage. These people may be identified via a bio-psycho-social based assessment.

Due to the mechanosensitivity and ischaemosensitivity of an AIGS and the innervated connective tissue sheath, a skilled assessment of the physical health of peripheral nerves should allow detection of the presence of an AIGS. Skills in handling, both physical and communicative, are critical and are emphasised in the examination sections.

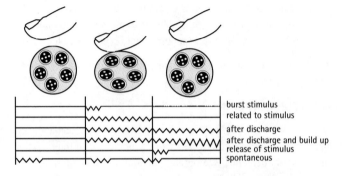

burst stimulus
related to stimulus

after discharge
after discharge and build up
release of stimulus
spontaneous

3.10 Features of mechanosensitivity in an abnormal impulse generating site. With a physical stimulus such as compression, a variety of responses may occur.

PERIPHERAL INPUT TO THE CNS

Neurones never act alone. The nervous system will not allow inflammation and abnormal impulse generating sites to go unnoticed. Inflammation in tissues will lead to increased responsiveness of dorsal horn neurones (eg. Hylden et al. 1989; Neugebauer and Schaible 1990; Grubb et al. 1993). When C fibres are repeatedly stimulated, a short term increase in dorsal horn neurone responsiveness will occur (Mendell and Wall 1965), known as the "wind-up" phenomenon. Further long term changes in the CNS will occur with input from injured nerves (eg. Basbaum and Wall 1976; Devor and Wall 1981; Devor and Seltzer 1999). The intensity and amount of afferent input is important for CNS changes (Svendsen et al. 1998). In experimental states, when ectopic activity is prevented from reaching the spinal cord, the central sensitisation will fade (Sheen and Chung 1993).

The degree of inhibition exerted by the CNS depends on the amount of C fibre afferent input (Schaible et al. 1991). Thus the CNS is "in phase" with afferent input and it makes it understandable how a loss of afferent input lifts the descending inhibitory controls and may lead to odd and bizarre pain states and consequent behaviours. Animals whose nervous systems were treated by capsaicin at birth had reduced C fibre input and reduced power in their descending inhibitory control systems (Cervero and Laird 1996).

Consider also that a multiplier effect might occur. For example a crush injury of the hand will create an afferent impulse barrage, which will also sensitise the DRG and thus create another barrage. The DRG cells will fire spontaneously and repeatedly when activated by thermal and mechanical stimuli (Gallego et al. 1987; Gurtu and Smith 1988).

The somatosensory system is not alone in signalling. The eyes, the ears and the nose have specialised receptors which provide the brain with information about the environment. The immune system also signals the brain. Pro-inflammatory cytokines such as tumour necrosis factor alpha (TNF alpha) and interleukins IL-1 and IL-6 are thought to be key brain communicators (Watkins et al. 1995; Watkins and Maier 2000). These are discussed in the next chapter.

CHAPTER SUMMARY

I have proposed in this chapter that manual therapists take a closer look at the total phenomenon of pain. This is because there is a great difference between the status of tissue healing and the amount and nature of pain reported by patients. Therefore while an understanding of tissue healing is important it is believed that an understanding of pain mechanisms is also important. Using known neurobiology and associated animal and human models, it is proposed that pattern recognition may allow identification of mechanisms related to pain.

In this chapter, the mechanisms of nociceptive and peripheral neurogenic pain and associated clinical patterns are presented.

These are exciting and challenging times for the manual therapy professions. I believe that the pain science world is handing extremely valuable information to clinicians. We now have a greater understanding of the behaviour of pain states and we are becoming aware of the molecular targets of manual therapy. Read on now to the next chapter. Here the central mechanisms and influences of the autonomic endocrine and immune systems are discussed.

REFERENCES CHAPTER 3

Ali Z, Ringkamp M, Hartke TV, et al. (1999) Uninjured C-fiber nociceptors develop spontaneous activity and alpha adrenergic sensitivity following L6 spinal nerve ligation in the monkey. Journal of Neurophysiology 81: 455-466.

Amir M, Michaelis M & Devor M (1999) Membrane potential oscillations in dorsal root ganglion neurons: role in normal electrogenesis and neuropathic pain. Journal of Neuroscience 19: 8589-8596.

Amir R & Devor M (1993) Ongoing activity in neuroma afferents bearing retrograde sprouts. Brain Research 630: 283-288.

Asbury AK & Fields HL (1984) Pain due to peripheral nerve damage: an hypothesis. Neurology 34: 1587-1590.

Baker M & Bostok H (1992) Ectopic activity in demyelinated spinal root axons of the rat. Journal of Physiology 451: 539-552.

Basbaum AI & Wall PD (1976) Chronic changes in the response of cells in adult cat dorsal horn following partial deafferentation: the appearance of responding cells in a previously non-responsive region. Brain Research 116: 181-204.

Bennett GJ (1999) Does a neuroimmune interaction contribute to the genesis of painful peripheral neuropathies. Proceedings of the National Academy of Science 96: 7737-7738.

Bevan S & Yeats J (1991) Protons activate a cation conductance in a sub-population of rat dorsal root ganglion neurones. Journal of Physiology 433: 145-161.

Birder LA & Perl ER (1999) Expression of alpha2-adrenergic receptors in rat primary afferent neurones after peripheral nerve injury or inflammation. Journal of Physiology (London) 515: 533-542.

Boden SD, Davis D, Dina TS, et al. (1990) Abnormal magnetic-resonance scans of the lumbar spine in asymptomatic subjects: A prospective investigation. Journal of Bone and Joint Surgery 72A: 403-408.

Bossut DF, Shea VK & Perl ER (1996) Sympathectomy induces adrenergic excitability of cutaneous C-fiber nociceptors. Journal of Neurophysiology 75: 514-517.

Bove GM & Light AR (1995) Calcitonin gene-related peptide and peripherin immunoreactivity in nerve sheaths. Somatosensory and Motor Research 12: 49-57.

Bove GM & Light AR (1997) The nervi nervorum. Pain Forum 6: 181-190.

Butler DS (1991) Mobilisation of the Nervous System, Churchill Livingstone, Melbourne.

Butler DS (1994) The upper limb tension test revisited. In: Grant R (ed.) Physical Therapy of the Cervical and Thoracic Spines, 2nd edn. Churchill Livingstone, New York.

Butler DS (1998) Integrating pain awareness into physiotherapy - wise action for the future. In: Gifford LS (ed.) Topical Issues in Pain, NOI Press, Falmouth.

Calixto JB, Cabrini DA, Ferreira J, et al. (2000) Kinins in pain and inflammation. Pain 87: 1-5.

Calvin WH, Devor M & Howe JF (1982) Can neuralgias arise from minor demyelination? spontaneous firing, mechanosensitivity, and afterdischarge from conduction axons. Experimental Neurology 75: 755-763.

Campbell JN, Meyer RA & Raja SN (1992) Is nociceptor activation by alpha-1 adrenoreceptors the culprit in sympathetically maintained pain? American Pain Society Journal 13: 344-350.

Campero M, Serra J, Marchettini P, et al. (1998) Ectopic impulse generation and autoexcitation in single myelinated afferent fibres in patients with peripheral neuropathy and positive sensory symptoms. Muscle Nerve 21: 1661-1667.

Carlton SM & Coggeshall RE (1999) Inflammation-inducd changes in peripheral glutamate receptor populations. Brain Research 820: 63-70.

Cervero F & Laird JMA (1996) From acute to chronic pain: mechanisms and hypotheses. In: Carli G & Zimmermann M (eds.) Towards the Neurobiology of Chronic Pain, Elsevier, Amsterdam.

Chahl L & Ladd R (1976) Local oedema and general excitation of cutaneous sensory recpetors produced by electrical stimulation of the saphenous nerve in the rat. Pain 2: 25-34.

Chen C, Cavanaugh JM, Ozaktay AC, et al. (1997) Effects of phospholipase A2 on lumbar nerve root structure and function. Spine 22: 1057-1064.

Chen Y & Devor M (1998) Ectopic mechanosensitivity in injured sensory axons arises from the site of spontaneous electrogenesis. European Journal of Pain 2: 165-178.

Cherkin DC (1998) Primary care research on low back pain. Spine 23: 1997-2002.

Chung K, Kim HJ, Na HS, et al. (1993) Abnormalities of sympathetic innervation in the area of an injured peripheral nerve in a rat model of neuropathic pain. Neuroscience Letters 162: 85-88.

Craig AD (1999) Functional anatomy of supraspinal pain processing with reference to the central pain syndrome. In: Max M (ed.) Pain 1999 - An Updated Review, IASP Press, Seattle.

Daemen MA, Kurvers HA, Kitslaar PJ, et al. (1998) Neurogenic inflammation in an animal model of neuropathic pain. Neurological Research 20: 41-45.

Davis KD, Treede RD, Raja SN, et al. (1991) Topical application of clonadine relieves hyperalgesia in patients with sympathetically maintained pain. Pain 47: 309-317.

Devor M & Seltzer Z (1999) Pathophysiology of damaged nerves in relation to chronic pain. In: Wall PD & Melzack R (eds.) Textbook of Pain, 4th edn. Churchill Livingstone, Edinburgh.

Devor M & Wall PD (1981) Plasticity in the spinal cord sensory map following peripheral nerve injury in rats. Journal of Neuroscience 1: 679-684.

Deyo RA (1993) Practice variations, treatment fads, rising disability: do we need a new clinical research paradigm? Spine 18: 2153-2162.

Dickenson AH (1996) Pharmacology of pain transmission and control. In: Campbell JN (ed.) Pain 1996 - An Updated Review, IASP Press, Seattle.

Dray A (1995) Inflammatory mediators of pain. British Journal of Anaesthesia 75: 125-131.

Drummond PD, Finch PM & Gibbins I (1996) Innervation of hyperalgesic skin in patients with complex regional pain syndrome. The Clinical Journal of Pain 12: 222-231.

Dyck PJ (1993) Quantitative severity of neuropathy. In: Dyck PJ & Thomas PK (eds.) Peripheral Neuropathy, 2nd edn. W.B. Saunders, Philadelphia.

Ebertz JM, Hirshman C, Kettelkamp NS, et al. (1987) Substance-P induced histamine release in human cutaneous mast cells. Journal of Investigative Dermatology 88: 682-685.

Eliav E, Herzberg U, Ruda MA, et al. (1999) Neuropathic pain from an experimental neuritis of the rat sciatic nerve. Pain 83: 169-182.

England JD, Happel LT, Liu ZP, et al. (1998) Abnormal distributions of potassium channels in human neuromas. Neuroscience Letters 255: 37-40.

Fitzgerald M & Lynn B (1997) The sensitization of high threshold mechanoreceptors with myelinated axons by repeated heating. Journal of Physiology (London) 365: 549-563.

Franson RC, Saal JS & J.A. S (1992) Human disc phospholipase A2 is inflammatory. Spine 17 (Suppl): S129-S132.

Gallego R, Ivorra I & Morales A (1987) Effects of central or peripheral axotomy on membrane properties of sensory neurones in the petrosal ganglia of the cat. Journal of Physiology (London) 391: 39-56.

Gifford L & Butler D (1997) The integration of pain sciences into clinical practice. The Journal of Hand Therapy 10: 86-95.

Gifford LS (1997) Pain. In: Pitt-Brooke J, Reid H, Lockwood J et al. (eds.) Rehabilitation of Movement, WB Saunders, London.

Gifford LS (1998) Tissue and input related mechanisms. In: Gifford LS (ed.) Topical Issues in Pain, NOI Press, Falmouth.

Grubb BD, Stiller RU & Schaible HG (1993) Dynamic changes in the receptive field properties of spinal cord neurons with ankle input in rats with chronic unilateral inflammation in the ankle region. Experimental Brain Research 92: 441-452.

Gurtu S & Smith PA (1988) Electrophysiological characteristics of hamster dorsal root ganglion cells and their response to axotomy. Journal of Neurophysiology 59: 408-423.

Habler H-J, Janig W & Koltzenburg M (1987) Activation of unmyelinated afferents in chronically lesioned nerves by adrenaline and excitation of sympathetic efferents in the cat. Neuroscience Letters 82: 35-40.

Hagermark O, Hokfelt T & Pernow B (1978) Flare and itch induced by substance P in human skin. Journal of Investigative Dermatology 71: 233-235.

Haldeman S (1990) Presidential address, North American Spine Society: Failure of the pathology model to predict back pain. Spine 15: 718-724.

Handwerker HO & Reeh PW (1991) Pain and inflammation. In: Bond MR, Charlton IE & Woolf CJ (eds.) Pain Research and Clinical Management, Elsevier, Amsterdam.

Howe JF, Loeser JD & Calvin WH (1977) Mechanosensitivity of dorsal root ganglia and chronically injured axons: a physiological basis for radicular pain of nerve root compression. Pain 3: 25-41.

Hromada J (1963) On the nerve supply of the connective tissue of some peripheral nervous system components. Acta Anatomica 55: 343-351.

Hulsebosch CE & Coggeshall RE (1981) Quantitation of sprouting of dorsal root axons. Science 213: 1020-1021.

Hylden JL, Nahin RL, Traub RJ, et al. (1989) Expansion of receptive fields of spinal lamina 1 projection neurones in rats with unilateral adjuvant-induced inflammation. The contribution of dorsal horn mechanisms. Pain 37: 229-243.

Janig W (1996) The puzzle of "reflex sympathetic dystrophy": Mechanisms, hypotheses, open questions. In: Janig W & Stantin-Hicks M (eds.) Reflex Sympathetic Dystrophy: A Reappraisal, IASP Press, Seattle.

Janig W, Levine JD & Michaelis M (1996) Interaction of sympathetic and primary afferent neurons following nerve injury and tissue trauma. In: Kumazawa T, Kruger L & Mizumura K (eds.) Progress in Brain Research, 113. The Polymodal Receptor; A Gateway to Pathological Pain, Elsevier, Amsterdam.

Jensen MC, Brant-Zawadzki MN, Obuchowski N, et al. (1994) Magnetic resonance imaging of the lumbar spine in people without back pain. The New England Journal of Medicine 331: 69-73.

Junger H & Sorkin LS (2000) Nociceptive and inflammatory effects of subcutaneous TNFalpha. Pain 85: 145-151.

Kang JD, Georgescu HI, McIntyre-Larkin L, et al. (1995) Herniated cervical intervertebral discs spontaneously produce matrix metalloproteinases, nitric oxide, interleukin-6, and prostaglandin E2. Spine 20: 2373-2378.

Kang JD, Georgescu HI, McIntyre-Larkin LM, et al. (1996) Herniated lumbar intervertebral discs spontaneously produce matrix metalloproteinases, nitric oxide, interleukin-6 and prostaglandin E2. Spine 21: 271-7.

Kolston J & Lisney SJW (1993) A study of vasodilator responses evoked by antidromic stimulation of A delta afferent fibers supplying normal and reinnervated rat skin. Microvascular Research 46: 143-147.

Koltzenburg M (1999) The changing sensitivity in the life of the nociceptor. Pain Supplement 6: S93-S102.

Kruger L (1996) The functional morphology of thin sensory axons: some principles and problems. In: Kumazawa T, Kruger L & Mizumura K (eds.) The Polymodal Receptor: A Gateway to Pathological Pain, Elsevier, Amsterdam.

Kuslich SD, Ulstrom CL & Michael CJ (1991) The tissue origin of low back pain and sciatica. Orthopedic Clinics of North America 22: 181-187.

Leadbetter WB, Buckwalter JA & Gordon SL eds. (1990) Sports-induced Inflammation, American Academy of Orthopedic Surgeons, Park Ridge, Illinois.

Levine JD & Reichling DB (1999) Peripheral mechanisms of inflammatory pain. In: Wall PD & Melzack R (eds.) Textbook of Pain, 4th edn. Churchill Livingstone, Edinburgh.

Lewis T (1942) Pain, Macmillan, New York.

Liu X, Eschenfelder S, Blenk KH, et al. (2000) Spontaneous activity of axotomised afferent neurons after L5 spinal nerve injury in rats. Pain 84: 309-318.

Loeser JD (1985) Pain due to nerve injury. Spine 10: 232-235.

Loh L & Nathan PW (1978) Painful peripheral states and sympathetic blocks. Journal of Neurology, Neurosurgery and Psychiatry 41: 664-671.

Lundborg G (1988) Nerve Injury and Repair, Churchill Livingstone, Edinburgh.

Mackinnon SE & Dellon AL (1988) Surgery of the Peripheral Nerve, Thieme, New York.

Maggi CA & Meli A (1988) The sensory-efferent function of capsaicin-sensitive neurones. General Pharmacology 19: 1-43.

Magni G, Marchetti M, Moreschi C, et al. (1993) Chronic musculoskeletal pain and depressive symptoms in the national health and nutrition examination. 1. Epidemiologic follow up-study. Pain 53: 163.

Matzner O & Devor M (1987) Contrasting thermal sensitivity of spontaneously active A and C fibres in experimental nerve-end neuromas. Pain 30: 373-384.

McLachlan EM, Janig W, Devor M, et al. (1993) Peripheral nerve injury triggers noradrenergic sprouting within dorsal root ganglia. Nature 363: 534-536.

Mendell LM & Wall PD (1965) Responses of single dorsal horn cells to peripheral cutaneous unmyelinated fibres. Nature 206: 97-99.

Mense S (1996) Group III and IV nociceptors in skeletal muscle: are they specific or polymodal? In: Kumazawa T, Kruger L & Mizumura K (eds.) Progress in Brain Research, Vol. 113, Elsevier, Amsterdam.

Mogil JS, Yu L & Basbaum AI (2000) Pain genes?: natural variation and transgenic mutants. Annual Review of Neuroscience 23: 777-811.

Moskowitz MA (1984) The neurobiology of vascular head pain. Annals of Neurology 16: 157-168.

Moskowitz MA (1993) The trigeminovascular system. In: Olesen J, Tfelt-Hansen P & Welch KMA (eds.) The Headaches, Raven Press, Ltd., New York.

Neary D & Ochoa RW (1975) Sub-clinical entrapment neuropathy in man. Journal of the Neurological Sciences 24: 283-298.

Neugebauer V & Schaible HG (1990) Evidence for a central component in the sensitization of spinal neurones with joint input during development of acute arthritis in a cat's knee. Journal of Neurophysiology 64: 299-311.

Nilsson J, von Eular AM & Dalsgaard C-J (1985) Stimulation of connective tissue cell growth by substance P and substance K. Nature 315: 61-63.

Nordin M, Nystrom B, Wallin U, et al. (1984) Ectopic sensory discharges and paresthesiae in patients with disorders of peripheral nerves, dorsal roots and dorsal columns. Pain 20: 231-245.

Nystrom B & Hagbarth KE (1981) Microelectrode recordings from transected nerves in amputees with phantom limb pain. Neuroscience Letters 27: 211-216.

Ochoa J (1993) Guest editorial: Essence, investigation and management of "neuropathic" pains: hopes from acknowledgement of chaos. Muscle & Nerve 16: 997-1008.

Ochoa J & Mair WGP (1969) The normal sural nerve in man. Acta Neuropathologica 13: 197-216.

Ochoa J & Torebjork E (1983) Sensations by intraneural microstimulation of single mechanoreceptor units innervating the human hand. Journal of Physiology 342: 633-654.

Ochoa JL, Cline M, Dotson R, et al. (1987) Pain and paresthesias provoked mechanically in human cervical root entrapment (sign of Spurling). Single sensory unit antidromic recording of ectopic, bursting, propagated nerve activity. In: Pubols LM & Sessle BJ (eds.) Effects of Injury on Trigeminal and Spinal Somatosensory Systems, Liss, New York.

Perl ER (1999) Causalgia, pathological pain, and adrenergic receptors. Proceedings of the National Academy of Science USA 96: 9664-7667.

Peterson CK, Bolton JE & Wood AR (2000) A cross-sectional study correlating lumbar spine degeneration with disability and pain. Spine 25: 218-223.

Raja SN, Abatzis V, Hocasek SJ, et al. (1998) Role of alpha adrenoceptors in neuroma pain in amputees. American Society of Anesthesiology 89.

Raja SN, Meyer RA, Ringkamp M, et al. (1999) Peripheral neural mechanisms of nociception. In: Wall PD & Melzack R (eds.) Textboook of Pain, 4th edn. Churchill Livingstone, Edinburgh.

Ramer MS, Thompson SWN & McMahon SB (1999) Causes and consequences of sympathetic basket formation in dorsal root ganglia. Pain Suppl 6: S111-S120.

Raminsky M (1978) Ectopic generation of impulses and cross-talk in spinal nerve roots of "dystrophic" mice. Annals of Neurology 3: 351-357.

Rappaport ZH & Devor M (1994) Trigeminal neuralgia: the role of self sustaining discharge in the trigeminal ganglion. Pain 56: 127-138.

Redford EJ, Hall SM & Smith KJ (1995) Vascular changes and demyelination induced by the intraneural injection of tumour necrosis factor. Brain 118: 869-878.

Reeh PW & Kress M (1995) Effect of classic algogens. Seminars in Neuroscience 7: 221-226.

Rempel D, Dahlin L & Lundborg G (1999) Pathophysiology of nerve compression syndromes: response of peripheral nerves to loading. Journal of Bone and Joint Surgery 81A: 1600-1610.

Ro LS & Jacobs JM (1993) The role of the saphenous nerve in experimental sciatic nerve mononeuropathy produced by loose ligatures: a behavioural study. Pain 52: 359-369.

Saal JS, Franson RC, Dobrow R, et al. (1990) High levels of inflammatory phospholipase A2 activity in lumbar disc herniation. Spine 15: 674-678.

Sann H & Pierau FK (1998) Efferent functions of C-fiber nociceptors. Zeitschrift fur Rheumatologie 57 (Suppl 2): 8-13.

Sato J & Perl ER (1991) Adrenergic excitation of cutaneous pain receptors induced by peripheral nerve injury. Science 251: 1608-1610.

Sauer SK, Bove GM, Averbeck B, et al. (1999) Rat peripheral nerve components release calcitonin gene-related peptide and prostaglandin E2 in response to noxious stimuli: evidence that the nervi nervorum are nociceptors. Neuroscience 92: 319-325.

Schaible HG, Neugebauer V, Cervero FA, et al. (1991) Changes in tonic descending inhibition of spinal neurones with articular input during the development of acute arthritis in the cat. Journal of Neurophysiology 66: 1021-1032.

Schaible HG & Schmidt RF (1988) Time course of mechanosensitivity changes in articular afferents during a developmental experimental arthritis. Journal of Neurophysiology 60: 2180-2185.

Schmidt RF (1996) The articular polymodal nociceptor in health and disease. In: Kumazama T, Kruger L & Mizumura K (eds.) Progress in Brain Research, Vol 113, Elsevier, Amsterdam.

Schmidt RF, Schaible KM, Heppelmann B, et al. (1994) Silent and active nociceptors: structure, functions and clincial implications. 7th World Congress on Pain , IASP Press,

Serra J (1999) Overview of neuropathic pain syndromes. Acta Neurologica Scandinavica (Suppl) 173: 7-11.

Sheen K & Chung JM (1993) Signs of neuropathic pain depend on signals from injured fibers in a rat model. Brain Research 61: 62-68.

Shinder V & Devor M (1994) Structural basis of neuron-to-neuron cross excitation in dorsal root ganglia. Journal of Neurocytology 23: 515-531.

Shu X-Q & Mendell LM (1999) Neurotrophins and hyperalgesia. Proceedings of the National Academy of Science USA 96: 7693-7696.

Sluka KA, Willis WD & Westlund KN (1995) The role of dorsal root reflexes in neurogenic inflammation. Pain Forum 4: 141-149.

Small JR, Scadding JW & Landon DN (1996) Ultrastructural localization of sympathetic axons in experimental rat sciatic nerve neuromas. Journal of Neurocytology 25: 573-582.

Smith KJ & McDonald WI (1980) Spontaneous and mechanically evoked activity due to cental demyelinating lesion. Nature 286: 154-155.

Smyth M & Wright V (1958) Sciatica and the intervertebral disc. Journal of Bone and Joint Surgery 40A: 1401-1418.

Sorkin LS, Xiao W-H, Wagner R, et al. (1997) Tumor necrosis factor alpha induces ectopic activity in nociceptive primary afferent fibres. Neuroscience 81: 255-262.

Sotgiu ML & Biella G (1997) Role of input from saphenous afferents in altered spinal processing of noxious signal that follows sciatic nerve constriction in rats. Neuroscience Letters 223: 101-104.

Steen KH, Issberner U & Reeh PH (1995) Pain due to experimental acidosis in human skin: evidence for non-adapting nociceptor excitation. Neuroscience Letters 199: 29-32.

Steen KH & Reeh PW (1993) Sustained graded pain and hyperalgesia from harmless experimental tissue acidosis in human skin. Neuroscience Letters 154: 113-116.

Steen KH, Steen AE, Kreysel HW, et al. (1996) Inflammatory mediators potentiate pain induced by experimental tissue acidosis. Pain 66: 163-170.

Sugawara O, Atsuta Y, Iwahara T, et al. (1996) The effects of mechanical compression and hypoxia on nerve roots and dorsal root ganglia. Spine 21: 2089-2094.

Sunderland S (1978) Nerves and Nerve Injuries, 3rd edn. Churchill Livingstone, Melbourne.

Svendsen F, Tjolsen A & Hole K (1998) AMPA and NMDA receptor-dependent spinal LTP after nociceptive tetanic stimulation. Neuroreport 9: 1185-1190.

Tal M & Bennett GJ (1994) Extra-territorial pain in rats with a peripheral neuropathy: mechano-hyperalgesia and mechano-allodynia in the territory of an uninjured nerve. Pain 57: 375-382.

Tal M & Eliav E (1996) Abnormal discharge originates at the site of nerve injury in experimental constriction neuropathy in the rat. Pain 64: 511-518.

Vallbo AB, Hagbarth KE, Torebjork HE, et al. (1979) Somatosensory, proprioceptive, and sympathetic activity in human peripheral nerves. Physiological Review 59: 919-957.

van Wingerden BAM (1995) Connective Tissue in Rehabilitation, Verlag-Vaduz Liechtenstein, Scipro.

Verhaak PF, Kerssens JJ, Dekker J, et al. (1998) Prevalence of chronic benign pain disorder among adults: a review of the literature. Pain 77: 231-239.

Waddell G (1998) The Back Pain Revolution, Churchill Livingstone, Edinburgh.

Waldmann R, Champigny G, Bassilana F, et al. (1997) A proton-gated cation channel involved in acid sensing. Nature 386: 173-177.

Wall PD (1996) The mechanisms by which tissue damage and pain are related. In: Campbell JN (ed.) Pain 1996- An Updated Review, IASP Press, Seattle.

Wall PD (1999) Pain, the Science of Suffering, Weidenfield & Nicholson, London.

Wall PD & Devor M (1983) Sensory afferent impulses originate from dorsal root ganglia and chronically injured axons: a physiological base for the radicular pain of nerve root compression. Pain 17: 321-339.

Wall PD & Gutnick M (1974) Ongoing activity in peripheral nerves: the physiology and pharmacology of impulses originating from a neuroma. Experimental Neurology 43: 580-593.

Wall PD & Melzack R eds. (1999) Textbook of Pain, 4th edn. Churchill Livingstone, Edinburgh.

Watkins LR & Maier SF (2000) The pain of being sick: implications of immune-to-brain communication for understanding pain. Annual Review of Psychology 51: 29-57.

Watkins LR, Maier SF & Goehler LE (1995) Immune activation: the role of pro-inflammatory cytokines in inflammation, illness responses and pathological pain states. Pain 63: 289-302.

Westlund KN (1999) Introduction to the basic science of pain and headache for the clinician: anatomical concepts. In: Max M (ed.) Pain 1999-An updated review, IASP Press, Seattle.

Woo SLY & Buckwalter JA eds. (1988) Injury and Repair of the Musculoskeletal Soft Tissues, American Academy of Orthopedic Surgeons, Park Ridge, Illinois.

Woolf CJ, Bennett GJ, Doherty M, et al. (1998) Towards a mechanism-based classification of pain. Pain 77: 227-229.

Zochodne DW, Theriault M, Sharkey KA, et al. (1997) Peptides and neuromas: calcitonin gene related peptide, substance P, and mast cells in a mechanosensitive human sural neuroma. Muscle & Nerve 20: 875-880.

CHAPTER 4

CENTRAL SENSITIVITY, RESPONSE AND HOMEOSTATIC SYSTEMS

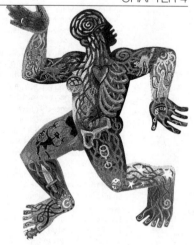

INTRODUCTION - CENTRAL SENSITIVITY CONCEPT

PROCESS OF SENSITIVITY CHANGES IN THE DORSAL HORN
CHANGES IN THE BRAIN
DESCENDING CONTROL SYSTEMS
A PROPOSED PATTERN OF CENTRAL SENSITIVITY
CLINICAL THOUGHTS

IMMUNE, ENDOCRINE, MOTOR AND SYMPATHETIC SYSTEMS AS RESPONSE AND BACKGROUND SYSTEMS

INTRODUCTION

AUTONOMIC/NEUROENDOCRINE SYSTEM

THE HYPOTHALAMUS–PITUITARY–ADRENAL AXIS (HPA)
SYMPATHETIC NEURAL AXIS AND SYMPATHETIC ADRENAL AXIS
SYMPATHETIC NERVOUS SYSTEM AND PAIN
THE PARASYMPATHETIC NERVOUS SYSTEM
MOTOR SYSTEM AS AN OUTPUT SYSTEM

IMMUNE SYSTEM

BASIC APPARATUS

THOUGHTS FOR CLINICIANS

REFERENCES CHAPTER 4

INTRODUCTION - CENTRAL SENSITIVITY CONCEPT

Pain mechanisms related to tissues and to peripheral nerves were discussed in the previous chapter. In this chapter, pain mechanisms related to the central nervous system and to response and homeostatic systems such as the autonomic and immune systems are discussed.

The setting of the central nervous system (CNS) varies within and between all of us. What tickles during one hour may not tickle the next; what is painful in one situation may not be painful in another. The value of another person's touch varies enormously from person to person. The nervous system's responses to a specified input is dynamic. The central sensitivity concept proposes that the CNS sensitivity or activation threshold is set lower, and thus stimuli which would not normally be able to access central neurones can now have an effect (Hardy et al. 1952; Woolf 1991). This is not just a sensitivity to physical stimuli, it is also a sensitivity to our thoughts and feelings. These psychological inputs will collide with the physically derived inputs and undergo a bilateral parallel processing in which the threshold exerted on any inputs will be lowered. This processing involves environmental input as well. As Hinde (1998) reminds us in a beautiful essay, the environment is not just something out there, it is also something which we create by choice and coping style. The environment that the person in pain occupies is different to the environment that the non-sufferer lives in.

Central sensitivity concepts are not new. For many years there have been suggestions that pain produced by innocuous stimulation around an injury site is central in origin. There is now plenty of evidence to support this contention (for a review see Doubell et al. 1999). Changes in the response properties of the multi-receptive wide dynamic range (WDR) neurones in the CNS are considered a key part (eg. Willis 1993; Treede and Magerl 1995). There are three ways in which central sensitisation will be manifested in CNS neurones. First the threshold of firing will be reduced, secondly there will be an increase in the responsiveness of neurones and thirdly, the receptive field of the neurone will increase (eg. Cook et al. 1987; Hoheisel and Mense 1989; Neugebauer and Schaible 1990; Woolf and King 1990; Simone et al. 1991; Hu et al. 1992; Woolf and Salter 2000).

PROCESS OF SENSITIVITY CHANGES IN THE DORSAL HORN

The process of sensitisation can be followed in the dorsal horn (or the medullary horn in the case of facial input), as long as this does not trivialise the role of higher CNS centres. Similar biological processes to that outlined in the dorsal horn are known to occur in the brain. Essentially, the dorsal horn goes through modes or states of operation. The state or mode that the horn (read entire nervous system) is in will determine the sensory perception. These states are a particularly useful and clinically relevant way for clinicians to engage neuroplasticity and link it to clinical decision making strategies. Shifting modes or preventing new modes should be the biological basis of therapy. Four states are discussed - normal, suppressed, sensitised and reorganised. These states are based on work performed and reviewed by Woolf (1994) and Woolf and Doubell et al. (1999).

NORMAL STATE (STATE 1)

In the normal state, any innocuous input such as light touch, pressure, vibration or warmth will be perceived to be that stimulus. Our nervous systems can extract the particular defining features of the various inputs. Feature extraction also applies to noxious inputs. This is normal physiological pain which usually serves an adaptive and useful purpose. The defining feature of the normal state is that input will equal output. Glutamate and substance P are the key transmission chemicals. Glutamate will activate an AMPA (alpha-amino-3-hydroxy-5-methyl-4-isoxozole-proprionic acid) receptor and substance P will activate a neurokinin 1 (NK1) receptor (eg. Yoshimura and Nishi 1993). This is illustrated in figure 4.1.

SUPPRESSED STATE (STATE 2)

Sometimes, inputs that would be expected to hurt don't hurt. This feature can be quite spectacular. Occasionally newspapers run amazing stories and pictures of people walking to hospital with a spear or stake impaled and reporting no pain. A person could be intent on finishing a particular sporting event and a serious injury may not be felt. Farm accidents involving machinery can be horrific. Yet severely injured workers may report that there was no pain at the time of the accident. We all probably know or have heard of similar stories. This ability to stop pain is a great survival feature and it enables flight or fight reactions. Immediate pain, commensurate with the extent of injury from a severe farm injury would probably mean that that person would go into shock and faint and perhaps die. Somehow the nervous system makes an executive decision, based on complex processing including past and future responses, that pain can be kept at bay for a later date. Stopping the pain of severe trauma must involve an extremely powerful biological process. In the suppressed state, this will be due in part to peripheral inputs but far more powerful effects will come from the endogenous pain control mechanisms in the brain and spinal cord.

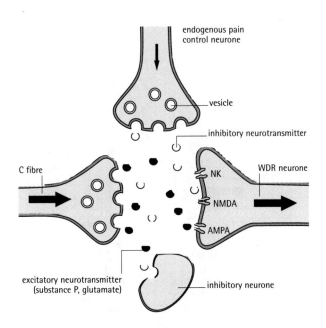

4.1   The control state of the dorsal horn (state 1). C fibre input creates a commensurate output in a wide dynamic ranging neurone (WDR). Substance P targets a neurokinin receptor (NK) and amino acids target an AMPA receptor. The NMDA receptor is closed. See text for details.

Note that in figure 4.2, the focus is now on the descending control systems. The release of an inhibitory chemical such as gamma-aminobutyric acid (GABA), enkephalin or serotonin can act presynaptically (therefore less excitatory transmitter released) or postsynaptically thus reducing dorsal horn activity. The inhibitory interneurones help. They also contain GABA and/or glycine and can have an inhibitory effect both pre and postsynaptically (Doubell et al. 1999).

We can take a lot of therapeutic power from observation of the suppressed dorsal horn state. Alteration of input from the periphery is the basis of transcutaneous electrical nerve stimulation (TENS). An awareness of the powerful endogenous pain control system should make it a target for pain management. Here, for example, is where distraction, positive thoughts, knowledge and healing environments come into play, in addition to drugs that mimic its actions. Patients can be made aware of the powerful pain control system they have within themselves.

INCREASED SENSITIVITY STATE (STATE 3)

The third mode discussed by Doubell et al. (1999) is the sensitised state. It gets a bit complex here, so take your time (Fig. 4.3). An incoming barrage of C fibre inputs from an abnormal impulse generating site, area of inflammation or acidic tissues will cause a release of more excitatory amino acids such as glutamate and aspartate, and also peptides such as substance P and dynorphin into the horn. Glutamate will activate AMPA receptors and with increasing sensitivity, eventually both pre and postsynaptic N-methyl-D-aspartate (NMDA) receptors will be activated (eg. Chen and Huang 1992). You can follow this in figure 4.3.

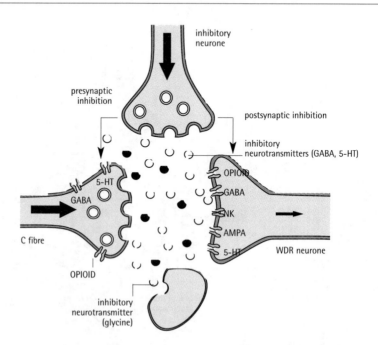

4.2   *The suppressed state of the dorsal horn (state 2). At the synapse, pre and postsynaptic inhibition reduces sensitivity. Inhibitory neurotransmitters eg. serotonin (5-HT), GABA, opioids and enkephalin are released from descending inhibitory neurones and GABA and glycine are released from inhibitory interneurones. These neurotransmitters target specific receptors. In this state there is both a reduction in excitatory neurotransmitters and a reduction in sensitivity of the postsynaptic membrane.*

The postsynaptic NMDA receptor is critical here. Normally (state 1) it is plugged with a magnesium ion and glutamate is unable to unplug the ion channel. Once the membrane is depolarised however, the NMDA channels unplug allowing ions, in particular, calcium to enter the WDR neurone. The opening of G protein metabotrophic receptors allows further calcium to stream into the cell. Recall in chapter 2 that a metabotrophic receptor could stay open for minutes. With all this calcium streaming into the cell, the activation of protein kinase C (PKC) causes phosphorylation of the NMDA receptor. PKC stimulates the attachment of phosphates to the NMDA receptor and makes it undergo the phosphorylation process. Phosphorylation essentially makes the receptor open for longer, stops the magnesium block at resting membrane potentials and produces long lasting changes in synaptic efficacy (Yu et al. 1997). We now have a leaky membrane with enhanced calcium flux. Long term changes in calcium can activate transcription factors which alter gene expression and thus more or different ion channels may be synthesised. The NMDA receptor has been a target for various drugs. Ketamine, dextromethorphan, memantine and the opioids such as methadone and dextropropoxyphene are NMDA receptor antagonists (Hewitt 2000). However the complexity of signalling is such that according to Besson (1999) a "magic bullet" for pain is unlikely.

With the sensitive leaky membrane and excitatory chemicals in the synaptic cleft, various other neuromodulators and transmitters such as nitric oxide and prostaglandins now come into play and make something of a chemical cascade. The gas nitric oxide (NO) (not the laughing gas, nitrous oxide) could also induce further transmitter release and thus participate in the induction of further sensitisation (Aimar et al. 1998; Harley 1998). Brain-derived

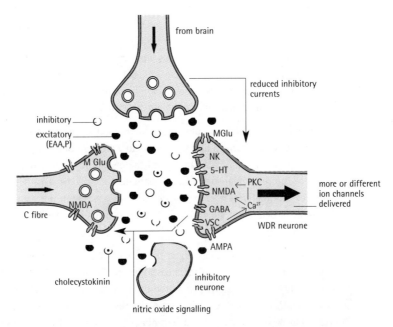

4.3   The sensitised state of the dorsal horn (state 3). At the synapse, input is now magnified. Excitatory amino acid (EAA) and substance P release is increased due to reduced inhibition at the presynaptic membrane, nitric oxide inducing more transmitter release and augmentation by positive feedback receptors such as NMDA and metabotropic glutamate receptors. At the postsynaptic membrane, the magnesium block is removed from the NMDA receptor. With increasing sensitivity, voltage sensitive ion channels (VSC) and metabotrophic receptors (M Glu) open. Calcium streaming will activate protein kinase PKC which will phosphorylate the NMDA receptor keeping it open. Increased expression of excitatory receptors may follow.

neurotrophic factor (BDNF) is another powerful modulator of sensory processing in the horn and brain (Kerr et al. 1999; McMahon and Bennett 1999). With G protein gated glutamate receptors and NMDA receptors open, messenger systems are engaged allowing further expression of excitatory receptors following gene upregulation. Dormant receptors may open. Increased levels of cholecystokinin (CCK), a neuromodulator which has antiopioid effects will enhance the sensitive soup in the synapse (Baber et al. 1989). The overall effect is clearly excitatory. The receptors and new receptors of the WDR neurones of the dorsal horn will react accordingly (Fig. 4.3) and supraspinal centres will have already begun to process response and escape behaviours.

Remember convergence now (chapter 2). Many peripheral neurones will synapse on one central neurone. Subthreshold components of the receptive field may now be engaged (Woolf 1991), leading to a spread of pain into other dermatomes or the other side. Contralateral sensitivity post unilateral injury frequently occurs in animal nerve constriction models (Colvin et al. 1996; Pither et al. 1999), and any aware clinician knows that nerve injuries such as nerve root disorders and carpal tunnel syndrome frequently have repercussions for the other side.

There is also recent evidence showing that some A fibres undergo a phenotype change, and will begin to express substance P and other excitatory modulators so that low intensity stimulation will produce or maintain dorsal horn changes (Noguchi et al. 1995; Neumann et al. 1996). This may be a process, allied by easily depolarised CNS neurones by which altered proprioceptive input could contribute to a maintained pain state following nerve injury and peripheral inflammation.

Overall though, the pain system now has a lower activation threshold. Inputs such as light touch and gentle movements via activation of low threshold afferents such as the large A beta fibres can now evoke pain (eg. Cook et al. 1987; LaMotte et al. 1991; Woolf 1991; Torebjork et al. 1992). It also means that a noxious input can now be magnified and made more intense and last for longer. This is all normal and part of the nervous system's grand design for survival. If this sensitivity makes the person limp, rest, avoid certain activities or take useful medication, this can be helpful for healing, at least initially.

This process of sensitivity should return to normal once the afferent input and central modulating effects return to normal. Presumably a chemical history of the event will remain in some neurones and pathways to remind the person of how he/she dealt with the afferent barrage for future comparisons. In some patients though, the sensitivity seems to persist. An example of this may be a man at 6 weeks post whiplash, with the symptoms not settling and work problems beginning. He may have just decided to engage a lawyer. The patient is on the cusp of chronicity.

Consider some clinical examples where the sensitivity to input is likely to be from the central nervous system. Sometimes a headache is so severe that just touching the hair hurts. Touching hair is merely large fibre activation, but in this situation, it has the ability now to link into the pain system. Or consider the clinical situation, say in chronic low back pain, where it doesn't matter what or where you touch or examine, it all seems to hurt. In this state consideration should go to the activation threshold that the CNS offers the input, not just the inputs related to a particular tissue. In this state, the once precise feature extraction of state 1 is now distorted. Think now about the patient who says that when her shirt collar rubs it hurts. It could be skin of course (primary hyperalgesia) but it is more likely CNS changes (secondary hyperalgesia). A recent neurodynamics based research study is of interest here. Kelley and Jull (1998), interested in the complication of arm pain following breast surgery, examined the impact of breast surgery on an Upper Limb Neurodynamic Test 2 (chapter 12) in 20 patients. Compared to preoperative measurements, at 6 weeks after the operation there was increased mechanosensitivity to the test as judged by loss of range of the shoulder abduction component and variance in symptoms. Unexpectedly, the range of abduction was reduced bilaterally. The authors suggested that central mechanisms may be involved. This is certainly biologically plausible, especially considering the environment and meaning of such surgery. In addition, as summarised by Coderre and Katz (1997), contralateral mechano and thermosensitivity as measured by flexion reflex thresholds commonly occurs post injury in animal studies. It is not necessarily abolished by local anaesthesia of the injured tissue, suggesting central mechanisms are involved. An explanation of the findings of Kelley and Jull (1998) may also involve a generalised immune based sensitivity increase as discussed later in this chapter.

The figures (4.1,4.2 and 4.3) and the discussion may give the impression that the firing of one neurone is necessary for pain perception. It is more likely that groups of neurones would need to fire to cause a perception of sensory change. (deCharms and Merzenich 1996).

MAINTAINED AFFERENT BARRAGE, CNS INFLUENCES, MORPHOLOGICAL CHANGE (STATE 4)

The question arises - what if the afferent barrage continues, or what if the barrage occurs in the presence of an already sensitised or injured cord, or if that person's normal coping mechanisms are impaired? Here, in some people, it appears that long lasting changes in the dorsal horn neurones can occur.

For the process of central sensitivity to continue, it seems that there must be a persistent driver from the periphery to maintain the central sensitivity set up by the initial injury (Coderre and Katz 1997). This may be one or a combination of A fibre phenotype changes, persistent dorsal root ganglion discharge, persistent inflammation, supraspinal influences, gene transcriptional changes in dorsal horn neurones, or inflammation in the dorsal horn and DRG. Behavioural responses to the initial injury such as maladaptive beliefs, fears and attitudes surely contribute as well (chapter 7). Resprouting in the dorsal horn could be yet another reason.

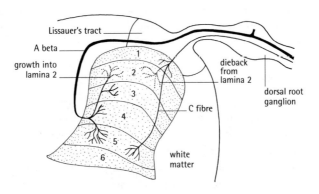

4.4   *The dorsal horn of the spinal cord. The C fibres terminate in lamina 1,2 and 5. The A beta fibres terminate in lamina 3,4 and 5. With peripheral nerve injury, there may be C fibre die back and A beta fibres now sprout into lamina 2.*

The dorsal horn is highly ordered into laminae (Fig. 4.4). Normally the C and A delta fibres terminate in the first, second and fifth lamina and A beta fibres terminate in lamina 3, 4 and 5. Dieback of the central terminals of C fibres occurs following nerve injury (eg. Castro-Lopes et al. 1990). The vacant space is taken up by A beta fibre terminals which normally terminate in the deeper laminae, but now sprout into lamina 2 (eg. Woolf et al. 1992; Koeber et al. 1995; Mannion et al. 1996; Nakamura and Myers 1999; Kohama et al. 2000). The sprouting will also occur in response to partial dorsal root ganglion injury (Nakamura and Myers 2000). Note that these are uninjured A beta fibres which sprout. If the processes of the sensitised state continue, there is now an even greater chance of non-noxious input being eventually perceived as pain. This sprouting has been shown to occur within two weeks of nerve injury in the rat (Doubell et al. 1999).

There are a number of additional processes that could occur and contribute to long term and perhaps irreversible dorsal horn changes. Persistent high levels of the excitatory amino acids, especially glutamate, can lead to excitotoxicity and cell death (Ikonomidou and Turski 1995). In particular, inhibitory interneurones may die (Seltzer et al. 1991). These inhibitory neurones normally contain GABA and/or glycine. This could be thought of as a loss of the more reflexive subconscious pain control system, making the person more under the control of the more voluntary control system from brain centres.

There is another class of neurones in the dorsal horn known as nociceptive specific neurones (NS). These are not as common as the WDR cells and they have a very high firing threshold. However in the presence of excitatory chemicals and probably influenced by the changes in WDR cells, these cells phosphorylse. Their terminals now behave like the more easily fired WDR neurones (Cook et al. 1987). To the brain, it is still a high threshold warning based input into the overall processing of the pain experience.

CHANGES IN THE BRAIN

A sensitive group of neurones in the dorsal horn will cause signalling changes in the brain. Brain processing changes probably occur at the same time as nerve or cord injury (Albe-Fessard et al. 1985) or well before if the environment suggests danger. Input from the horn to supraspinal centres will be carried by neurones in the anterolateral system on the opposite side of the spinal cord, with many fibres peeling away to go to numerous brain areas such as the periaqueductal grey region or the reticular formation. Signalling related to deep tissue nociception may be carried by the dorsal columns (Willis and Westlund 1997). There are other pathways such as the spinohypothalamic tract which will carry nociceptive information directly to the limbic system (Giesler et al. 1994; for a review see Craig and Dostrovsky 1999). PET scanning and functional MRI have revealed that numerous areas of the brain have altered activity during painful experiences (see chapter 2).

The same processes which have been identified in the dorsal horn during mode 3 and 4 are known to occur in the brain. This includes receptor upregulation, receptive field changes in the cortex, and excitotoxicity. Hippocampal cells are particularly vulnerable to persistent high levels of cortisol and glutamate. NMDA receptors are widespread throughout the CNS and so is the protein tyrosine kinase (PTK) which regulates its functions. Any receptor upregulation in the dorsal horn for example, will cause upregulation in the hippocampus (Yu and Salter 1999) and other centres. A similar chemical cascade as in the horn, leading to gene expression and production of new and different ion channels seems likely.

DESCENDING CONTROL SYSTEMS

Any discussion on the role of the brain must include the powerful descending control systems. As part of the distributed processing in the brain, a network exists which can exert a facilitatory or inhibitory effect on the pain transmission neurones in the dorsal horn via opioids, serotonin and noradrenaline. For details on the pathways and actions, see Fields and Basbaum (1999). While many brain areas are involved, the most studied pathway is the periaqueductal grey (PAG), rostral ventromedial medulla (RVM) pathway. The PAG has many links throughout the brain and its component neurones act to integrate ascending nociceptive input with information from the limbic system. Most of the projections to the spinal cord arise via the RVM and terminate in lamina 1, 2 and 5 of the spinal cord. In addition, pain modulating neurones in the PAG and NRM have near total body receptive fields (Oliveras et al. 1990) and high collateralisation within the RVM, suggesting a global rather than anatomically discrete control over pain transmission (Fields and Basbaum 1999). Various studies have shown that neutral contextual clues can alter activity in nociceptive neurones in the dorsal horn in the absence of a noxious stimulus (eg. Bushnell et al. 1985; Duncan et al. 1987). You, the therapist may well be a cue to heightened or decreased descending control merely by your presence.

The endogenous pain control systems of the brain will come into play depending on the meaning of the pain. Threat of injury will usually activate the system (Fields and Basbaum 1999). Noxious cutaneous input will also (Le Bars et al. 1997), which may explain the pain relief from powerful stinging linaments, cupping and strong manual techniques. The endogenous pain control systems probably also form an important part of placebo analgesia.

Pain intensity can be altered by expectation and learning. As you may have experienced, pain sometimes goes shortly after making your appointment with a health professional. There are therefore clinical variables related to the descending control systems which are worth manipulating. These could be interactional, environmental and psychological and in some cases, treating pain with pain.

A PROPOSED PATTERN OF CENTRAL SENSITIVITY

This is a proposed pattern based on known pathobiology and clinical observations, to alert clinicians that a maladaptive process of central sensitivity may be occurring. It may help identify patients who are shifting state, from 1 to 3 or 1 to 4. Central sensitivity occurs in all pain states. In some, the features become more obvious. It is in chronic pain where central sensitivity is likely to be more of a clinical feature.

AREA AND DESCRIPTION

The following pain areas, descriptions and clinical scenarios may relate to central sensitivity:

• Symptoms are often not within neat anatomical or dermatomal boundaries.

• Any original pain may have spread.

• In the case of multiple area symptoms, pains may be linked in that they either occur together, or the patient has one pain or the other pain.

• The contralateral side to the initial pain may be painful, though rarely as much as the initially injured side. There can be mirror pains, which are hard to explain in terms of primary hyperalgesia.

• Clinicians may "chase the pain". This is a common practice in manual therapy. For example, back pains may ease but then the patient complains of thoracic pains. It is almost as though the pain processing networks need to include a somatic component.

• There could be unexpected sudden stabs of pain.

• Patients may say "it has a mind of its own". The pain is called "it" suggesting that it has lost the neat stimulus/response relationships of familiar, and to the patient, understandable tissue based pains.

BEHAVIOUR

The behaviour of the pain state may provide clues to a central mechanism. For example:

• The perception of pain is ongoing. If pain persists past known healing times of tissues and a comprehensive subjective evaluation reveals no occupational provocation, disease or other reason for pain maintenance, then a central mechanism could be suspected.

• Summation. A number of repeated similar activities evoke pain, for example, using a computer, an exercise bike, or interpreters using sign language.

• The stimulus/response relationship is distorted. The pain state worsens or is evoked at variable times after the input. This could be after 10 seconds or even after a day or so. Most clinicians are familiar with the often uncomfortable situation where they examine a patient and then pain starts a short time after the examination.

• Responses to treatment and input are unpredictable. What may appear a successful treatment technique one day may not be successful the next. There is a pattern though, where traditional manual therapy may help for a day or two, but then symptoms invariably return.

• It could be that every movement hurts, yet there may be no great range of movement loss. These patients are often labelled as "irritable" or "unstable". I believe that it is more likely that patients present with instability of symptoms rather than instability of structure. In routine physical examination, such as a straight leg raise, a patient may complain of pain, yet you the therapist may feel no resistance. It is as though the movement has touched a memory rather than a damaged tissue.

• Patients may say "it hurts when I think about it".

OTHER FEATURES

There are other features which could be a part of a central sensitivity pattern:

• These pains can be cyclical, with perhaps more in winter, and perhaps at anniversaries or reminders of traumatic times in life.

• With the CNS dysregulation, changes in response and background homeostatic systems such as the autonomic, endocrine, motor and immune systems are likely. Sometimes these responses may be overt in some systems, for example, focal dystonias of the hand in musicians, central contributions to complex regional pain syndromes (CRPS), or sickness responses in the case of the immune system.

• There may be links to traumatic and multiple traumatic events in life. These events could be during childhood or around the injury time.

• This state may be associated with anxiety and depression.

• "Miracle cures" are possible. Every clinician has hopefully had a "miracle" in the clinic. If there is a sudden, dramatic and apparently miraculous relief of severe and long lasting symptoms from little input, then the pathobiological mechanisms are unlikely to be from local tissues. Miracles are great, but they are even better if you have some idea of why they happened. It is more likely a central change involving some alteration in cognitions and emotions.

• Central sensitivity is likely to be involved in syndromes such as fibromyalgia, myofascial syndrome, reflex sympathetic dystrophy, chronic low back pain and post-whiplash pain syndromes, in fact anywhere pain persists or the word "syndrome" is attached to a piece of anatomy.

I can recall many patients I assessed many years ago and thinking "what on earth is going on here." On reflection, central sensitivity was probably part of the pain state and my operational framework was entirely peripheralist.

CLINICAL THOUGHTS

Central sensitisation, a likely biological state involved in many chronic pain sufferers is a dangerous situation for the individual. Inputs are now magnified and even previously non-painful inputs may be perceived as pain. The brain will process inputs as threatening and respond with an appropriate stress and behavioural response. These responses could be due to pain inputs from damaged and/or deconditioned tissues, but also inputs from healthy tissues, for example secondary hyperalgesia. Put another way, the brain may be operating on faulty data. The signal of sensitivity, whether primary or secondary, is naturally interpreted as a warning of potential harm. It may cause an alteration of function which is not necessary and ultimately harmful to the individual. Somehow, that patient must be able to function while experiencing pain. Education on the non-damaging nature of the pain would seem a logical first step.

Peripheral and central mechanisms are unlikely to be mutually exclusive and a management approach should consider targeted both processes. However, it should also become evident that a relentless diagnostic and therapeutic hunt for sources of nociception while the patient's presentation is dominated by a central sensitivity state may prove fruitless and worsen a disorder. This is particularly so if it leads to the reinforced belief that there is still something in the tissues which should be found. There may be peripheral pain generators identified by skilled examination, but they should not be the sole focus of attention. Hence a physical assessment based on reasoned pathobiological mechanisms in operation is suggested.

The sensitivity evoked from physical tests such as palpation, straight leg raise or a muscle test must be interpreted in the light of likely operant mechanisms. False positives in regard to tissue damage seem likely. In a patient with a sensitive upper limb neurodynamic test, the nerves, muscles, fascia and joints may be quite normal, however in the presence of altered processing in cord and brain, the perceptual output is pain. False positives may also occur with the structural differentiation process used with nerve injury (chapter 10). A straight leg raise test may cause buttock symptoms and the addition of ankle dorsiflexion could increase that buttock symptom. The current interpretation of this is that the dorsiflexion increases mechanical loading on nerve, nerve root or meninges and thus pain increases. However in the presence of a sensitised nervous system, the addition of ankle dorsiflexion could be the addition of normal or slightly noxious input which simply adds to the afferent barrage. The clinical consequence here is that physical examination is best considered as a test of sensitivity first, and then this is broken down to consider tissues and pain processing components. Perhaps a key clinical link here is that "…..a particular stimulus can clearly not be used as a predictor of the sensation that will be elicited without knowing what mode the system is in" (Doubell et al. 1999).

A clinical reasoning approach is the basis of the management strategies in this book. Neurobiology does enhance knowledge of the targets of therapy, but it also enhances the interactional aspects of the clinical reasoning process. It may mean that a clinician can listen to a pain and disability report, making sense of the symptoms which 10 years ago may have been considered impossible or too weird to be real.

Manual therapy includes many basic skills vital to the management of central sensitivity. These include skilled subjective and physical evaluation, knowledge of exercise therapy, time with patients for education, and skills to identify and rectify altered afferent input into the nervous system. The new skills (for some) of nervous system assessment, educating patients about neuroscience, paced movement, more active control giving therapies and more judicious application of techniques are the next step.

IMMUNE, ENDOCRINE, MOTOR AND SYMPATHETIC SYSTEMS AS RESPONSE AND BACKGROUND SYSTEMS

INTRODUCTION

The nervous system processes and gives value to any input. Sometimes this value judgment is visibly expressed via the sympathetic (eg. sweating, redness) or the motor system (spasm, withdrawal, learnt movement patterns). The responses of other systems such as the immune and endocrine systems remain hidden, at least initially, but could be measured. Nervous system response computations are extremely complex, individual and situation specific. They are usually survival driven but often disturbed by novel modern psychosocial demands.

The systems involved often work synergystically. Although considered as response systems, these systems are also closely associated background homeostatic systems, operating at the same time as signalling in the peripheral and central nervous systems.

Systems such as the endocrine, immune, motor and autonomic are foremost protective systems, yet while they can protect and heal, something which requires considerable power, they can also damage, especially in states of maintained stress and pain. Clinical patterns from the activities of these systems are not as obvious as say, peripheral neurogenic pain. There is much synergystic activity between systems, and like all pathobiological mechanisms they will always be in action. In extreme states, the systems will become evident, for example the motor system in focal dystonia, the sympathetic nervous system in complex regional pain syndrome and the endocrine and immune system in Cushing's disease and rheumatoid arthritis. Chronic pain probably involves maladaptive responses in all systems.

A useful way to link things together is to look at the integrated actions of the stress response, remembering that pain is probably the ultimate stressor. Stress biology has only recently been associated with the neurobiology of pain (eg. Gifford 1998; Melzack 1999; Melzack 1999).

Such links and use of the clinical consequences are long overdue. Useful general references include Fink (2000), Sapolsky (1994) Lovallo (1997) and Martin (1997).

AUTONOMIC/NEUROENDOCRINE SYSTEM

Pain and stress will activate three key circuits - the hypothalamus-pituitary-adrenal axis (HPA), the sympathoadrenal axis (SA) and the sympathetic neural axis. These are the peripheral limbs of the stress system. The central components are located in the brainstem and hypothalamus. These axes are linked to other brain areas with interests in survival such as the amygdala, multiple cortical areas and the motor system. These three circuits will respond to a variety of signalling including blood borne, sensory, limbic and circadian signals. The circuits will also respond to immune mediated inflammatory molecules such as tumour necrosis factor alpha and the interleukins 1 and 6.

Pain nearly always acts a stressor. The activities of these stress systems will also be integrated into the overall CNS processing of pain.

THE HYPOTHALAMUS-PITUITARY-ADRENAL AXIS (HPA)

Paired adrenal glands, perched on top of the kidneys and essential for life are two of the key structures (Fig. 4.5). They have a central medulla and outer cortex. Both areas function in times of stress, but secrete different chemicals; adrenaline and noradrenaline from the medulla (sympathoadrenal axis) and corticosteroids (cortisol) from the cortex. The cortex is part of the HPA axis.

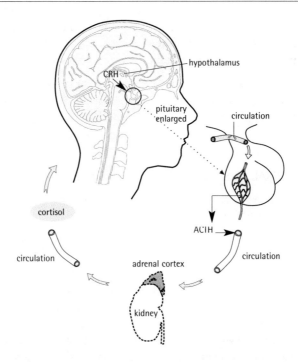

4.5   The hypothalamus-pituitary-adrenal axis. The stimulated hypothalamus secretes corticotropin-releasing hormone (CRH) into the anterior pituitary, stimulating it to release adrenocorticotropic hormone (ACTH) into the bloodstream. In response the adrenal glands will release cortisol which has widespread effects on body tissues. Cortisol will cross the blood brain barrier and inhibit further release of CRH. Cortisol is also a powerful immunoregulator.

Cortisol secretions are activated by the adrenocorticotropic hormone (ACTH) secreted into the blood from the anterior pituitary gland. ACTH secretions, matched by cortisol secretions are high in the morning, low in the evening but stimulated by all forms of stress over 24 hours. Forms of stress such as pain, injury, thoughts, feelings, deeds of others, memories and environmental changes are signalled via corticotrophin releasing hormone (CRH) from the hypothalamus to the pituitary gland (Fig. 4.5). The actions of CRH are inhibited by blood cortisol levels which are sampled by the hypothalamus. A feedback system is therefore in operation. CRH neurones and noradrenergic neurones innervate and stimulate each other in the brain, thus linking the stress systems (Chrousos 1995).

CORTISOL

It is the adrenal cortex and its secretion cortisol which are particularly critical to life. Almost all tissues of the body have receptors for cortisol, including the brain. Cortisol gets a bad rap as a stress chemical, but it is vital to life. It maintains cardiovascular and metabolic homeostasis, in particular stimulating protein catabolism and glycogen synthesis - vital energy for dealing with emergencies. In addition, cortisol can cross the blood brain barrier and effect brain structures, one result being mood changes including depression. Cortisol can also exert regulatory effects on the inflammatory and immune responses through the inhibition of cytokine action and production. For reviews, see Lovallo (1997), Fink (2000) and Sternberg and Gold (1997).

In an emergency, cortisol shuts down activities not needed for survival and enhances those that are. Hence the inflammatory and immune systems, digestive and reproductive systems are shut down. With the proverbial tiger confrontation, reproduction, digestion, and wound healing are not high priorities - they can wait for later. Energy goes to systems which can help avoid the stress and contribute to survival, such as the cardiovascular system, brain and muscles, ie. be smart, think clearly and perhaps run very fast.

A chronic excess of cortisol as in chronic pain or stress poses problems. Cushing's syndrome (chronic hypercortisolism) is an extreme example. The features include immunosuppression, osteoporosis, cardiovascular disease, depression and insulin resistance (Whitehouse 2000). More subtle cases of tissue degeneration, mood swings, slow tissue healing and susceptibility to infection may be noted by clinicians managing patients with chronic pain.

SYMPATHETIC NEURAL AXIS AND SYMPATHETIC ADRENAL AXIS

The HPA axis is closely linked to the sympathetic nervous system (SNS) by links from the hypothalamus to the locus ceruleus, a key sympathetic nervous system control network in the brainstem. The SNS is also mobilised in times of stress, it innervates immune organs as well as nearly every tissue in the body. Stimulation will evoke arousal, fear and readiness.

The SNS also plays a role in the stress response and body homeostatic function. A well known figure demonstrating the sympathetic nervous system is in figure 4.6. Note that this one is slightly different from most in that it acknowledges that muscles, joints, skin and the connective tissue sheaths of the nervous system have a sympathetic innervation. The sympathetic nervous system output to the entire body emerges from spinal levels T1 to L3. The paired trunks are continuous, connective tissue sheathed preganglionic structures, and are known to evoke pain if stimulated (Walker and Nulson 1948; Echlin 1949). One preganglionic sympathetic neurone will diverge onto 15 or more postganglionic neurones (Wolf 1941). Its physical health may be of interest to manual therapists (chapter 15). This part of the nervous system is very glandular - noradrenaline can dribble out of numerous varicosities along the postganglionic fibres (chapter 3).

Although sympathetic responses are usually widespread (eg. total limb or body sweating), the sympathetic nervous system has varying layers of control from local organ to the brain (Lovallo and Sollers 2000). Local organ control allows, for example, blood flow adjustments to muscles, another control layer is ganglionic mechanisms which regulate the output of the postganglionic neurones and then the brain and hypothalamus regulate the entire system. The first two respond more to physiological challenges, the brain responds more to psychological stress.

The sympathoadrenal axis is a powerful part of the sympathetic nervous system. Note in figure 4.6 that the adrenal medulla receives a direct sympathetic preganglionic innervation from the spinal cord. This allows secretion of adrenaline and a little noradrenaline directly and rapidly into the bloodstream. This is known as the sympathetic adrenal axis.

ADRENALINE/NORADRENALINE

Mental and physical effects and psychosocial conditions evoke adrenaline and noradrenaline secretions. Mental stress causes more adrenaline secretion whereas physical stress, linked with more physical activity and blood pressure homeostasis evokes more noradrenaline (Lundberg 2000).

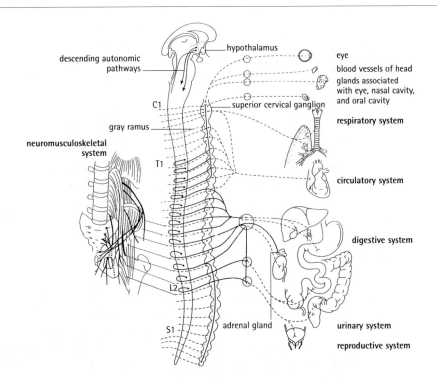

4.6   The sympathetic neural and adrenal axes. Hatched lines are postganglionic fibres. Solid lines are preganglionic fibres. Adapted from Noback et al. (1996).

Both adrenaline and noradrenaline prepare us for action. They stimulate cardiovascular responses, blood is shunted to the heart, muscles and brain and away from the digestive system and skin. They promote increased levels of glucose and free fatty acids. More oxygen is available, sweating occurs to cool the body and make it slippery. Via its immune organ innervation, these catacholamines can modulate inflammation. Adrenaline is immunosuppressive by altering lymphocyte production from the spleen. These are useful secretions for an emergency, but like cortisol, maintained high levels lead to the risk of cardiovascular disease and tissue damage.

Normal or threshold levels of adrenaline do not exist. Levels may double during mild stress such as daily work. Severe stress with emotional demands may cause levels to rise 10 times the resting level for that person. Novel inputs and anticipation markedly raise adrenaline levels (Lundberg 2000). However an increased level of adrenaline does not necessarily mean pain. While the levels surely contribute, an upregulated sensory system involving inflammation and adrenoceptors will be necessary for adrenaline and noradrenaline to access the pain system.

SYMPATHETIC NERVOUS SYSTEM AND PAIN

The sympathetic nervous system can contribute to the sensitivity of inflamed tissues and it can also contribute to the sensitivity of damaged nerves. This can be seen spectacularly with increases in pain if adrenaline is injected into patients with nerve injuries such as a neuroma (Chabal et al. 1992; Raja et al. 1998). However adrenaline injected into a person with no nerve injury will be painless.

The sympathetic nervous system is essentially a motor system. To cause pain it must somehow activate the afferent system, especially C and A delta fibres or A beta fibres if the CNS is sensitised. Understanding this pain comes back to receptors. Adrenaline itself does not hurt, it needs receptors attached to nociceptors to contribute to pain or it must contribute to a chemical soup which activates nociceptors. There are thus three places where adrenaline may activate the afferent system. These are contributions to inflammatory soup, contributions to an AIGS or influences due to adrenoceptor upregulation at the DRG. Adrenaline can act as a central excitatory neurotransmitter, thus it may contribute to the magnification of afferent input. There are more details in chapter 3. Review also figure 3.9.

The stress chemicals such as noradrenaline and cortisol could also contribute to input via destructive effects on tissues. Persistent high level bathing by cortisol and catecholamines appears to have a deleterious effect on connective tissues (Oxlund and Manthorpe 1982; Curwin et al. 1988; Eyre 1990). Noradrenaline pathways in the brain are also closely linked to negative emotional states.

THE PARASYMPATHETIC NERVOUS SYSTEM

Often forgotten with the excitement of the sympathetic nervous system is the parasympathetic nervous system. "Flight and fight" has reminded generations of students about the role of the sympathetic nervous system. The catch cry of the parasympathetic nervous system - "rest and digest" was also proposed by Cannon (Kandel et al. 1995), and is just as important for students and patients to understand. Usually these two systems balance each other. The parasympathetic nervous system is more operational at rest when it repairs and heals the tissue traumas of the day.

It may be worthwhile telling patients about this healing and helping system, particularly when talking about sleep health and the need for some patients to introduce relaxation as a coping strategy.

MOTOR SYSTEM AS AN OUTPUT SYSTEM

Muscles can be inflamed, acidic and weak and hence be potent sites of high threshold input into the CNS. There are secondary effects of damaged muscle also, for example joint instability or a change of the container tissue around a peripheral nerve, all of which could contribute to primary or secondary hyperalgesia.

The motor system can also be conceptualised as a response system. Motor responses to pain and stress include weakness, spasm, changes in facial expressions and tone of voice, muscle imbalances, loss of quality and range of movement, loss of variety of movement selections etc. To some degree these changes are a product of the physical health of the muscles, but they are also products of central processing and are essentially coping mechanisms. Like the increased cortisol in acute stress, some spasm and muscle tension (eg. Knost et al. 1999), even a change in tone of voice are useful in acute pain and injury if it enables optimal management. If they persist then these once useful behaviours become maladaptive and destructive to outcome.

A hyperactive sensory system will have repercussions for the motor system (Woolf 1984) as well as the other output systems. Like the sympathetic nervous system, there are local responses such as spasm and ill-health of collagen. There are also observable changes in patterns of gross movement and postures as people cope. These are often conceptualised as muscle imbalance syndromes. The decreased movement options available and the learned habits of the chronic pain sufferer may lead to deconditioning.

Muscles will react to thoughts. The cortical activity which occurs at the thought of a movement is similar to the cortical activity when the movement occurs (Lotze et al. 1999). In an experimental situation, patients with chronic low back pain who discussed pain episodes had elevated EMG activity compared to those exposed to neutral stimuli (Flor et al. 1992). Powerful psychophysiological influences on motor behavior include fear of movement, fear of reinjury and fear of pain (for recent reviews see Vlaeyen et al. 1995; Crombez et al. 1999; Vlaeyen and Crombez 1999).

The straight leg raise (SLR) is one of the key neurodynamic tests (chapter 11). McCracken et al. (1993) showed that anxiety related to pain was a predictor of pain level and range of SLR movement in chronic low back pain patients.

IMMUNE SYSTEM

BASIC APPARATUS

The days of considering the immune system as a separate system to the nervous system are gone and there are now well defined multilevel and reciprocal links between the immune system and the nervous system. For reviews of the immune system and pain see Watkins (2000), Watkins and Maier (1999), Black (1995) and Sternberg and Gold (1997).

The immune system comprises organs (bone marrow, thymus, lymph nodes and spleen) and various cells (T cells, B cells, natural killer cells, macrophages and neurotrophils). It also comprises messenger molecules known as the cytokines, which allow communication between cells. Sternberg and Gold (1997) note that the immune and nervous systems are quite similar in that they possess sensory elements which receive information from the body and the environment, and they possess motor elements to carry out responses. The cytokines fulfill that role and are of particular interest here.

CYTOKINES

Cytokines are produced in response to various physical and emotional stressors. They have a critical role in infection control and can powerfully contribute to inflammation and pain. Some cytokines are anti-inflammatory and some are pro-inflammatory, making something of a balance. The identified pro-inflammatory cytokines are interleukin-1 (IL-1), interleukin-6 (IL-6) and Tumour Necrosis Factor Alfa (TNF alpha), called TNF alpha because it will cause a haemorrhaging necrosis of tumours if injected into animals. It's apparently powerful stuff. The anti-inflammatory ones include IL-4, IL-10 and IL-13. If a human is injected with IL-1, fever, headache, joint and muscle pain will ensue (Dinarello 1999). IL-1 also stimulates prostaglandin and phospholipase A2 synthesis as part of a contribution to the chemical cascade of inflammation. For reviews, see Marshall (2000) and Watkins (1999).

The immune system is powerfully regulated by the peripheral and central nervous systems, although this signalling is not all one way. Any CNS activation via physical and psychological

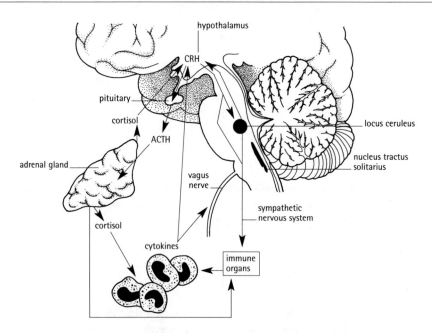

4.7   *Brain, immune and sympathetic nervous system interaction. Immune cells such as macrophages produce cytokines which influence the brain via the vagus nerve to the nucleus tractus solitarius and the bloodstream to the hypothalamus. The hypothalamus secretes corticotropin-releasing hormone (CRH) into the anterior pituitary, stimulating it to release adrenocorticotropic hormone (ACTH) into the bloodstream which stimulates the adrenal glands to produce cortisol. Cortisol back to the brain regulates CRH. CRH influences the locus ceruleus and thus the sympathetic nervous system which innervates immune organs and regulates inflammatory responses. Adapted from Sternberg and Gold (1997)*

stressors may result in immunity changes (Ligier and Sternberg 2000). Activation of the HPA axis and the sympathetic nervous system axes will effect immunity primarily by release of cortisol. See figure 4.7. The sympathetic nervous system also modulates the immune response through its innervation of the immune organs such as the spleen and lymph nodes. Peripheral nerve responses such as substance P (Dickerson et al. 1998) will activate pro-inflammatory cytokines.

The proinflammatory cytokines IL-1, IL-6 and TNF alpha can also signal the nervous system in a number of ways. Cytokine signalling can occur through its stimulatory effects on inflammatory soup and in damaged peripheral nerve as discussed in chapter 3. Cytokines have an influence in the brain also, but these large proteins have some difficulty crossing the blood-brain barrier. They require a leaky section to pass. Another mode of the signalling is thought to involve sensory paraganglia attached to the vagus nerve (Maier et al. 1998; Watkins and Maier 2000). The vagus nerve terminates in the nucleus tractus solitarius which has links to many areas such as the hippocampus and hypothalamus. Glia in the spinal cord and brain will respond to immune signalling by synthesising and releasing IL-1 and thus stimulating the release of further neuroactive substances such as nitric oxide, NGF and excitatory amino acids such as glutamate. Interleukin 1 can potentiate secretion of corticotrophin releasing factor and thus a stress response. (Watkins et al. 1994; Watkins and Maier 2000). The brain is perhaps the most prolific endocrine organ in the body (Sternberg and Gold 1997).

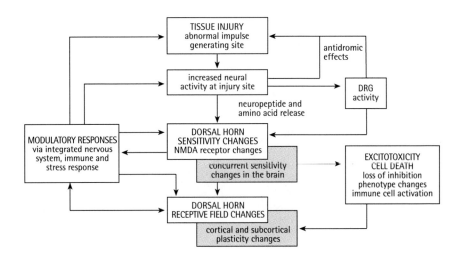

4.8   The neurobiology of pain - an overall summary of chapters 3 and 4.

THOUGHTS FOR CLINICIANS

Much is made of our stress response systems having to function in the age of computers, bureaucracy, new diseases, pollution and job stress, all with a design based on the needs of many thousands of years ago. As Nesse and Young (2000) suggest, we may have forgotten that the ancestral physical stresses of no police, no food resources, no laws, rampant diseases and predators were are also extremely powerful.

The majority of research articles about pain mechanisms state that their hope is that the findings may lead to improved pharmacological interventions. Only a few look at other options and realise that the non-drug management potential is also increasing and the side effects may be less. In addition to improving tissue health, cardiovascular fitness and applying various movement enhancement strategies, there are a number of psychosocial variables which can be manipulated by movement based therapists as a management strategy or to enhance a physical strategy. For example, optimism, motivation, coping methods, an understanding of the meaning of pain, and social support will all, to some degree, protect against the psychological, cardiovascular, endocrine and immune effects of stress. The reasoning models proposed in chapters 6 and 7 should allow integration of all pain mechanisms. In figure 4.8, there is a summary of the pain mechanisms. This links the peripheral mechanisms (chapter 3) with the central and response mechanisms in this chapter.

REFERENCES CHAPTER 4

Aimar P, Pasti L, Carmignoto G, et al. (1998) Nitric oxide-producing islet cells modulate the release of sensory neuropeptides in the rat substantia gelatinosa. Journal of Neuroscience 18: 10375-10388.

Albe-Fessard DG, Berkley KJ, Kruger L, et al. (1985) Diencephalic mechanisms of pain sensation. Brain Research 356: 217-296.

Baber NS, Dourish CT & Hill TR (1989) The role of CCK caerulein and CCK antagonists in nociception. Pain 39: 307-328.

Besson JM (1999) The neurobiology of pain. Lancet 353: 1610-1615.

Black PH (1995) Psychoneuroimmunology: brain and immunity. Science & Medicine 2: 16-27.

Bushnell MC, Duncan GH, Dubner R, et al. (1985) Attentional influences on noxious and innocuous cutaneous heat detection in humans and monkeys. Journal of Neuroscience 5: 1103-1110.

Castro-Lopes JM, A. C, Grant G, et al. (1990) Ultrastructural changes in the central scalloped (C1) primary afferent endings of synaptic glomeruli in the substantia gelatinosa Rolandi of the rat after peripheral neurotomy. Journal of Neurocytology 19: 329-327.

Chabal C, Jacobson L, Russell LC, et al. (1992) Pain response to perineuromal injection of normal saline, epinephrine and lidocaine into humans. Pain 49: 9-12.

Chen L & Huang L-Y, M. (1992) Protein kinase C reduces Mg2+ block of NMDA receptor channels as a mechanism of modulation. Nature 366: 521-523.

Chrousos GP (1995) The hypothalamic-pituitary-adrenal axis and immune-mediated inflammation. New England Journal of Medicine 332: 1351-1362.

Coderre TJ & Katz J (1997) Peripheral and central hyperexcitability. Behavioural and Brain Sciences 20: 404-419.

Colvin LA, Mark MA & Duggan AW (1996) Bilaterally enhanced dorsal horn postsynaptic currents in a rat model of peripheral neuuropathy. Neuroscience Letters 207: 29-32.

Cook AJ, Woolf CJ, Wall PD, et al. (1987) Expansion of cutaneous receptive fields of dorsal horn neurones following C-primary afferent fibre inputs. Nature 325: 151-153.

Craig AD & Dostrovsky JO (1999) Medulla to thalamus. In: Wall PD & Melzack R (eds.) Textbook of Pain, 4th edn. Churchill Livingstone, Edinburgh.

Crombez G, Vlaeyen JWS, Heuts PHTG, et al. (1999) Fear of pain is more disabling than pain itself. Evidence on the role of pain related fear in chronic back pain disability. Pain 80: 329-340.

Curwin SL, Vailas AC & Wood J (1988) Immature tendon adaptation to strenuous exercise. Journal of Applied Physiology 65: 2297-2301.

deCharms RC & Merzenich MM (1996) Primary cortical representations of sounds by the coordination of action potential timing. Nature 381: 610-613.

Dickerson C, Undem B, Bullock B, et al. (1998) Neuropeptide regulation of proinflammatory cytokine responses. Journal of Leukocyte Biology 63: 602-605.

Dinarello CA (1999) Overview of cytokines and their role in pain. In: Watkins LR & Maier SF (eds.) Cytokines and Pain, Birkhauser, Basel.

Doubell TP, Mannion R & Woolf CJ (1999) The dorsal horn: state dependent sensory processing, plasticity and the generation of pain. In: Wall PD & Melzack R (eds.) Textbook of Pain, 4th edn. Churchill Livingstone, Edinburgh.

Duncan GH, Bushnell MC, Bates R, et al. (1987) Task related responses of monkey medullary dorsal horn neurons. Journal of Neurophysiology 57: 289-310.

Echlin F (1949) Pain responses on stimulation of the lumbar sympathetic chain under local anaesthesia. Journal of Neurosurgery 6: 530-533.

Eyre DR (1990) The collagens of the musculoskeletal soft tissues. In: Leadbeater WB, Buckwalter JA & Gordon SL (eds.) Sports-induced Inflammation, American Academy of Orthopedic Surgeons, Rosemont,IL.

Fields HL & Basbaum AI (1999) Central nervous system mechanisms of pain modulation. In: Wall PD & Melzack R (eds.) Textbook of Pain, 4th edn. Churchill Livingstone, Edinburgh.

Fink G ed. (2000) Encyclopedia of Stress, Academic Press, San Diego.

Flor H, Birbaumer N, Schugens MM, et al. (1992) Symptom specific psychophysiological responses in chronic pain patients. Psychophysiology 29: 452-460.

Giesler GJ, Katter JT & Dado RJ (1994) Direct spinal pathways to the limbic system for non-nociceptive information. Trends in Neuroscience 17: 244-250.

Gifford LS (1998) Pain, the tissues and the nervous system. Physiotherapy 84: 27-33.

Hardy JD, Wolff HG & Goodell H (1952) Pain Sensations and Reactions, Haffner Publishing, New York.

Harley JA (1998) Gases as neurotransmitters. Essays in Biochemistry 33: 79-91.

Hewitt DJ (2000) The use of NMDA-receptor antagonists in the treatment of chronic pain. Clinical Journal of Pain 16 (2 Suppl): S73-S79.

Hinde RA (1998) Humans and human habitats: reciprocal influences. In: Cartledge B (ed.) Mind, Brain and Environment, Oxford University Press, Oxford.

Hoheisel U & Mense S (1989) Long term changes in discharge behaviour of cat dorsal horn neurones following noxious stimulation of deep tissues. Pain 36: 239-247.

Hu JW, Sessle BJ, Raboisson P, et al. (1992) Stimulation of craniofacial muscle afferents induced prolonged facilitatory effects in trigeminal nociceptive brainstem neurones. Pain 48: 53-60.

Ikonomidou C & Turski L (1995) Excitotoxicity and neurodegenerative diseases. Current Opinion in Neurobiology 8: 377-396.

Kandel ER, Schwartz JH & Jessell TM (1995) Essentials of Neural Science and Behaviour, Appleton & Lange, Norwalk.

Kelley S & Jull G (1998) Breast surgery and neural tissue mechanosensitivity. Australian Journal of Physiotherapy 44: 31-37.

Kerr BJ, Bradbury EJ, Bennett DL, et al. (1999) Brain-derived neurotropic factor modulates nociceptive sensory inputs and NMDA-evoked responses in the rat spinal cord. Journal of Neuroscience 19: 5138-5148.

Knost B, Flor H, Birbaumer N, et al. (1999) Learned maintenance of pain: muscle tension reduces central nervous system processing of painful stimulation in chronic and subchronic pain patients. Psychophysiology 36: 755-764.

Koeber HR, Mimics K & Mendell LM (1995) Properties of regenerated primary afferents and their functional connections. Journal of Neurophysiology 73: 693-702.

Kohama I, Ishikawa K & Kocsis JD (2000) Synaptic reorganisation in the substantia gelatinosa after peripheral nerve neuroma formation: aberrant innervation of lamina II neurons by A beta afferents. Journal of Neuroscience 20: 1538-1549.

LaMotte RH, Shain CN, Simone DA, et al. (1991) Neurogenic hyperalgesia: Psychophysical studies of underlying mechanisms. Journal of Neurophysiology 66: 190-211.

Le Bars D, Dickenson AH & Besson JM (1997) Diifuse noxious inhibitory control (DNIC). 11. lack of effect on non-convergent neurones, supraspinal involvement and theoretical implications. Pain 6: 305-327.

Ligier S & Sternberg EM (2000) Immune response. In: Fink G (ed.) Encyclopedia of Stress, Academic Press, San Diego.

Lotze M, Montoya P, Erb M, et al. (1999) Activation of cortical and cerebellar motor areas during executed and imagined hand movements: an fMRI study. Journal of Cognitive Neuroscience 11: 491-501.

Lovallo WR (1997) Stress and Health, Sage Publications, Thousand Oaks.

Lovallo WR & Sollers JJ (2000) Autonomic Nervous System. In: Fink G (ed.) Encyclopedia of Stress, Academic Press, San Diego.

Lundberg U (2000) Catecholamines. In: Fink G (ed.) Encyclopedia of Stress, Academic Press, San Diego.

Maier SF, Goehler LE, Fleshner M, et al. (1998) The role of the vagus nerve in cytokine-to-brain communication. Annals of the New York Academy of Science 840: 289-300.

Mannion RJ, Doubell TP, Coggeshall RE, et al. (1996) Collateral sprouting of injured afferent A fibres into the superficial dorsal horn of the adult rat spinal cord after topical capsaicin treatment to the sciatic nerve. Journal of Neuroscience 16: 5189-5195.

Marshall GD & Rossio JL (2000) Cytokines. In: Fink G (ed.) Encyclopedia of Stress, Academic Press, San Diego.

Martin P (1997) The Sickening Mind, Harper-Collins, London.

McCracken LM, Gross RT, Sorg PJ, et al. (1993) Prediction of pain in patients with chronic low back pain: effects of inaccurate prediction and pain-related anxiety. Behaviour Research and Therapy.

McMahon SB & Bennett DLH (1999) Trophic factors and pain. In: Wall PD & Melzack R (eds.) Textbook of Pain, 4th edn. Churchill Livingstone, Edinburgh.

Melzack R (1999) From the gate to the neuromatrix. Pain Suppl 6: S121-S126.

Melzack R (1999) Pain and stress: a new perspective. In: Gatchel RJ & Turk DC (eds.) Psychosocial factors in pain, Guildford Press, New York.

Nakamura S & Myers RR (1999) Myelinated afferents sprout into lamina 2 of L3-5 dorsal horn following chronic constriction nerve injury in the rat. Brain Research 818: 285-290.

Nakamura SI & Myers RR (2000) Injury to dorsal root ganglia alters innervation of spinal cord dorsal horn lamina involved in nociception. Spine 25: 537-542.

Ness RM & Young EA (2000) Evolutionary origins and functions of the stress response. In: Fink G (ed.) Encyclopedia of Stress, Academic Press, San Diego.

Neugebauer V & Schaible HG (1990) Evidence for a central component in the sensitization of spinal neurones with joint input during development of acute arthritis in a cat's knee. Journal of Neurophysiology 64: 299-311.

Neumann S, Doubell TP, Leslie TA, et al. (1996) Inflammatory pain hypersensitivity mediated by phenotypic switch in myelinated primary sensory neurones. Nature 384: 360-364.

Noback CR & Demerest (1996) Human Nervous System: Structure and Function, Williams & Wilkins, Baltimore.

Noguchi K, Kawai Y, Fukuoka T, et al. (1995) Substance P produced by peripheral nerve injury in primary afferent sensory neurons and its effect on dorsal column nucleus neurons. Journal of Neuroscience 15: 7633-7643.

Oliveras J-L, Martin G, Montagne J, et al. (1990) Single unit activity at ventromedial medulla level in the awake, freely moving rat: effects of noxious heat and light tactile stimuli on convergent neurones. Brain Research 506: 19-30.

Oxlund H & Manthorpe R (1982) The biomechanical properties of tendon and skin as influenced by long term glucocorticoid treatment and food restriction. Biorheology 19: 631-646.

Pither GM, Ritchie J & Henry JL (1999) Nerve constriction in the rat: model of neuropathic, surgical and central pain. Pain 83: 37-46.

Raja SN, Abatzis V, Hocasek SJ, et al. (1998) Role of alpha adrenoceptors in neuroma pain in amputees. American Society of Anesthesiology 89.

Sapolsky RM (1994) Why Zebras Don't Get Ulcers, Freeman, New York.

Seltzer Z, Beilin BZ, R. G, et al. (1991) The role of injury discharge in the induction of neuropathic pain behaviour in rats. Pain 46: 327-336.

Simone DA, Sorkin LS & Oh U (1991) Neurogenic hyperalgesia: Central neuron correlates in responses of spinothalamic tract neurones. Journal of Neurophysiology 66: 228-246.

Sternberg EM & Gold PW (1997) The mind-body interaction in disease. Scientific American 7 Special Issue- Mysteries of the Mind: 8-17.

Torebjork HE, Lundberg LER & LaMotte RH (1992) Central changes in processing of mechanoreceptive input in capsaicin-induced secondary hyperalgesia in humans. Journal of Physiology 448: 765-780.

Treede RD & Magerl W (1995) Modern concepts of pain and hyperalgesia: Beyond the polymodal C nociceptor. New in Physiological Sciences 10: 216-228.

Vlaeyen JWS & Crombez G (1999) Fear of movement/(re)injury, avoidance and pain disability in chronic low back pain patients. Manual Therapy 4: 187-195.

Vlaeyen JWS, Kole-Snijders AMJ, Boeren RGB, et al. (1995) Fear of movement/(re)injury in chronic low back pain and its relation to behavioural performance. Pain 62: 363-372.

Walker AE & Nulson F (1948) Electrical stimulation of the upper thoracic portion of the sympathetic chain in man. Archives of Neurology and Psychiatry 59: 559-560.

Watkins LR & Maier SF (1999) Cytokines and Pain, Birkhaüser, Basel.

Watkins LR & Maier SF (2000) The pain of being sick: implications of immune-to-brain communication for understanding pain. Annual Review of Psychology 51: 29-57.

Watkins LR, Wiertelak EP, Goehler LE, et al. (1994) Characterization of cytokine-induced hyperalgesia. Brain Research 654: 15-26.

Whitehouse BJ (2000) Adrenal cortex. In: Fink G (ed.) Encyclopedia of Stress, Academic Press, San Diego.

Willis WD (1993) Mechanical allodynia. A role for sensitized tract cells with convergent input from mechanoreceptors and nociceptors. American Pain Society Journal 2: 23-33.

Willis WD & Westlund KN (1997) Neuroanatomy of the pain system and the pathways that modulate pain. Journal of Clinical Neurophysiology 14: 2-31.

Wolf GA (1941) The ratio of preganglionic neurons to postganglionic neurons in the visceral nervous system. Journal of Comparative Neurology 75: 235-243.

Woolf CJ (1984) Long term alteration in the excitability of the flexion reflex produced by peripheral tissue injury in the chronic decerebrate rat. Pain 18: 325-343.

Woolf CJ (1991) Generation of acute pain: central mechanisms. British Medical Bulletin 47: 523-533.

Woolf CJ (1994) The dorsal horn: state dependent sensory processing and the generation of pain. In: Wall PD & Melzack R (eds.) Textbook of Pain, 3rd edn. Churchill Livingstone, Edinburgh.

Woolf CJ & King AE (1990) Dynamic alterations in cutaneous mechanoreceptive fields of dorsal horn neurones in rat spinal cord. Journal of Neuroscience 10: 2717-2726.

Woolf CJ & Salter MW (2000) Neuronal plasticity: increasing the gain in pain. Science 288: 1765-1768.

Woolf CJ, Shortland P & Coggeshall RE (1992) Peripheral nerve injury triggers central sprouting of myelinated afferents. Nature 355: 75-77.

Yoshimura M & Nishi S (1993) Blind patch-clamp recordings from substantia gelatinosa neurons in adult rat spinal cord slices: pharmacological properties of synaptic currents. Neuroscience 53: 519-526.

Yu XM, Askalan R, Keil GJ, et al. (1997) NMDA channel regulation by channel-associated protein tyrosine kinase Src. Science 275: 674-678.

Yu XM & Salter MW (1999) Src, a molecular switch governing gain control of synaptic transmission mediated by N-methyl-D-aspartate receptors. Proceedings of the National Academy of Science USA 96: 7697-7704.

CHAPTER 5

NEURODYNAMICS

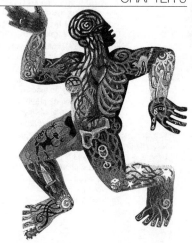

LINKS BETWEEN SYSTEMS

INTRODUCTION - NEURODYNAMICS

NEURODYNAMICS - OPERATING DEFINITIONS

GROSS MOVEMENTS AND THE NERVOUS SYSTEM

THE CONTINUUM OF THE NERVOUS SYSTEM

DYNAMIC NEUROANATOMY

NEURAL CONNECTIVE TISSUES - FABULOUS DESIGN FOR MOVEMENT

THE MENINGES
CONNECTIVE TISSUES OF THE NERVE ROOT COMPLEX
PERIPHERAL NERVE CONNECTIVE TISSUES
THE CONNECTIVE TISSUE/NEURAL TISSUE RELATIONSHIPS IN A NERVE
ATTACHMENTS AND SURROUNDINGS OF THE NERVOUS SYSTEM
SENSITIVITY AND THE NEURAL CONNECTIVE TISSUES

SPACES AND FLUIDS

EPIDURAL SPACE
SUBARACHNOID SPACE AND CEREBROSPINAL FLUID
AXOPLASM

BLOODTHIRSTY NEURONES REQUIRE A MOBILE BLOOD SUPPLY

NEURONES UNFOLD, UNRAVEL AND STRETCH

BRAIN AND SPINOMEDULLARY ANGLE
SPINAL CORD
NERVE ROOTS AND PERIPHERAL NERVES

CLINICAL NEURODYNAMICS

RELATIONSHIP TO JOINT AXES AND NEURAL CONTAINER
EXTENT OF MOVEMENT AND STRAIN
ORDER OF MOVEMENT AND THE ACCUMULATION OF LOAD
EFFECT OF ELONGATION AND PRESSURE ON BLOOD SUPPLY
VARIABLE DIRECTIONS
BEST NEURAL REST POSITION
CHANGES IN DAMAGED NERVOUS SYSTEMS

SUMMARY

REFERENCES CHAPTER 5

LINKS BETWEEN SYSTEMS

It is a jump from the molecular biology presented in the previous chapters to this chapter on gross functional neuroanatomy. Scientists deal with a small portion of the nervous system, medical specialists deal with sections of the body. Movement based therapists need knowledge of gross anatomy down through levels of anatomy and systems to some molecular biology. Unfortunately in science, the links between the levels of anatomy and physiology are rarely made and we are often left with many questions. For example, what is the relationship between an abnormal impulse generating site which we know to be mechano and chemosensitive, and a nerve, say the ulnar nerve, which bends 140 degrees during elbow flexion? And when the extraordinary dynamics of the spinal cord, associated fluids and membranes are revealed, what is the place of dorsal horn based receptor changes and abnormal processing? What do we do to neural structures when we move them and attempt to give to them back what they once had in terms of physical health and sensitivity? There are many questions that are difficult to answer. Let's now consider gross functional neuroanatomy to bring sensitivity closer to the clinic and the realm of the movement based therapist.

INTRODUCTION – NEURODYNAMICS

Next time you are at the ballet, watching a sports event, or a contortionist busking in the street, take a moment to marvel at the physical demands placed upon the nervous system and contemplate how the nervous system copes with these physical forces. If it cannot move, glide and stretch, then the nervous system's cardinal function of conduction will be useless.

Optimal communication in all situations is the main function of the nervous system. The complexity of electrochemical communication is remarkable enough, however the fact that it must be achieved in a sensitive, reactive and plastic structure which is continually sliding, stretching, rubbing and angulating during movement has been neglected. This concept of biomechanics of the nervous system or "neurodynamics" as Shacklock (1995) called it, is relatively new, and has only recently begun to be incorporated into medicine and physiotherapy, although by no means universally (Breig 1978; Elvey 1986; Maitland 1986; Rydevik et al. 1989; Butler 1991; Selvaratnam et al. 1994; Shacklock 1995; Gifford 1998).

NEURODYNAMICS – OPERATING DEFINITIONS

"Neural tension test" is the usual term referring to the examination of the physical abilities of the nervous system. It has limitations. I have embraced the term "neurodynamic test" (Shacklock 1995). "Neurodynamic" is more encompassing than "tension". It allows a shift away from pure mechanical thoughts to include physiological issues. It also allows inclusion of the plasticity changes in the nervous system.

The study of neurodynamics means the study of the mechanics and physiology of the nervous system and how they relate to each other (Shacklock 1995).

A neurodynamic test aims to test the mechanics and physiology of a part of the nervous system. For example, a mechanical component of an SLR would be the ability of the sciatic nerve tract to move and strain in relation to surrounding tissues such as lower lumbar discs. The physiological components may relate to blood flow, ion channel activity, inflammation and representational changes in the CNS of the sciatic nerve, leg and its movement.

Neurodynamic testing should not just be an analysis of the lengthening (stretching) and sliding (gliding) abilities of neural structures. It should also include the ability of the nervous system to cater to the changes in interfacing structures.

GROSS MOVEMENTS AND THE NERVOUS SYSTEM

Like most gymnasts and many athletes, the woman illustrated in figure 5.1 exhibits extraordinary flexibility and she has no fear of movement. Her soft tissues and joints are extremely mobile. Her neural tissues must also be endowed with comparable mechanical abilities to allow her to achieve these movements. From spinal extension to flexion, her spinal canal may be up to 9 cm longer (Inman and Saunders 1942; Louis 1981). When she puts her head down, her brain stem will elongate a centimetre or more (Breig 1960). To achieve the straight leg raise, her sciatic nerve must somehow adapt to a length change in the tissues around the nerve of at least 12% (eg. Beith et al. 1995). If she lifted her arm above her head, the tissues encircling her median nerve could be nearly 20% longer (eg. Zoech et al. 1991). The median nerve must stretch and slide to adapt. Her nervous system will not only slide about her body, up to 2 cm in relation to surrounding tissues in some parts (Wright et al. 1996), but pressures will double, even quadruple (Pechan and Julis 1975). This is all part of normal movement. The essential electrochemical processes involved in communication must occur during a remarkable array and variety of body movement. The communicating tissues must be also be physically healthy.

Most readers and their patients will not have the range of movement of the model in figure 5.1. However, the extent of neural movements will still be proportional to the surrounding tissue movement in much less mobile people. Our patients may have additional demands on the system. There may be tight muscles that nerves must slide through, scar linking the nervous system to surrounding tissues, the system may have been overstretched, pinched, swollen and could contain an abnormal impulse generating site. Our patients may be frightened to move their bodies for fear of pain and reinjury.

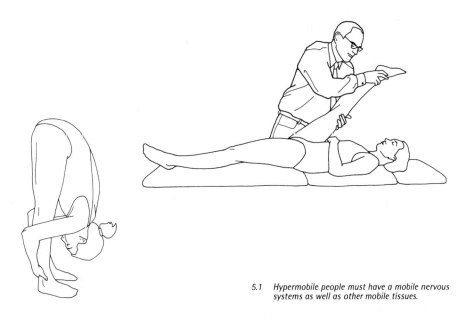

5.1   *Hypermobile people must have a mobile nervous systems as well as other mobile tissues.*

Elongation of the nervous system can be quite dramatic, but there are two other impressive mechanical features. One is its ability to handle compressive forces such as the ulnar nerve flattening on the humerus at the elbow during elbow flexion, or the pinching forces which may occur during spinal extension when intervertebral foramina become smaller around nerve roots. Second is that the nervous system adapts to shortening, for example the meninges and spinal cord need to fold a little, as the cervical spine goes from flexion to extension.

There is nothing new about neurodynamics. Hamstring stretches have always placed unrecognised physical demands upon the sciatic tract. Tai Chi and Quigong are probably the most commonly performed exercise programmes on earth. They must involve considerable nervous system movements with the added benefit of composed mental states. Yoga, most athletic stretching and martial arts all involve varying degrees of nervous system mobilisation as well as mobilisation of other tissues. What is new is the attempted inclusion of neurodynamics and pathodynamics of neural tissues into manual therapy models. At the heart of it is the question, "what are the sources and mechanisms of the patient's pain state and resultant disability?"

THE CONTINUUM OF THE NERVOUS SYSTEM

This is the key concept in neurodynamics. Textbooks, traditional teaching and library referencing systems usually cut the nervous system into sections such as peripheral, central and autonomic. Once divided like that, it can be hard to put it all together again. Yet all functions of the nervous system are dependent in some way on other parts of the system. The electrical, mechanical and chemical connectedness of the nervous system is unique among the organs and to alter one of these features will affect the others.

The implication of this kind of continuity is that mechanical, electrical and chemical changes in one part of the nervous system can have far reaching effects on other parts and that the mechanical, electrical and chemical events are related. Consider a person who has posterior knee pain in the slump position (Fig. 5.2) (chapter 11). It is the case in asymptomatic subjects and frequently in those suffering neurogenic spinal and leg pain, that cervical extension rapidly relieves the leg pain evoked in the slump test and the subject is able to extend her knee further. Sometimes only a small amount of cervical extension is necessary to alter the leg pain. We don't know why the pain relief occurs, but it could be due to alterations in the pressure in

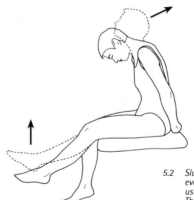

5.2   *Slump test. In an asymptomatic individual, evoked hamstring and spinal symptoms will usually disappear with cervical extension. The knee can usually be extended further.*

peripheral nerves - perhaps at nerve root or nerve trunk level, thus allowing mechano and ischaemo sensitive ion channels to close and protective motor responses to ease. Without knowledge of neuroanatomy, consideration of the continuum and sensitivity of the nervous system, this common phenomenon which is useful for clinical diagnosis, would be difficult to explain.

To fully appreciate this neural connectedness and its clinical consequences, note that there are significant design features in the nervous system related to movement. Not only are there strong and well distributed connective tissues, but neurones and related blood vessels have design features that allow normal function in loaded, unloaded and compressed positions. These anatomical design features are described and discussed in the next few sections.

DYNAMIC NEUROANATOMY

Appreciating that the design of the nervous system must include a place for its own mechanical abilities will foster a better appreciation of mechanosensitivity in the system and allow integration of the peripheral and central neurobiology discussed in chapters 3 and 4. I have discussed and illustrated mechanical design features in detail in "Mobilisation of the Nervous System" (Butler 1991) and there are excellent reviews elsewhere (eg. Sunderland 1978; Lundborg 1988; Rydevik et al. 1989; Rossitti 1993; Millesi et al. 1995; Shacklock 1995; Gifford 1998; Rempel et al. 1999). What follows in this chapter is an updated summary.

Within our neuroanatomical design there must be features that allow:

• sliding, gliding and strain, eg. the sciatic nerve as you touch your toes.

• return from an elongated position to a shortened position eg. cervical meninges from flexion to extension.

• compression, eg. the ulnar nerve compressing on the humerus during elbow flexion.

• strength, eg. the sciatic nerve during a football kick.

• jolting, eg. meninges, cord and brainstem during a whiplash.

• repetitive forces, eg. the median nerve in the carpal tunnel of a musician.

• bending, eg. the tibial nerve at the knee in full knee flexion.

• some selectivity of fluids and chemicals which have access to neurones.

The dynamic neuroanatomy section looks at neural connective tissue design, the effects of movement on the fluids and spaces of the nervous system, the mobile blood supply to neurones, and how neurones usually have remarkable adaptations to physical forces.

NEURAL CONNECTIVE TISSUES - FABULOUS DESIGN FOR MOVEMENT

The connective tissues of the nervous system provide the neurones and glia with protection from undesired forces and chemicals. The neural connective tissues are connected through the body, from the cranial dura and spinal dura to the filum terminale and the connective tissue sheath of peripheral nerves. These strong but sensitive connective tissues also have connections to surrounding somatic tissues.

THE MENINGES

Three different connective tissue membranes make up the meninges surrounding the spinal cord and brain - the dura, arachnoid and pia maters (Fig. 5.3).

DURA MATER

The outermost layer, the dura mater is by far the toughest and strongest. It consists primarily of collagen fibres aligned in the longitudinal axis, but also obliquely and in layers (Rogers and Payne 1961; Tunturi 1977; Patin et al. 1993; Runza et al. 1999). Dura is elastic too. The elastin content of the spinal dura varies from about 7% in the ventral aspect to double that amount in the posterior aspect (Nagakawa et al. 1994). The variation in elastic content is necessary considering that when the dura is fully loaded in spinal flexion, the posterior dura will be more heavily loaded than the anterior dura. Spinal dura mater has considerable strength in the longitudinal axis, more than in the transverse direction (Haupt and Stoept 1978; Zarzur 1996). If dura mater tears, for example from trauma or accidental durotomy, it will often tear in the longitudinal axis, due to this design feature.

ARACHNOID AND PIA MATER

Far more delicate than the dura, the arachnoid and pia mater, embryologically once one membrane, are collectively known as the leptomeninges (Fig. 5.3). They are comprised of a mesh or lattice of collagen fibres. This allows some "telescoping" during elongation and compressive movements (Breig 1978), providing some protection to the neural tissues they surround. The pia

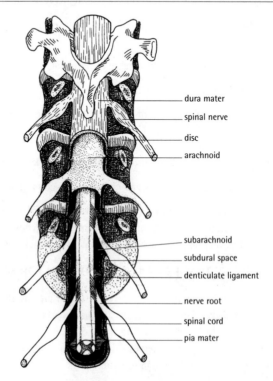

dura mater
spinal nerve
disc
arachnoid

subarachnoid
subdural space
denticulate ligament
nerve root
spinal cord
pia mater

5.3   *Diagrammatic cutaway section of the meninges and spinal cord. From Butler DS (1991) Mobilisation of the Nervous System, Churchill Livingstone, Edinburgh, with permission.*

mater is a continuous bilayered tissue enveloping the cord and brain and providing a barrier control between neural tissue and the cerebrospinal fluid. The arachnoid mater lines the inner dural theca. The many "tight cell" junctions in the leptomeninges point to their role as a controlling barrier to fluid and ion movement (Haines et al. 1993). This barrier is not complete though. Peptide hormones and immune molecules can gain access to the brain in some areas - essential for communication between the endocrine, immune and nervous systems.

CONNECTIVE TISSUES OF THE NERVE ROOT COMPLEX

The term "root" is concise and well established, though Raushning (1997) suggests it would be better to consider the term "root complex" for this part of the nervous system. I agree. The root complex is composed of structurally and physiologically dissimilar elements - the root sleeve, the motor and ventral roots soaked in CSF, the highly vascularised and reactive dorsal root ganglion and the spinal nerve. These neural elements have a varying relationship with surrounding tissues depending on the spinal level.

In figure 5.4, the connective tissues of the nerve root complex and their relationship to neural tissues are demonstrated. Nerve roots involve the meninges, lack Schwann cells and receive at least half of their nutrition from the circulating cerebrospinal fluid. Peripheral nerve epineurium is continuous with the dura. The perineurium splits into two, most of it merges with the dura mater, but a few layers merge with pia mater to make a sheath for the nerve root (Haller and Low 1971). The endoneurium also merges with the pia mater of the nerve

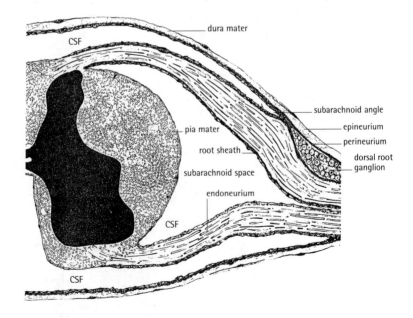

5.4   The nerve root complex and the relationship of the connective tissues with neural elements. The roots are bathed in cerebrospinal fluid (CSF). Note how the elongative forces are taken away from the roots by the split perineurium and the dura. From Haller FR, Low FN (1971) The fine structure of the peripheral nerve sheath in the subarachnoid space in the rat and other laboratory animals. American Journal of Anatomy 131: 1-20, with permission.

roots. Not shown in figure 5.4 are links from the dura to epidural tissues, allowing elongative forces to be further dissipated to the wall of the spinal canal (Sunderland 1978).

Other than the weak connective tissue sheath and some supportive CSF, nerve roots appear weak (Rydevik et al. 1984). There is no epineurium and very little perineurium. The weakness to compressive forces is obvious as is the loss of membranes which may limit chemical infiltration into the root. In addition the nerve fibres are parallel in nerve roots and the twisted arrangement of fascicles seen in nerve trunks is absent (Murphy 1977). So the nerve root complex appears to withstand elongative forces. Birth paralysis, for example usually occurs at the brachial plexus and not at nerve root level. However, compressive forces such as pinching from zygapophyseal joints in spinal extension may not be so easily fended off (chapter 15).

The dorsal root ganglion is a more mechanosensitive structure than the root (Hanai et al. 1996), and it would seem that in normal circumstances the bony protection offered in the intervertebral foramen makes it an ideal location.

PERIPHERAL NERVE CONNECTIVE TISSUES

Peripheral nerves are tough and strong. The three major connective tissue constituents in peripheral nerve - epineurium, perineurium and the endoneurium, are all exhibited clearly in figure 5.5. Note also the sheath around the nerve, referred to as the mesoneurium (Smith 1966) or paraneurium (Millesi et al. 1995). This tissue allows a nerve to glide alongside adjacent tissues, plus it can contract in an "accordion like arrangement" (Smith 1966). This gliding layer obviously facilitates movement. It is probably the tissue responsible for the hard cord like nerve felt slipping away when palpated (see chapter 8). However, with injury, it may become fibrotic and shrink like a tight stocking (Millesi et al. 1995). External neurolysis is a surgical operation which usually frees the nerve from fibrotic mesoneurium. Early movement post trauma may limit the fibrosis.

EPINEURIUM

Most peripheral nerve connective tissue is epineurium. During movement it slides in relation to surrounding tissues and the mesoneurium. Epineurium has two distinct layers; an outer external epineurium with vascular components in it and an internal epineurium which keeps fascicles apart and facilitates interfascicular gliding (Fig. 5.5). Interfascicular gliding is

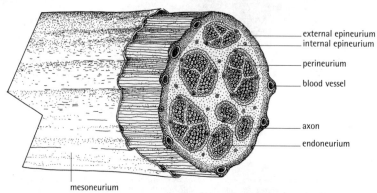

external epineurium
internal epineurium

perineurium

blood vessel

axon

endoneurium

mesoneurium

5.5   *The peripheral nerve connective tissues. From Butler DS (1991) Mobilisation of the Nervous System, Churchill Livingstone, Edinburgh, with permission.*

necessary when a nerve has to bend (Millesi 1986) which the ulnar nerve does to great extremes during flexion of the elbow and the tibial nerve does during knee flexion. Thus peripheral nerve has an extraneural (nerve and surrounding tissues) and an intraneural (fascicle on epineurium) gliding surface. Epineurium embeds the fascicles and cushions them from external trauma.

Lymph channels accompany the arteries of the nerve trunk (Sunderland 1978) and there is a well developed lymphatic network in the epineurium. However there are no lymph channels inside the perineurium. This can be a problem if inflammation gains access inside the fascicles. There are also fat deposits in peripheral nerve, particularly in the sciatic nerve at the buttocks. These deposits probably have a cushioning role (Sunderland 1978).

PERINEURIUM AND ENDONEURIUM

The perineurium is the connective tissue sheath surrounding the bundles of nerve fibres and forming fascicles (Fig. 5.5). It is multilayered, with up to 15 layers and overlapping cells and "tight junctions"(Thomas and Olsson 1984) similar to those seen in the arachnoid mater. The perineurium has a very important role as a diffusion barrier, controlling fluids and ions which come in contact with the neural tissues. The health of these connective tissues is clearly important for nerve function. Perineurial collagen fibres run parallel to the nerve fibres, although there are some oblique and circular running bundles which probably stop the nerve from kinking at acute angles (Thomas 1963). Perineurium is a strong tissue and it keeps its contents under some pressure. If a small cut is placed in it, the nerve fibres contained will "mushroom" out (Lundborg 1988).

The endoneurial tube surrounds myelinated fibres or a group of unmyelinated fibres. This is a distensible elastic structure made up of closely packed collagen tissue. The endoneurial space provides an optimal environment for nerve fibres. There is a fluid in here, under some pressure (endoneurial fluid pressure). Control of pressure and ionic balance in the fluid is necessary for health of the nerve, but endoneurial fluid pressure and contents will change quickly with nerve compression (Lundborg 1988).

THE CONNECTIVE TISSUE/NEURAL TISSUE RELATIONSHIPS IN A NERVE

Approximately half of a peripheral nerve is connective tissue sheath, however the range is from 21% in the ulnar nerve at the elbow to 81% in the sciatic nerve in the buttocks (Sunderland 1978). These variations should sound like an adaptive protective mechanism - the ulnar nerve is well protected from mechanical forces in the ulnar groove, whereas the sciatic nerve needs some adaptive protection, given the time humans sit on it.

The number of fascicles in a nerve at any one cross section varies enormously. For example at the posterior knee crease, the common peroneal nerve has approximately 8 fascicles, however a few centimetres distal where the nerve wraps around the head of the fibula, approximately 16 fascicles are present (Sunderland and Bradley 1949). When the number of fascicles increases, the cross sectional area devoted to connective tissues increases.

The fascicles of a peripheral nerve form a twisted or plexiform arrangement to allow the right combination of sensory, motor and autonomic fibres for a particular branch (Sunderland 1978). This gives the nerve strength and probably allows some dissipation of forces away from neurones. The plexiform arrangement does not exist in nerve roots and is much less towards the terminals of nerves (Jabaley et al. 1980).

Can you see that peripheral neurogenic symptoms may be determined by gross anatomy just as much as the molecular biology discussed in chapter 3? It appears likely that tingling and symptoms from the conducting fibres are more likely to come from areas where there are less fascicles and less connective tissue, such as the ulnar nerve at the elbow. There is a diagram illustrating this (figure 8.3) in the chapter on nerve palpation.

Thinking of the length of the entire nervous system, the nerve roots have 6 times as much collagen as the spinal cord, but a peripheral nerve has five times as much collagen as the nerve root (Stodieck et al. 1986).

ATTACHMENTS AND SURROUNDINGS OF THE NERVOUS SYSTEM

The nervous system has a variable anatomical relationship with its surrounding parts. This is defined in terms of spaces and connections and it requires consideration when pain states involving signs of altered neurodynamics are evaluated.

MENINGEAL CONNECTIONS

Inside the cranium, the dura mater is loosely adhered to the periosteum in the central portion of the cranial bones and tightly adhered at the suture levels (Murzin and Goriunov 1979). There is a firm attachment at the level of the foramen magnum, the nerve roots are also a form of attachment and at the caudal end, the external filum terminale attaches the dural theca to the coccyx. The filum terminale is a thin elastic band and according to Tani et al. (1987) is a likely buffer to cord overstretch. It is possible that both coccygeal pain and headache has a mechanical contribution from the meninges. Clinical support for this may come from positive slump tests.

The dura mater is also anchored along its anterior aspect to the anterior and anterolateral aspect of the spinal canal by meningovertebral ligaments, sometimes referred to as Hofmann's ligaments or dural ligaments (Hofmann 1898; Spencer et al. 1983; Tencer et al. 1985; Wiltse et al. 1993; Bashline et al. 1996) (Fig. 5.6, 5.7). These ligaments are best represented in the lumbar spine, (Blikra 1969; Scapinelli 1990), to the point of being able to stop side to side migration of extruded lumbar disc herniation. The studies of Tencer et al (1985) found that the meningovertebral ligaments, nerve roots and trunks were of equal importance in the dissipation of forces. These ligaments are innervated, and may also be responsible for symptoms if movement causes them to pull on inflamed posterior longitudinal ligaments or the outer annuli of discs (Parke and Watanabe 1990; Kuslich et al. 1991). The meningovertebral ligaments must be part of the neuromeningeal structures mobilised when movement is restored post trauma or post spinal surgery.

From the posterior dura to the ligamentum flavum, a septum (dorsomedial septum) has been shown to be a consistent feature (Parkin and Harrison 1985; Blomberg 1986; Savolaine et al. 1988) (Fig. 5.7). These are longer attachments than the anterior meningovertebral ligaments, and are likely to play a part (perhaps restraining) in the postero-anterior movement of the dural theca in the spinal canal during flexion and extension movements. Sometimes, epidural injections may not have the desired effect. These attachments may prevent a complete bathing of the dura by the infiltrate.

Inside the dural theca and on the lateral aspect, the pia forms a septum and then continues laterally to join onto the denticulate ligaments. There are 21 pairs of these ligaments and they act to keep the cord central in the dural theca. Abnormal forces on the denticulate ligaments are thought to tense the pia mater and perhaps cause a tensile field in a small section of cord (Breig 1978) The other internal dural connection is via the subarachnoid trabeculae. They form channels for the CSF to flow in, and are thought to dampen pressure waves in the CSF (Nicholas and Weller 1988) (Fig. 5.7).

A connection exists between the rectus capitis posterior muscle and the dura mater between the occiput and the atlas (Von Lanz 1929; Hack et al. 1995; Rutten et al. 1997). This connection may assist in limiting dural infolding during extension (Hack et al. 1995; Rutten et al. 1997). Alternatively, it could also act to provide static and dynamic proprioceptive feedback to the CNS, particularly since this muscle contains a large number of proprioceptors (Rutten et al. 1997). Stretches of the cervical extensor muscles therefore load the cervical neuromeningeal tissues, via the upper cervical flexion position and possibly via this muscle connection.

PERIPHERAL NEURAL CONNECTIONS

The peripheral nervous system is also connected to the somatic tissue in a variable way. There are some areas where peripheral nerve is firmly connected to the somatic tissue nerve and in other areas where it is quite slack. Compare, for example, the mobility of the ulnar nerve in the ulnar groove, or the terminal branches of the peroneal nerve in the foot to the peroneal nerve at the head of the fibula. Variable connections are probable contributors to the non-uniform movement of the nervous system. Some anatomical research in this area could provide assistance with the interpretation of symptoms related to neural tissue.

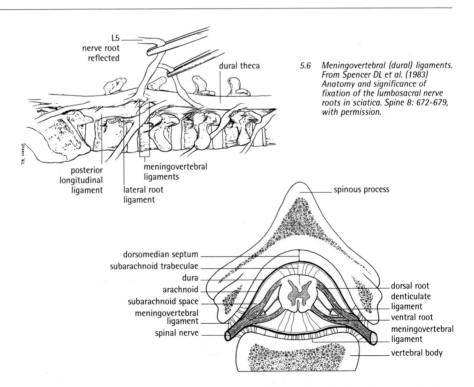

5.6   *Meningovertebral (dural) ligaments. From Spencer DL et al. (1983) Anatomy and significance of fixation of the lumbosacral nerve roots in sciatica. Spine 8: 672-679, with permission.*

5.7   *Diagrammatic transverse section of the cord and spinal canal showing the intra and extradural connections. From Butler DS (1991) Mobilisation of the Nervous System, Churchill Livingstone, Edinburgh, with permission.*

SYMPATHETIC TRUNK CONNECTIONS

From a movement perspective, the sympathetic trunks, rami and ganglia are of interest. They are closely associated with discs and costovertebral joints, especially in the lower thorax. You can review the segmental anatomy and the relationship of the sympathetic nervous system with local joints in figure 5.8. The trunk is also a continuous structure. It is covered by a dense epineurium which forms a capsule at each ganglion (Harati 1993).

If the sympathetic trunk is aligned alongside the skeleton, then potential for deformation and perhaps injury from trauma and postural changes seem possible. Note the anterior view in figure 5.9A. The superior cervical ganglion is attached anteriorly at the C1-2 level, a joint which rotates markedly. The middle cervical ganglion is around C5-C6, an area prone to arthritic changes post injuries. Then both trunks shift laterally to lie on the first rib at the stellate ganglion. It then sits on or lateral to the costovertebral joints. Lateral flexion of the spine would appear likely to elongate the sympathetic trunk on the contralateral side. In figure 5.9B, the trunk is viewed from the side. The most noteworthy mechanical features are that forward head postures and thoracic spinal flexion would probably load the trunks. Arthritic changes of the costovertebral joints are very common and have been shown to compromise the sympathetic trunks (Nathan 1987).

SENSITIVITY AND THE NEURAL CONNECTIVE TISSUES

It would be a healthy advantage for an organ with such mechanical abilities as the nervous system to be sensitive to movement, and not be reliant on neighbouring tissues to warn of

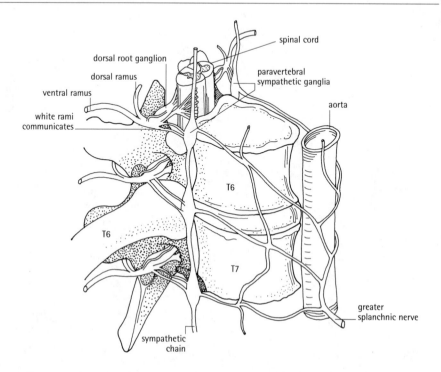

5.8   *The sympathetic trunk and its relationship to the disc, costovertebral joints, cord and nerve root complex.*
Adapted from Harati Y (1993) Anatomy of the spinal and peripheral autonomic nervous system. In: Low PA (ed)
Clinical Autonomic Disorders, Little, Brown and Company, Boston.

potential injury. In addition, a tissue that is injured requires adaptable sensitivity to allow the most appropriate behavior for healing. The innervation of the connective tissues allows this.

MENINGEAL INNERVATION

The meninges are innervated. In the cranium, the trigeminal nerve innervates the dura and blood vessels of all but the posterior cranial fossa. The remainder of the dural theca is innervated by the sinuvertebral nerve which passes via the foramen magnum from the upper three cervical segments. Sinuvertebral nerves are tiny, hardly visible to the unaided eye. They emerge distal to the dorsal root ganglion from a union of a somatic root off the ventral ramus and a sympathetic root from the grey ramus communicantes, or sometimes a sympathetic ganglion (Fig. 5.10). The nerve then returns into the spinal canal as a number of strands (Edgar and Nundy 1966). The sinuvertebral nerve innervates the nerve root sheath, periosteum, epidural contents and the spinal canal (Hovelaque 1927; Bridge 1959; Kimmel 1961; Edgar and Nundy 1966; Edgar and Ghadially 1976; Bogduk 1983; Cuatico et al. 1988; Groen et al. 1988; Kallakuri et al. 1998). The thoracic meninges and root sleeves are not as richly innervated as the cervical and lumbar meninges (Cuatico et al. 1988), but neither are they subjected to as much movement (Breig 1978).

Dural innervation density is richer in the superficial dural layers than those deeper, perhaps suggesting a need to warn of irritant chemicals more than mechanical forces. The ventral aspect of the dura mater has a much richer innervation than the dorsal aspect and towards the dorsal midline the dura may be completely insensitive (Groen et al. 1988). Cyriax noted

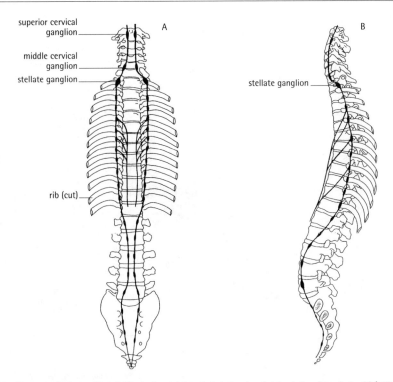

5.9   The sympathetic trunk in relation to the skeleton. A. Anterior view, B. lateral view. From Butler DS (1991) Mobilisation of the Nervous System, Churchill Livingstone, Edinburgh, with permission.

that lumbar puncture into the posterior dura was not painful (Cyriax 1978). There are suggestions from experimental work in man that the dura is more sensitive around blood vessels (Penfield and McNaughton 1940; Wirth and van Buren 1971). Cranial dura is more richly innervated than spinal dura (Kumar et al. 1996). If the midline fusion theory (chapter 2) holds true, then the meninges may be represented by neurones in the brain which have bilateral receptive fields.

CLINICAL FEATURES OF MENINGEAL INNERVATION

We don't know a lot about dural pain. Presumably, since it is innervated it can be a source of pain, particularly if it is inflamed (McCarron et al. 1987; Kuslich et al. 1991). There are reports of pain produced from noxious stimuli to the dura mater (Penfield and McNaughton 1940; Feindel et al. 1960; Wirth and van Buren 1971). A particularly noxious stimulus may be inflammatory material produced by injured discs (McCarron et al. 1987; MacMillan et al. 1991; Olmarker et al. 1993). The sensation of spinal stiffness has also been attributed to the dura mater (El Mahdi et al. 1981). Each sinuvertebral nerve will supply 4 or more spinal segments, sometimes 8 segments. Cyriax (1978) suggested that symptoms from dural irritation may be felt over a wide non-dermatomal area.

When the meninges are inflamed and sensitised, the mechanism of pain is nociceptive. Despite the intimate relationship of the neural connective tissue with neurones, meningeal or connective tissue sheath pain is still nociceptive and thus would be expected to behave in the ischaemic/inflammatory patterns outlined in chapter 3. Neurodynamic tests are very likely to

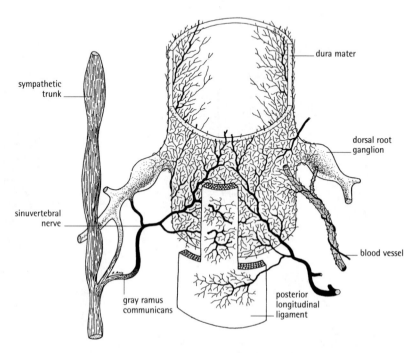

5.10 Sinuvertebral nerve and the innervation of the dura mater. From Butler DS (1991) Mobilisation of the Nervous System, Churchill Livingstone, Edinburgh, with permission.

evoke symptoms from sensitive meninges even at some distance from the point of initial movement. For example, it seems possible that passive neck flexion may evoke thoracic or lumbar pain of meningeal origin.

It is worth noting that the innervation of the meninges is designed for movement. Terminals are twisted and in coiled bundles (Groen et al. 1988) meaning that when healthy dura is stretched, there are minimal forces on the presumed mechanosensitive nerve endings. This is another example of neural design for a mechanical function.

LEPTOMENINGES

Less well studied than the larger dura are the leptomeninges. Bridge (1959) noted nerves running longitudinally in the pia mater though not the arachnoid. Janig (1990) has recently identified an innervation to both membranes. There are mechanoreceptors in the pial ligaments (the small ligaments which attach the anterior spinal artery to the linea splendens) These mechanoreceptors may serve as a form of tension monitoring mechanism (Parke and Whalen 1993).

PERIPHERAL NERVE CONNECTIVE TISSUE SHEATH

Sunderland (personal communication 1989) commented that the innervation of the connective tissue sheath of peripheral nerve was an area which needed greater study. Recently there has been a greater focus in this area. These tissues have an intrinsic innervation, the nervi nervorum from local axonal branching. There is also an extrinsic vasomotor innervation by autonomic fibres from approximating perivascular plexuses (Thomas and Olsson 1984; Dhital et al. 1986; Lincoln et al. 1993). Free nerve endings and Paccinian corpuscles have been observed in all three of the sheaths (Hromada 1963; Thomas and Olsson 1984). Bove et al. (1995; 1997), and Sauer et al. (1999) have shown that the epineurium and perineurium contain a plexus of unmyelinated nerve fibres containing neuropeptides such as substance P and calcitonin gene related peptide. This suggests that the nervi nervorum participates in neurogenic inflammation.

The connective tissues of the dorsal roots and dorsal root ganglia are innervated by fibres originating in the dorsal root ganglia (Pedersen et al. 1956; Hromada 1963; Edgar and Nundy 1966; Parke and Watanabe 1990).

The nervi nervorum must also handle severe mechanical distortion as a peripheral nerve goes through the normal bending and stretching demands of daily movements. Inflammation and scarring in the epineurium or pathological attachments of the nerve to surrounding tissues may well cause symptoms during movement, especially if the nerve contains an abnormal impulse generating site. The perception of nervi nervorum pain may not be entirely local as the nervi nervorum has receptive fields in distal tissues (Bove and Light 1995). Clinicians with good palpation skills (chapter 8) may be able to identify sensitive areas of connective tissue sheath.

SPACES AND FLUIDS

Spaces are not really spaces as they are usually filled with fluids, fat and blood vessels. These contents also change shape and size with movement.

EPIDURAL SPACE

The epidural space (Fig. 5.7) varies depending on the spinal canal level. It is smallest at the T6 spinal level (Dommisse 1975) and in the cervical spinal canal at the C5-6 level (Parke 1988).

The lumbar spinal canal is larger than the thoracic canal and becomes triangular in the lower lumbar spine. The major feature of the epidural space is the internal vertebral venous plexus, which is occasionally damaged during trauma and in rare instances, during epidurals and lumbar puncture. There are also fat deposits in the posterior recess and in the intervertebral foramina, (Parkin and Harrison 1985). The amount of fat is regulated by the space available and in spinal stenosis, the amount of fat diminishes. Substances which enter the epidural space may not be excluded from neurones, as epidurally applied substances such as corticosteroids have a direct route via arachnoid villi and capillaries in nerve roots (Byrod et al. 1995).

SUBARACHNOID SPACE AND CEREBROSPINAL FLUID

Between the arachnoid and the pia mater in the brain and spinal cord is the subarachnoid space, filled with flowing cerebrospinal fluid (CSF). CSF is a colourless water like fluid which forms continually from plasma in the choroid plexus - the capillary loops which protrude into the ventricles of the brain. CSF provides oxygen and metabolites to cord and nerve roots and also removes carbon dioxide and waste before draining into the venous system via the arachnoid villi. CSF also cushions the central nervous system by enabling some shock absorption during rapid movements and by providing a mechanical bouyancy. CSF has often been referred to as the "water cushion" of the brain. Remember too, that brain density is only slightly greater than CSF (Westmoreland et al. 1994). The CSF cushion is sometimes lost during dural puncture and consequently traction forces on cranial dura and blood vessels increase and may cause symptoms (Spielman 1982; Vandam 1992). This may include a descent of cerebellar tonsils towards or into the foramen magnum. Body movement helps move CSF. In normal subjects a sudden increase in thoracic pressure can produce enough pressure to force 8ml of CSF into the brain (du Boulay et al. 1972). With cervical flexion, the shape of the ventricles changes and probably helps CSF flow (Breig 1960).

An intermediate leptomeningeal layer has been described by Nicholas and Weller (1988) and along with the subarachnoid trabeculae, may serve to dampen pressure waves in the cerebrospinal fluid during movements. Normal movement, healthy meninges and surrounding tissues surely assists the distribution of CSF.

AXOPLASM

The cytoplasm of peripheral nerves is known as axoplasm. We often forget that a tibial nerve neurone could be over a metre long and that it has to bend and stretch while the internal workings of the cell have to function. Cytoplasm moves in all cells, but here in the long axon it is a particularly vital process, as the axon must be kept physically healthy and the ion channels and neurotransmitters have to be delivered to the cell membranes.

From the cell body of a peripheral axon and travelling distally, there is a fast flow of 100-400 mm per day, sometimes up to 1000 mm per day. There is also a much slower flow of around 6 mm per day in the same axon. The fast flow carries material such as ion channels and neurotransmitters bound for the cell membrane. The slow flow carries cytoskeletal proteins and neurofilaments. The slow flow essentially looks after the physical health of the axon. A retrograde transport (200 mm per day) also occurs. This carries unused anterograde material, and exogenous material taken up by the nerve terminals such as neurotrophic factors and sometimes viruses. The retrograde flow thus has a signalling function, allowing the nucleus to respond to disturbances in the chemical environment at the neurone terminals (Donnerer et al. 1992). "Molecular motors" in the axon such as kinesin and dynein have the ability to transform energy into physical movement and power vesicles and organelles. A close up view of these molecular motors reveals that they have "little feet" which walk the cellular material along the axon, a bit like a treadmill. Axonal tranport is nicely described by Delcomyn (1998), Kandel (1995), Lundborg (1988) and (Ochs 1984), among others.

Movement based therapists should be aware that the flow of axoplasm may be diminished or stop due to ischaemia or physical constriction (Ochs 1984; Dahlin and McLean 1986). Mammalian axoplasm is quite viscous, about 5 times that of water (Haak et al. 1976). Axoplasm also has thixotrophic properties, that is, it flows better when it is kept moving (Baker et al. 1977). I often tell patients about "nerve juice" and how it loves movement. Diabetes has a well known association with nerve entrapment (eg. Hurst et al. 1985). In experimental diabetes, nerves are more susceptible to compression. The fast axoplasmic flow becomes particularly sluggish (Dahlin et al. 1987)

BLOODTHIRSTY NEURONES REQUIRE A MOBILE BLOOD SUPPLY

Neurones are very bloodthirsty. The brain and spinal cord have a combined mass of about 1.5 kilograms which is about 2% of body mass, yet they consume about 20% of the available oxygen in circulating blood (Dommisse 1994).

If the blood supply to the nervous system is to be adequate in all postures and movements, then there must be some morphological adaptation in the vasa nervorum to handle it. The general pattern of blood supply to neural tissues is to have extrinsic vessels supplying feeder vessels, which in turn supply an intraneural system. The feeder vessels usually have some slack to accommodate movement and if a feeder vessel is injured, the intraneural supply often has enough reserve to supply all neurones.

There are a number of intricate adaptive mechanisms to enable a good blood supply in any position or posture. In the spinal cord, the longitudinal blood vessels which are tortuous and slack at rest (extension) will straighten and narrow when loaded (flexion). The transverse running vessels will shorten and wrinkle with longitudinal loading. (Breig et al. 1966; Breig 1978). The nerve root complex ensures its blood supply during movements by a complex system of T-bars to allow blood shunting, and coiled, twisted arteries to allow stretch and yet still provision of blood (Parke and Watanabe 1985).

Peripheral nerves have a well developed microvascular system and multiple feeder vessels (Lundborg 1988). Feeder vessels often have a reserve length to go "around corners" as the ulnar nerve does during elbow flexion. In between fascicles, arteries have some slack to allow intrafascicular sliding. For greater details of the circulatory supply to the nervous system, especially in a physical sense, consult Dommissee (1994), Lundborg (1988) and Butler (1991) and the work of Parke and Watanabe (1985).

NEURONES UNFOLD, UNRAVEL AND STRETCH

Neurones and glia, although reliant on the connective tissues are not without their own physical resources.

BRAIN AND SPINOMEDULLARY ANGLE

The brain effectively floats in the cerebrospinal fluid and will move in relation to the skull box during normal movements and the odd bumps on the head that everyone gets. For this it is well protected by the cranial meninges and the skull. Due to the continuum of the nervous system, cervical movements have a significant mechanical effect on brain structures. When the head and spine are moved, the shape of the brain stem and spinal cord changes (Breig 1960; Breig 1978). The brainstem could be a centimetre and a half longer from cervical extension to flexion. In addition, the 12th to the 5th cranial nerves are pulled tight to their exit zones in the base of the skull (Breig 1960; Rossitti 1993). There are no denticulate ligaments between the connective tissues of the brain and the neural elements. The cranial nerves, in particular the large trigeminal nerve may actually assist in anchoring the brainstem in the posterior fossa (Rossitti 1993).

The ventricles change dimensions during movement. The floor of the fourth ventricle becomes longer and narrower during cervical flexion and shorter and wider during extension. In extension the choroid plexus bulges further into the ventricle (Breig 1960).

The spinomedullary angle undergoes considerable change during head and neck movements. In 18 asymptomatic subjects measured by magnetic resonance imaging (MRI), the spinomedullary angle in flexion ranged from 1 to 32 degrees with an average of 14 degrees (Doursounian et al. 1989). The angle is closely related to movements at the craniocervical junction. The medulla oblongata moves forward during flexion and in the mid cervical spine will come to rest against the skeleton of the spinal canal. The circumference of the medulla oblongata is 4 mm greater in extension compared to flexion (Breig 1960).

There are increasing reports of a relationship of mild brain injury and chronic pain (eg. Ettlin et al. 1992; Andary et al. 1997). The cingulate and hippocampal gyri, important areas in pain processing, may be particularly susceptible in an injury such as whiplash (Duckett and Duckett 1993). Brainstem areas may also be vulnerable considering the forces placed on them by cervical movements.

On a different pitch, a little known fact is that the dendritic spine of a hippocampal neurone can wriggle up to 30% of its length. This may assist in synapse formation (Fischer et al. 1998). Never doubt the mechanical abilities of the nervous system.

SPINAL CORD

The centrode of the spinal motion segment is close to the middle of the disc (Gertzbein et al. 1985). Therefore, in spinal flexion, the posterior spinal cord columns will be loaded more than the anterior columns. This also means that they must contract more during spinal extension (Breig 1978; Yuan et al. 1998). When the spine is laterally flexed, the tracts on the convex side will be stretched more than those on the concave. This sounds potentially dangerous for the affected neurones but along with protection from the connective tissues, the neural tissues have their own protection. Neurones in the spinal cord are arranged in folds and spirals, which straighten as the spinal cord elongates and refolds as the cord shortens. This mechanism, along with neuromeningeal movements in relation to the spinal canal, protects the cord during movement. In addition, during flexion movements, the cord will take the "shortest route" and thus move anteriorly in the canal.

The cervical spinal cord is particularly stretchy. From extension to flexion, the cord is approximately 20% longer (Breig 1960). From the neutral position to the flexed position, the cord is approximately 10% longer (Reid 1960; Margulies et al. 1992; Yuan et al. 1998). From extension to flexion the sagittal diameter of the cervical cord is nearly 30% less (Muhle et al. 1998), thus significant intraneural pressure increases must occur.

Transmission of tension in the neural tissues of the spinal canal is quite remarkable. It needs to be, because from spinal extension to flexion, the spinal canal could be between 5-9 cm longer (Inman and Saunders 1942; Breig 1960; Louis 1981). The posterior canal wall lengthens approximately 3 time more than the anterior wall (Babin and Capesius 1976). Cervical flexion will create mechanical changes in neural tissues of the lumbar spine (Breig 1978). Any flexion of the spine, by elongating the canal will place a strain on the contained cord, roots and meninges. (Smith 1956; Reid 1960; Louis 1981).

The link between the cord movement and the processing changes and fluid accumulations which occur at the dorsal horn are not known nor considered. The nervous system usually adapts superbly to the movement, although intra-canal pathological changes such as a spondylitic bar may have clinical repercussions. Since the spinal cord is designed for movement, it is probably healthy to move it. Maybe movement of the spinal cord may be one way of dispersing accumulated excitatory neurotransmitters and enhancing CSF movements.

NERVE ROOTS AND PERIPHERAL NERVES

Nerve roots, like spinal cord, receive much of their nutrition from the CSF. Like the rest of the nervous system, nerve roots are not static. They move within the CSF and in relation to surrounding tissues, although well protected by the neural connective tissues. As Weinstein suggests (1997) it is the micromotion which allows the root to keep its mechanical properties and receive nutrition, which is lost with tissue irritation and resultant fibrosis from disc pathology or stenosis. Of greater clinical concern here, as discussed earlier, is the adaptation of the roots to compressive and pinching forces.

In the slack position, peripheral axons run a slightly undulatory course in the endoneurium and the fascicles spiral in the epineurium. These features and the interfascicular sliding will assist tension transmission. In a gross sense, so will the design of the brachial plexus. An elongative force on one nerve, say the ulnar nerve, will be transmitted to numerous cervical nerve roots complexes (Butler 1991; Kleinrensink et al. 2000).

CLINICAL NEURODYNAMICS

For the remainder of this chapter, key clinical issues related to the remarkable excursion and strain of the nervous system are discussed.

RELATIONSHIP TO JOINT AXES AND NEURAL CONTAINER

Neurodynamic tests evolved because clinicians listened to patients' stories about mechanisms of injury, of pain aggravating and easing positions and they looked at the relationship of neural tissues to joint axes. In many cases research followed the clinical observations. Take the upper limb neurodynamic test 1 (chapter 12) for example. To challenge the physical health of the median nerve, extension of the fingers (Rempel et al. 1997), wrist extension and forearm supination (Rempel et al. 1998), elbow extension, shoulder abduction and cervical lateral flexion away from the test side (1995; Kleinrensink et al. 2000) are desired test components all on the basis of the relationship of the nerve to joint axes. It should not be difficult for clinicians to make up their own neurodynamic tests and vary the suggested base tests in chapters 11 and 12.

The tissues adjacent to nerves need closer analysis. Sometimes they form a tunnel around nerve and the movement of these adjacent tissues will also place stretch or compressive forces upon nerve. The concept of a "neural container" (Shacklock 1995) or "mechanical interface" (Butler 1991) is helpful. In the case of a patient with a carpal tunnel syndrome associated with a sensitive upper limb neurodynamic test, I would be interested in the health of the neural container in the entire upper limb and neck. Some clinical situations may be "container dependent" (eg. cervical extension pinching nerve root), or "neural dependent" (eg. cervical flexion straining nerve root).

The nervous system is sometimes associated with very mobile neighbouring tissues. For example, in the carpal tunnel, during wrist and finger flexion, the median nerve has a movement relationship with the flexor tendons. With active finger flexion, proximal sliding of the median nerve at the wrist occurs at 43% of the rate of sliding of the flexor tendons (Szabo et al. 1994).

Some "containers," by virtue of proximity to major neural structures or of involvement in injury, will be more important than others. In general, from the neutral position, spinal flexion increases the size of the spinal canal and intervertebral foramina. Spinal extension will decrease the size. In the lumbar spine, from flexion to extension, the cross sectional area of the lumbar spinal canal gets smaller by approximately 16% (Schonstrom et al. 1989), much of it due to posterior bulging of discs and forward bulging of the interflaval fat pad (Penning 1992). Contralateral lateral flexion and rotation will increase the size of the foramina (eg. Penning and Wilmink 1987; Schonstrom et al. 1989; Yoo et al. 1992; Inufusa et al. 1996). Where there are degenerative joints, there will be less space and a greater likelihood of pinching forces applied to nerves and blood vessels (Panjabi et al. 1983).

Container/nerve relationships are discussed further in chapter 15.

EXTENT OF MOVEMENT AND STRAIN

Movement of nerves and neuromeningeal tissues during limb and trunk movement have been described by a number of researchers. Most of the focus has been in the upper limb (McLellan and Swash 1976; Millesi 1986; Shaw Wilgis and Murphy 1986; Zoech et al. 1991; Szabo et al. 1994; Wright et al. 1996). Two studies are discussed.

The recent work by Wright et al. (1996) was a very neat and detailed study on 5 transthoracic cadavers (10 upper extremities). The cadavers were minimally dissected and all the upper limb joints and the neck position were controlled. Combinations of movements were found to have a profound effect on excursion and strain of the median nerve at the wrist and elbow. For example, from wrist extension to flexion, the median nerve will slide nearly 2 cm at the wrist. From experimenting with combinations of movements, these researchers concluded that a mean total of 35 mm of movement at the wrist and at the elbow was necessary to cater for daily activities. Just finger movements from extension to flexion will move the median nerve at the carpal tunnel about one centimetre and strain it 13%, depending on the position elsewhere. The findings in this study are similar to other upper limb studies such as Shaw Wilgis and Murphy (1986) and McLellan and Swash (1976).

Zoech et al. (1991), defining the median nerve as from the bracelet crease at the wrist to the upper border of the latissimus dorsi muscle, found that the difference in length of the nerve bed from wrist flexion and elbow flexion to wrist extension and elbow extension was approximately 100 mm. With the average length of nerve approximately 517 mm, this means that the median nerve must adapt to a length difference of approximately 19% during every day motions, such as hanging out washing on the line or a game of tennis. Only 22-23% of the adaptation is by elastic elongation, the remainder occurs by gliding and changing in undulations. Considering that in Zoech et al's. (1991) cadaver series, the shoulder was maintained at 90 degrees abduction, it is easy to extrapolate that similar movements and strains would occur in the upper limb neurodynamic test.

THE DYNAMIC ULNAR NERVE AT THE ELBOW

The ulnar nerve at the elbow provides an example of the aspects of neurodynamics described above. During elbow flexion, the nerve will be tractioned thus increasing intraneural pressure and flattening on the humerus. The ulnar nerve at the elbow may decrease in area by as much as 50% and elongate by nearly half a centimetre (Apfelberg and Larson 1973). The cubital tunnel is also up to 50% smaller in flexion compared to extension (Apfelberg and Larson 1973; Gelberman et al. 1998). In patients with ulnar neuropathy, the pressure within their cubital tunnels could be easily over 60 mmHg (Per Ohlin and Elmqvist 1985). Stretch of the retinaculum and movement of the olecranon away from the medial epicondyle by an average of 10 to 15 mm also contribute to pressure changes during flexion. In extension, the retinaculum bulges therefore allowing more space (O'Driscoll et al. 1991; Schuind et al. 1995).

The position of the wrist and shoulder will affect ulnar nerve dynamics at the elbow. Combining wrist extension and shoulder abduction with elbow flexion will significantly increase the intraneural pressure in the ulnar nerve at the cubital tunnel (Pechan and Julis 1975). Gelberman et al. (1998) noted in their cadaver studies that cutting the aponeurotic roof of the cubital tunnel did not alter the intraneural pressure significantly and they suggest that traction may be a dominant force. These traction forces as suggested by the Pechan and Julis study may have arisen some distance from the cubital tunnel.

These powerful physical forces upon neural tissues must now be considered in the light of the pathological changes involved in neuropathy. An abnormal impulse generating site, sensitive neural connective tissue sheath or sensitive tissues attached to the nervous system would be likely to react in response to these physical forces.

ORDER OF MOVEMENT AND THE ACCUMULATION OF LOAD

The sequences of movements involved in a soccer kick are different to the sequences in a kung fu kick. Knee extension comes before hip flexion in soccer and vice versa in the kung fu kick. The sequence of routine slump testing is different to a straight leg raise. Clinicians have noted that the sequence of joint movements used in a neurodynamic test, or any movement appears to effect the responses. For example, when slump testing, Maitland would commonly test neck flexion first and then add the slump components (Maitland 1985). I have often noted that in carpal tunnel syndrome, a better symptomatic response occurs when the technique is started at the wrist, and then elbow and shoulder components added (chapter 12). This may relate in part to Breig's (1978) idea of a "tissue borrowing" phenomenon, that is, the first movement tested "borrows" the neural tissue first and thus allows a better examination of it. If the nervous system in the rest of the limb is slackened, then presumably the first component tested will test the movement of the nerve and its relationship with surrounding structures better than if it was performed in a tension position. In physical examination it may be worthwhile applying different sequences of testing. The key principle is that the greatest challenge to a segment of neural tissue will occur when the adjacent joint to the nerve is loaded first in a sequence of testing (Shacklock 1995). Thus the most vigorous challenge to the terminal branches of the peroneal nerve on the dorsum of the foot, would occur when ankle plantar flexion was performed first, then the SLR performed. This feature is probably more consistent with focal peripheral neurogenic pain. Of course, with pathological changes, anything can happen.

Breig and Marions (1963) showed that in the lumbar region, neural structures slid cephalad when cervical flexion was performed. This contrasts with Louis (1981) who noted that lumbar neural movements were in a caudal direction when the whole spine was flexed. This underlines the complexity of neurodynamics.

These features have a number of clinical applications. First, loading the hypothesised site of neuropathy first and then adding load, may be a way of accessing a minor neuropathy (see "heel spurs", chapter 15). Second, it is a way of carefully examining a particularly sensitive person. In such cases, starting movements away from the site of symptoms, with the nervous system in the rest of the body unloaded should lessen the chance of aggravation, and in particular, easing anxiety. Third, altering order of movement may be a way of presenting movement differently and perhaps more acceptably to a nervous system used to the cue of a particular movement pattern (chapter 14.)

The accumulation of load is non-uniform. After all, if the median nerve had a consistent structure along its length, it should not matter what order the movement is taken up. However the varying connective tissue content, attachments and variable relationships to the container sees to that. For example, full spinal flexion will cause a 15% dural strain at L1-2, whereas at L5, the strain is approximately 30% (Louis 1981). With plantar flexion/inversion of the foot, the tightness of the terminal branches of the superficial peroneal nerve can be easily observed. Some of this loading will have transmitted proximally, perhaps to the sciatic nerve (Borges et al. 1981), although with less strain. The major clinical implication is that a variable order of movement evaluation may be needed for a more in depth physical evaluation of the physical health of the nervous system.

EFFECT OF ELONGATION AND PRESSURE ON BLOOD SUPPLY

A key tenet of neurodynamics is that a careful consideration of the physiological effects of mechanical forces on the nervous system is always required. There is a clear relationship between the strain placed on a nerve and the amount of blood available to the strained neurones. At approximately 6 to 8% strain, blood flow in a peripheral nerve will slow (Lundborg and Rydevik 1973; Ogata and Naito 1986). Nerve conduction will be adversely affected if this strain is held for an hour (Wall et al. 1992). Complete arrest of blood flow will occur at approximately 15% elongation (Ogata and Naito 1986).

Compressive forces will also easily alter blood flow. From experimental animal models, an extraneural pressure of only 20-30 mmHg may interfere with intraneural blood supply, impair axoplasmic flow and thus nerve function (Rydevik et al. 1981; Dahlin and McLean 1986;

Rempel et al. 1999). Pressures of 50 mmHg applied for 2 minutes will distort myelin sheaths and they may begin to split (Dyck et al. 1990). Similar pressures have been shown to alter nerve function in healthy human carpal tunnels. Nerve function begins to falter at approximately 30-40 mmHg and will usually begin to block at 30 mmHg less than diastolic pressure (Gelberman et al. 1983). This means that a person with high blood pressure will require greater pressures to effect the median nerve in the carpal tunnel than a person with low blood pressure. An association of carpal tunnel syndrome with treated hypertensive patients has been noted (Emara and Saadah 1988).

The effects of compression can last for some time. In one animal study, two hours of mild compression (30 mmHg) caused a rapid increase in endoneurial fluid pressures for at least 24 hours after the pressure was removed (Lundborg et al. 1983). With higher pressures held for a longer period, more long term changes such as endoneurial oedema, fibrin deposits, demyelination, axonal sprouting (at 1 week), and endoneurial invasion by mast cells were noted all in a dose response relationship (Powell and Myers 1986; Dyck et al. 1990). The pressure in the carpal tunnel of a healthy human is about 3 mmHg in the neutral position. In patients with carpal tunnel syndrome, the pressure in the neutral position is about 30 mmHg rising to 100 mmHg with wrist flexion (Gelberman et al. 1981; Werner et al. 1983). See Rempel et al. (1999) for a recent review.

Focal demyelination and slippage at nodes of Ranvier have often been noted at nerve compression sites (Ochoa and Marotte 1973; for review see Ochoa 1998). The bare axolemma is likely to provide an opportunity for ion channel upregulation (chapters 2 and 3). In addition, mechanical and physiological responses to peripheral nerve injury are known to occur at undamaged sites of the nerve. This is reviewed in the discussion on the "double crush syndrome in chapter 15.

Remember that responses to nerve compression are not all mechanical. For example, van Meeteren et al. (1997) have shown that recovery from a sciatic nerve crush lesion is slower in rats subjected to chronic intermittent stress.

CLINICAL THOUGHT

Earlier in this chapter, I made the comment that the nerve bed could be between 12% and 20% longer during a limb movement. The inference was that the peripheral nerve would stretch the same amount. However with the above data, one would expect symptoms to be provoked quite easily with limb movement even in healthy subjects. However this does not happen. To handle the loading, the nervous system both slides and stretches. For example, if you were to extend your wrist now with your elbow flexed, there would be considerable gliding and some strain of the median nerve, say for example, 5% at the wrist crease. This is not enough to alter blood flow and hence no symptoms of an ischaemic nature ensue, unless the position was held for a period of time. However, in this case, the median nerve has called upon its movement adaptation reserves in the rest of the arm, thus the forces are spread. If the nerve was entrapped, say at the elbow, then the forces may not be dissipated as far, and a greater strain may occur at the wrist, perhaps to the point of altered blood flow and thus symptoms may ensue. In patients of course, it also depends on the health status of the nerve at the wrist and CNS inhibitory/excitatory controls. (These thoughts have great clinical consequences related to the nervous system as a continuum.) Contributions to neural health issues at the wrist may arise from some distance away.

VARIABLE DIRECTIONS

A number of studies have shown that during body movements, the neuromeningeal tissues move in opposite directions (Smith 1956; Reid 1960; Louis 1981). This research was extrapolated to a "tension point" concept (Butler 1989; Butler 1991). Review figures 5.11A and 5.11B. The arrows represent the direction of neural movement in relation to surrounding structures. This variable direction was recently shown again using a motion tracking MRI technique. During cervical flexion, the upper cord moves caudad in the spinal canal and the lower cord moves cephalad (Yuan et al. 1998). Another way of viewing it, is that this illustrates a variable movement relationship between two mobile structures - the neuromeningeal tissues and the spinal canal. At the C5-6 level, during movement, the contained neuromeningeal tissues keep pace with movement at the spinal canal.

The clinical consequences of this reversal pattern are unknown. My feeling is that when the nervous system is sensitive or physically unhealthy, areas of reversal such as C5-6, T6 and L4-5 may be areas where symptoms may show first. This suggestion comes from observing many patients with probable nervous system involvement from whiplash, disc intrusion into the spinal canal and nerve root disorders. Here a pattern of low cervical, mid thoracic and low lumbar linked pains may follow. Neurodynamic tests are often sensitive. You may find a patient with a subtle lumbar nerve root disorder who puts her finger right on the tibial nerve at the knee crease during a SLR. This probably suggests some neurogenic involvement, not necessarily at the knee, but perhaps in the lumbar spine.

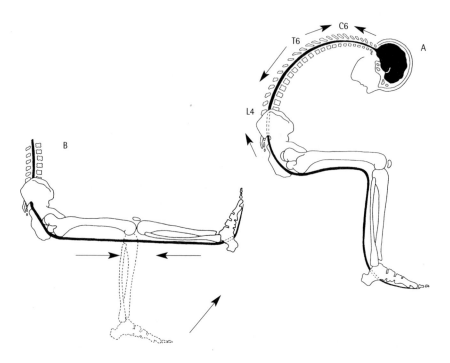

5.11   Postulated neural movements in relation to surrounding tissues. A. spinal canal from flexion to extension, B. straight leg raise. Adapted from Louis (1981) and Smith (1956). From Butler DS (1991) Mobilisation of the Nervous System, Churchill Livingstone, Melbourne, with permission.

BEST NEURAL REST POSITION

Is there a position which is best for rest of the nervous system? This will depend on the injury, disease or pain state of course. For example, the position which relieves pressure on one part of the nervous system may put increased load on another. A judgement will be necessary in relation to the container and to the loading on the nervous system.

The cervical spine is of particular interest. In injured states, too much flexion will load the neural elements yet extension will make the spinal canal smaller. Both movements could damage neural elements especially after acute trauma. An MRI study by De Lorenzo et al. (1996) of healthy volunteers showed that the optimal position (ie. most favourable cord/spinal canal ratio) was with the head elevated about 2 cm from the supine position. The position where pressure in the carpal tunnel is least is in a few degrees of extension and ulnar deviation (Weiss et al. 1995). The consideration may be useful for resting or splinting or even trying to find the most painfree position so that a person may be able to perform some gentler movements short of pain.

CHANGES IN DAMAGED NERVOUS SYSTEMS

There is little information available on the physical performance of damaged nervous systems. Neural movement and ability to strain is lost and is usually accompanied by an increase in sensitivity. There are a number of case studies where freeing of adhesions around neural tissues allowed better movement and a decrease in pain (eg. Fahrni 1966; Brown 1972; Lerman and Drasnin 1975; Sogaard 1983; Revel et al. 1988; Benson and Schutzer 1999). We presume that the physical health of the nerve must have been improved with resultant beneficial effects for neurophysiological processes. Chronically injured nerves have been shown to have altered biomechanical properties such as increased stiffness, increased strength and decreased elasticity (Beel et al. 1984).

Movements of damaged nerves have recently been studied in patients. Vall-Sole et al. (1995) compared latencies in the median nerve of carpal tunnel syndrome patients and controls, in wrist extension and flexion. Significant slowing was shown in the patient group suggesting that the lack of displacement is related to the altered nerve functioning. In another study of patients with bilateral carpal tunnel syndrome, reduced sliding of the median nerve was shown by ultrasound imaging (Nakamichi and Tachibana 1995).

Greening et al.(1999), via the medium of MRI, demonstrated reduced median nerve movement in the carpal tunnels of patients with upper limb overuse disorders. These three studies, all using different techniques are hopefully the beginning of many more.

SUMMARY

As stated at the beginning of this chapter, the links between the physical abilities of the nervous system and the biological processes which lead to pain and disability are only just emerging. When a patient presents with sensitive movements, we must be able to make some judgements about the sources and mechanisms of that sensitivity. Skilled clinical use of the science of neurodynamics can contribute.

For neurodynamics to find its place in the clinic, an open and uncorrupted clinical reasoning process using as much of this basic science knowledge as possible is necessary. The next two chapters attempt that.

REFERENCES CHAPTER 5

Andary MT, Crewe N, Ganzel SK, et al. (1997) Traumatic brain injury/chronic pain syndrome: A case comparison study. The Clinical Journal of Pain 13: 245-250.

Apfelberg DB & Larson SJ (1973) Dynamic anatomy of the ulnar nerve at the elbow. Plastic and Reconstructive Surgery 51: 76-81.

Babin E & Capesius P (1976) Etude radiologique des dimensions du canal rachidien cervical et de leurs variations au cours des epreuves fonctionelles. Annals of Radiology 19: 457-462.

Baker P, Ladds M & Rubinson K (1977) Measurement of the flow properties of isolated axoplasm in a defined chemical environment. Journal of Physiology 269: 10-11.

Bashline SD, Bilott JR & Ellis JP (1996) Meningovertebral ligaments and their putative significance in low back pain. Journal of Manipulative and Physiological Therapeutics 19: 592-596.

Beel JA, Groswald DE & Luttges MW (1984) Alterations in the mechanical properties of peripheral nerve following crush injury. Journal of Biomechanics 17: 185-193.

Beith ID, Robins EJ & Richards PR (1995) An assessment of the adaptive mechanisms within and surrounding the peripheral nervous system, during changes in nerve bed length resulting from underlying joint movement. In: Shacklock MO (ed.) Moving in on Pain, Butterworth-Heinemann, Australia.

Benson ER & Schutzer SF (1999) Posttraumatic piriformis syndrome. The Journal of Bone and Joint Surgery 81A: 941-949.

Blikra G (1969) Intradural herniated lumbar disc. Journal of Neurosurgery 31: 676-679.

Blomberg R (1986) The dorsomedian connective tissue band in the lumbar epidural space of humans: An anatomical study using epiduroscopy in autopsy cases. Anesthesia and Analgesia 65: 747-752.

Bogduk N (1983) The innervation of the lumbar spine. Spine 8: 286-292.

Borges LF, Hallett M, Selkoe DJ, et al. (1981) The anterior tarsal tunnel syndrome. Journal of Neurosurgery 54: 89-92.

Bove GM & Light AR (1995) Calcitonin gene-related peptide and peripherin immunoreactivity in nerve sheaths. Somatosensory and Motor Research 12: 49-57.

Bove GM & Light AR (1995) Unmyelinated nociceptors of rat paraspinal tissues. Journal of Neurophysiology 73: 1752-1762.

Bove GM & Light AR (1997) The nervi nervorum. Pain Forum 6: 181-190.

Breig A (1960) Biomechanics of the Central Nervous System, Almqvist and Wiksell, Stockholm.

Breig A (1978) Adverse Mechanical Tension in the Central Nervous System, Almqvist and Wiksell, Stockholm.

Breig A & Marions O (1963) Biomechanics of the lumbosacral nerve roots. Acta Radiologica 1: 1141-1159.

Breig A, Turnbull I & Hassler O (1966) Effects of mechanical stresses on the spinal cord in cervical spondylosis: a study on fresh cadaver material. Journal of Neurosurgery 25: 45-56.

Bridge CJ (1959) Innervation of spinal meninges and epidural structures. Anatomical Record 133: 533-561.

Brown BA (1972) Internal neurolysis in traumatic peripheral nerve lesions in continuity. Surgical Clinics of North AmericA 52: 1167-1175.

Butler DS (1989) Adverse mechanical tension in the nervous system: a model for assessment and treatment. Australian Journal of Physiotherapy 35: 227-238.

Butler DS (1991) Mobilisation of the Nervous System, Churchill Livingstone, Melbourne.

Byrod G, Olmarker K, Konno S, et al. (1995) A rapid transport route between the epidural space and the intraneural capillaries of the nerve roots. Spine 20: 138-143.

Cuatico W, Parker JC, Pappert E, et al. (1988) An anatomical and clinical investigation of spinal meningeal nerves. Acta Neurochirurgica 90: 139-143.

Cyriax J (1978) Mechanisms of symptoms: Dural pain. The Lancet: 919-921.

Cyriax J (1978) Textbook of Orthopaedic Medicine, 8th edn. Bailliere Tindall, London.

Dahlin LB, Archer DR & McLean WG (1987) Treatment with an aldose reductase inhibitor can reduce the inhibition of fast axonal transport following nerve compression in the streptozotocin-rat. Diabetologia 30: 414-418.

Dahlin LB & McLean WG (1986) Effects of graded experimental compression on slow and fast axonal transport in rabbit vagus nerve. Journal of Neurological Science 72: 19-30.

De Lorenzo RA, Olson JE, Boska M, et al. (1996) Optimal positioning for cervical immobilisation. Annals of Emergency Medicine 28: 301-308.

Delcomyn F (1998) Foundations of Neurobiology, W.H. Freeman, New York.

Dhital KJ, Lincoln J, Appenzeller O, et al. (1986) Adrenergic innervation of vasa and nervi nervorum of optic, sciatic, vagus and sympathetic nerve trunks in normal and steptozotocin-diabetic rats. Brain Research 367: 39-44.

Dommisse G (1975) Morphological apects of the lumbar spine and lumbosacral regions. Orthopedic Clinics of North America 6: 163-175.

Dommisse GF ed. (1994) The blood supply of the spinal cord and the consequences of failure. Grieve's Modern Manual Therapy, 2nd edn. Churchill Livingstone, Edinburgh.

Donnerer J, Schuligoi R & Stein C (1992) Increased content and transport of substance P and calcitonin gene-related peptide in sensory nerves innervating inflamed tissues: evidence for a regulatory function of nerve growth factor in vivo. Neuroscience 49: 693-698.

Doursounian L, Alfonso JM, Iba-Zizen MT, et al. (1989) Dynamics of the junction between the medulla and the cervical spinal cord: an in vivo study in the sagittal plane by magnetic resonance imaging. Surgical and Radiologic Anatomy 11: 313-322.

du Boulay G, O;Connell J, Currie JC, et al. (1972) Further investigations on pulsatile movements in the cerebrospinal fluid pathways. Acta Radiologica 13: 496-523.

Duckett S & Duckett S (1993) The neuropathology of the minor head injury syndrome. In: Mandel S, Thayer Sataloff R & Schapiro SR (eds.) Minor Head Trauma, Springer Verlag, New York.

Dyck PJ, Lais AC, Giannini C, et al. (1990) Structural alterations of nerve during cuff compression. Proceedings of the National Academy of Science 87: 9828-9832.

Edgar MA & Ghadially JA (1976) Innervation of the lumbar spine. Clinical Orthopedics and Related Research 115: 35-41.

Edgar MA & Nundy S (1966) Innervation of the spinal dura mater. Journal of Neurology, Neurosurgery, and Psychiatry 29: 530-534.

El Mahdi M, Latif F & Janko M (1981) The spinal nerve root innervation and a new concept of the clinicopathological interrelations in back pain and sciatica. Neurochirurgia 24: 137-141.

Elvey RL (1986) Treatment of arm pain associated with abnormal brachial plexus tension. The Australian Journal of Physiotherapy 32: 225-230.

Emara M & Saadah AM (1988) The carpal tunnel syndrome in hypertensive patients treated with beta-blockers. Postgraduate Medical Journal 64: 191-192.

Ettlin TM, Kischka U, Reichmann S, et al. (1992) Cerebral symptoms after whiplash injury of the neck: a neuropsychological study of whiplash injury. Journal of Neurology, Neurosurgery and Psychiatry 55: 943-948.

Fahrni WH (1966) Observations on straight leg-raising with special reference to nerve root adhesions. Canadian Journal of Surgery 9: 44-48.

Feindel W, Penfield W & McNaughton F (1960) The tentorial nerves and the localization of intracranial pain in man. Neurology 10: 555-563.

Fischer M, Kaech S, Knutti D, et al. (1998) Rapid actin based plasticity in dendritic spines. Neuron 20: 847-854.

Gelberman RH, Hergenroeder PT, Hargens AR, et al. (1981) The carpal tunnel syndrome: a study of canal pressures. Journal of Bone and Joint Surgery 63A: 380-383.

Gelberman RH, Szabo RM, Williamson RV, et al. (1983) Sensibility testing in peripheral nerve compression syndromes. An experimental study in humans. Journal of Bone and Joint Surgery 65A: 632-638.

Gelberman RH, Yamaguchi K & Hollstein SB (1998) Changes in interstitial pressure and cross-sectional area of the cubital tunnel and of the ulnar nerve with flexion of the elbow. Journal of Bone and Joint Surgery 80A: 492-501.

Gertzbein S, Seligman J, Holtby R, et al. (1985) Centrode patterns and segmental instability. Spine 10: 257-261.

Gifford LS (1998) Factors influencing movement - neurodynamics. In: Pitt-Brooke J, Reid H, Lockwood J et al. (eds.) Rehabilitation of Movement, WB Saunders, London.

Greening J, Smart S, Leary R, et al. (1999) Reduced movement of the median nerve in carpal tunnel during wrist flexion in patients with non-specific arm pain. Lancet 354: 217-218.

Groen GJ, Baljet B & Drukker J (1988) The innervation of the spinal dura mater: Anatomy and clincial implications. Acta Neurochirurgica 92: 39-46.

Haak RA, Kleinhaus FW & Ochs S (1976) The viscosity of mammalian nerve axoplasm measured by electron spin resonance. Journal of Physiology 263: 115-137.

Hack GD, Koritzer RT, Robinson WL, et al. (1995) Anatomic relation between the rectus capitis posterior minor muscle and the dura mater. Spine 20: 2484-2486.

Haines DE, Harkey HL & al-Mefty O (1993) The "subdural" space: a new look at an outdated concept. Neurosurgery 32: 111-120.

Haller FR & Low FN (1971) The fine structure of the peripheral nerve root sheath in the subarachnoid space in the rat and other laboratory animals. Journal of Anatomy 131: 1-20.

Hanai F, Matsui N & Hongo N (1996) Changes in responses of wide dynamic range neurons in the spinal dorsal horn after dorsal root or dorsal root ganglion compression. Spine 21: 1408-1415.

Harati Y (1993) Anatomy of the spinal and peripheral autonomic nervous system. In: Low PA (ed.) Clinical Autonomic Disorders, Little, Brown and Company, Boston.

Haupt W & Stoept E (1978) Uber die Dehnbarkeit und Reißfestigkeit der Dura mater spinalis des Menschen. Verhandlungen Anatomische Gesellschaft 72: 139-144.

Hofmann M (1898) Die befestigung der dura mater im wirbelcanal. Archives of Anatomy and Physiology: 403-412.

Hovelaque A (1927) Anatomie des nerfs craniens et rachidiens et du sisteme grand sympathetique chez l'homme, Gaston Doin et Cie, Paris.

Hromada J (1963) On the nerve supply of the connective tissue of some peripheral nervous system components. Acta Anatomica 55: 343-351.

Hurst LC, Weissberg D & Carroll RE (1985) The relationship of the double crush to carpal tunnel syndrome: (an analysis of 1,000 cases of carpal tunnel syndrome). Journal of Hand Surgery 10B: 202-205.

Inman VT & Saunders JBC (1942) The clinico-anatomical aspects of the lumbosacral region. Journal of Radiology 38: 669-678.

Inufusa A, An HS & Lim I (1996) Anatomic changes of the spinal canal and intervertebral foramen association with flexion-extension movements. Spine 21: 2412-2420.

Jabaley ME, Wallace WH & Heckler FR (1980) Internal topography of the major nerves of the forearm and hand. A current view. Journal of Hand Surgery 5: 1-18.

Janig W & Koltzenburg M (1990) Receptive properties of pial afferents. Pain 45: 300-309.

Kallakuri S, Cavanaugh JM & Blagoev DC (1998) An immunohistochemical study of innervation of lumbar spinal dura and longitudinal ligaments. Spine 23: 403-411.

Kandel ER, Schwartz JH & Jessell TM (1995) Essentials of Neural Science and Behaviour, Appleton & Lange, Norwalk.

Kimmel DL (1961) Innervation of spinal dura mater and dura mater of the posterior cranial fossa. Neurology: 800-809.

Kleinrensink GJ, Stoeckart R, Mulder PGH, et al. (2000) Upper limb tension tests as tools in the diagnosis of nerve and plexus lesions. Clinical Biomechanics 15: 9-14.

Kleinrensink GJ, Stoeckart R, Vleeming A, et al. (1995) Mechanical tension in the median nerve. The effects of joint positions. Clinical Biomechanics 10: 240-244.

Kumar R, Berger RJ, Dunsker SB, et al. (1996) Innervation of the spinal dura: myth or reality. Spine 21: 18-26.

Kuslich SD, Ulstrom CL & Michael CJ (1991) The tissue origin of low back pain and sciatica. Orthopedic Clinics of North America 22: 181-187.

Lerman VI & Drasnin HV (1975) Adhesive lesions of the nerve root in the dural oriface as a cause of sciatica. Surgical Neurology 4: 229-232.

Lincoln J, Milner P, Appenzeller O, et al. (1993) Innervation of normal human sural and optic nerves by noradrenaline and peptide-containing nervi vasorum and nervorum: effect of diabetes and alcoholism. Brain Research 632: 48-56.

Louis R (1981) Vertebroradicular and vertebromedullar dynamics. Anatomia Clinica 3: 1-11.

Lundborg G (1988) Nerve Injury and Repair, Churchill Livingstone, Edinburgh.

Lundborg G, Myers R & Powell H (1983) Nerve compression injury and increased endoneurial fluid pressure: a "miniature compartment syndrome". Journal of Neurology, Neurosurgery and Psychiatry 46: 1119-1124.

Lundborg G & Rydevik B (1973) Effects of stretching the tibial nerve of the rabbit. A preliminary study of the intraneural circulation and barrier function of the perineurium. Journal of Bone and Joint Surgery 55B: 390-401.

MacMillan J, Schaffer JL & Kambin P (1991) Routes and incidence of communication of lumbar discs with surrounding neural structures. Spine 16: 167-171.

Maitland G (1985) The slump test: examination and treatment. Australian Journal of Physiotherapy 31: 215-219.

Maitland GD (1986) Vertebral Manipulation, 6th edn. Butterworths, London.

Margulies SS, Meaney DF, Bilston LB, et al. (1992) In vivo motion of the human cervical spinal cord in extension and flexion. Proceeding of the International IRCOBI Conference on the Biomechanics of Impacts.

McCarron RF, Wimpee MW, Hudkins PG, et al. (1987) The inflammatory effect of nucleus pulposus: a possible element in the pathogenesis of low-back pain. Spine 12: 760-764.

McLellan DL & Swash M (1976) Longitudinal sliding of the median nerve during movements of the upper limb. Journal of Neurology, Neurosurgery, and Psychiatry 39: 566-570.

Millesi H (1986) The nerve gap: theory and clinical practice. Hand Clinics 2: 651-663.

Millesi H, Zoch G & Riehsner R (1995) Mechanical properties of peripheral nerves. Clinical Orthopedics and Related Research 314: 76-83.

Muhle C, Wiskirchen J, Weinert D, et al. (1998) Biomechanical aspects of the subarachnoid space and cervical cord in healthy individuals examinaed with kinematic magnetic resonance imaging. Spine 23: 556-567.

Murphy RW (1977) Nerve roots and spinal nerves in degenerative disk disease. Clinical Orthopedics and Related Research 129: 46-60.

Murzin VE & Goriunov VN (1979) Study of strength of fixation of dura mater to the cranial bones. Zhurnal Voprosy Neirokhirurgii Imeni 4: 43-47.

Nagakawa H, Mikawa Y & Watanabe R (1994) Elastin in the human posterior longitudinal ligament and spinal dura. A histologic and biochemical study. Spine 19: 2164-2169.

Nakamichi K & Tachibana S (1995) Restricted motion of the median nerve in carpal tunnel syndrome. Journal of Hand Surgery 20B: 460-464.

Nathan H (1987) Osteophytes of the spine compressing the sympathetic trunk and splanchnic nerves in the thorax. Spine 12: 527-532.

Nicholas DS & Weller RO (1988) The fine anatomy of the human spinal meninges. Journal of Neurosurgery 69: 276-282.

Ochoa J & Marotte L (1973) Nature of the nerve lesion underlying chronic entrapment. Journal of Neurological Science 19: 491-499.

Ochoa JL ed. (1998) Nerve fibre pathology in acute and chronic compression, 2nd edn. WB Saunders, Philadelphia.

Ochs S (1984) Basic properties of axoplasmic transport. In: Dyck PJ, Thomas PK, Lambert EH et al. (eds.) Peripheral Neuropathy, 2nd edn. WB Saunders, Philadelphia.

O'Driscoll SW, Horii E, Carmichael SW, et al. (1991) The cubital tunnel and ulnar neuropathy. Journal of Bone and Joint Surgery 73B: 613-617.

Ogata K & Naito M (1986) Blood flow of peripheral nerve: Effects of dissection, stretching and compression. Journal of Hand Surgery 11B: 10-14.

Olmarker K, Rydevik B & Nordborg C (1993) Autologous nucleus pulposus induces neurophysiologic and histologic changes in porcine cauda equina nerve roots. Spine 18: 1425-1432.

Panjabi MM, Takata K & Goel VK (1983) Kinematics of lumbar intervertebral foramen. Spine 8: 348-357.

Parke WW (1988) Correlative anatomy of cervical spondylotic myelopathy. Spine 13: 831-837.

Parke WW & Watanabe R (1985) The intrinsic vasculature of the lumbosacral spinal nerve roots. Spine 10: 508-515.

Parke WW & Watanabe R (1990) Adhesions of the ventral lumbar dura: an adjunct source of discogenic pain? Spine 15: 300-303.

Parke WW & Whalen JL (1993) The pial ligaments of the anterior spinal artery and their stretch receptors. Spine 18: 1542-1549.

Parkin IG & Harrison GR (1985) The topographical anatomy of the lumbar epidural space. Journal of Anatomy 141: 211-217.

Pechan J & Julis F (1975) The pressure measurement in the ulnar nerve: a contribution to the pathophysiology of cubital tunnel syndrome. Journal of Biomechanics 8: 75-79.

Penfield W & McNaughton F (1940) Dural headache and the innervation of the dura mater. Archives of Neurology and Psychiatry 44: 43-75.

Penning L (1992) Functional pathology of lumbar spinal stenosis. Clinical Biomechanics 7: 3-17.

Penning L & Wilmink JT (1987) Posture-dependent bilateral compression of L4 or L5 nerve roots in facet hypertrophy. Spine 12: 488-500.

Per Ohlin CO & Elmqvist D (1985) Pressures recorded in ulnar neuropathy. Acta Orthopaedica Scandinavica 56: 404-412.

Powell HC & Myers RR (1986) Pathology of experimental nerve compression. Laboratory Investigation 55: 91-100.

Rauschning W (1997) Anatomy and pathology of the cervical spine. In: Frymoyer JW (ed.) The Adult Spine: Principles and Practice, 2nd edn. Lippincott-Raven, Philadelphia.

Reid JD (1960) Effects of flexion-extension movements of the head and spine upon the spinal cord and nerve roots. Journal of Neurology, Neurosurgery, and Psychiatry 23: 214-221.

Rempel D, Bach JM, Richmond CA, et al. (1998) Effects of forearm pronation/supination on carpal tunnel pressure. Journal of Hand Surgery 23A: 38-42.

Rempel D, Dahlin L & Lundborg G (1999) Pathophysiology of nerve compression syndromes: response of peripheral nerves to loading. Journal of Bone and Joint Surgery 81A: 1600-1610.

Rempel D, Keir P, Smutz WP, et al. (1997) Effects of static fingertip loading on carpal tunnel pressure. Journal of Orthopedic Research 15: 422-426.

Revel M, Amor B, Mathieu A, et al. (1988) Sciatica induced by primary epidural adhesions. Lancet 1: 527-528.

Rossitti S (1993) Biomechanics of the pons-cord tract and its enveloping structures: an overview. Acta Neurochirurgica 124: 144-152.

Rutten HP, Szpak K & van Mameren H (1997) Letters. Spine 22: 924-928.

Rydevik B, Brown MD & Lundborg G (1984) Pathoanatomy and pathophysiology of nerve root compression. Spine 9: 7-15.

Rydevik B, Lundborg G & Bagge U (1981) Effects of graded compression on intraneural blood flow: An in-vivo study on rabbit tibial nerve. Journal of Hand Surgery 6: 3-12.

Rydevik B, Lundborg G & Skalak R (1989) Biomechanics of peripheral nerves. In: Nordin N & Frankel VH (eds.) Basic Biomechanics of the Musculoskeletal System, 2nd edn. Lea and Febiger, Philadelphia.: 75-87.

Sauer SK, Bove GM, Averbeck B, et al. (1999) Rat peripheral nerve components release calcitonin gene-related peptide and prostaglandin E2 in response to noxious stimuli: evidence that the nervi nervorum are nociceptors. Neuroscience 92: 319-325.

Savolaine ER, Pandja JB, Greenblatt EH, et al. (1988) Anatomy of the lumbar epidural space: new insights using CT-epidurography. Anesthesiology 68: 217-223.

Scapinelli R (1990) Anatomical and radiologic studies an the lumbosacral meningovertebral ligaments of humans. Journal of Spinal Disorders 3: 6-15.

Schonstrom N, Lindahl S, Willen J, et al. (1989) Dynamic changes in the dimension of the lumbar spinal canal: An experimental study in vitro. Journal of Orthopedic Research 7: 115-121.

Schuind FA, Goldschmidt D, Bastin C, et al. (1995) A biomechanical study of the ulnar nerve at the elbow. Journal of Hand Surgery 20B: 623-627.

Selvaratnam PJ, Matyas TA & Glasgow EF (1994) Noninvasive discrimination of brachial plexus involvement in upper limb pain. Spine 19: 26-33.

Shacklock M (1995) Neurodynamics. Physiotherapy 81: 9-16.

Shaw Wilgis EF & Murphy R (1986) The significance of longitudinal excursion in peripheral nerves. Hand Clinics 2: 761-766.

Smith CG (1956) Changes in length and position of the segments of the spinal cord with changes in posture in the monkey. Radiology 66: 259-265.

Smith JW (1966) Factors influencing nerve repair. Archives of Surgery 93: 335-341.

Sogaard I (1983) Sciatic nerve entrapment. Journal of Neurosurgery 58: 275-276.

Spencer DL, Irwin GS & Miller JAA (1983) Anatomy and significance of fixation of the lumbosacral nerve roots in sciatica. Spine 8: 672-679.

Spielman FJ (1982) Post lumbar puncture headache. Headache 22: 280-283.

Stodieck LS, Beel JA & Lutges MW (1986) Structural properties of spinal nerve roots: Protein composition. Experimental Neurology 91: 41-51.

Sunderland S (1978) Nerves and Nerve Injuries, 3rd edn. Churchill Livingstone, Melbourne.

Sunderland S & Bradley KC (1949) The cross sectional area of peripheral nerve trunks devoted to nerve fibres. Brain 72: 428-439.

Szabo RM, Bay BK, Sharkey NA, et al. (1994) Median nerve displacement through the carpal canal. Journal of Hand Surgery 19A: 901-906.

Tani S, Yamada S & Knighton RS (1987) Extensibility of the lumbar and sacral cord: pathophysiology of the tethered spinal cord in cats. Journal of Neurosurgery 66: 116-123.

Tencer AF, Allen BL & Ferguson RL (1985) A biomechanical study of thoracolumbar spine fractures with bone in the spinal canal: part 111. Mechanical properties of the dura and its tethering ligaments. Spine 10: 741-747.

Thomas PK (1963) The connective tissue of peripheral nerve: an electron microscope study. Journal of Anatomy 97: 35-44.

Thomas PK & Olsson Y (1984) Microscopic anatomy and function of the connective tissue components of peripheral nerve. In: Dyck PJ, Thomas PK, Lambert EH et al. (eds.) Peripheral Neuropathy, 2nd edn. Saunders, Philadelphia.

Valls-Sole J, Alvarez R & Nunez M (1995) Limited longitudinal sliding of the median nerve in patients with carpal tunnel syndrome. Muscle & Nerve 18: 761-767.

van Meeteren NL, Brakee JH, Helders PJ, et al. (1997) Functional recovery from sciatic nerve crush lesion in the rat correlates with individual differences in responses to chronic intermittent stress. Journal of Neuroscience Research 48: 524-532.

Vandam LD (1992) Symptoms following lumbar puncture may be related to decreased cerebrospinal fluid pressure and/or venous dilation. Anesthesiology 76: 321.

Von Lanz T (1929) Über die Rückenmarkshaute. 1. Die konstruktive form der harten haut des menschlichen rücken markes und ihrer bünder. Arch Entwickl Mech Org 118: 252-307.

Wall EJ, Massie JB, Kwan MK, et al. (1992) Experimental stretch neuropathy. Journal of Bone and Joint Surgery 74B: 126-129.

Weinstein JN (1997) Pain. In: Frymoyer JW (ed.) The Adult Spine: Principles and Practice, Lippincott-Raven, Philadelphia.

Weiss ND, Gordon L, Bloom T, et al. (1995) Position of the wrist associated with the lowest carpal-tunnel pressure: Implications for splint design. Journal of Bone and Joint Surgery 77A: 1695-1699.

Werner CO, Elmquist D & Ohlin T (1983) Pressure and nerve lesions in the carpal tunnel. Acta Orthopaedica Scandinavica 54: 312-316.

Westmoreland BF, Benaroch EE, Daube JR, et al. (1994) Medical Neurosciences, 3rd edn. Little, Brown and Company, Boston.

Wiltse LL, Fonseca AS, Amster J, et al. (1993) Relationship of the dura, Hofmann's ligaments, Batson's plexus and a fibrovascular membrane lying on the posterior surface of the vertebral bodies and attaching to the deep layer of the posterior longitudinal ligament. Spine 18: 1030-1043.

Wirth FP & van Buren JM (1971) Referral of pain from dural stimulation in man. Journal of Neurosurgery 34: 630-642.

Wright TW, Glowczewski F, Wheeler D, et al. (1996) Excursion and strain of the median nerve. Journal of Bone and Joint Surgery 78A: 1897-1903.

Yoo JU, Zou D, Edwards WT, et al. (1992) Effect of cervical spine motion on the neuroforaminal dimensions of human cervical spine. Spine 17: 1131-1136.

Yuan Q, Dougherty L & Margulies SS (1998) In vivo human spinal cord deformation and displacement in flexion. Spine 23: 1677-1683.

Zarzur E (1996) Mechanical properties of the human lumbar dura mater. Arquivos de Neuropsiquiatria 54: 455-460.

Zoech G, Reihsner R, Beer R, et al. (1991) Stress and strain in peripheral nerves. Neuro-Orthopedics 10: 73-82.

CHAPTER 6

CLINICIANS AND THEIR DECISIONS

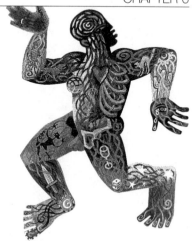

INTRODUCTION

REASONING AND EXPERTS – THE CURRENT STATE OF AFFAIRS

CLINICIANS, SCIENTISTS AND EVIDENCE
CLINICIAN/SCIENTIST RELATIONSHIPS
THE GREY ZONES OF MANUAL THERAPY PRACTICE

CLINICAL REASONING SCIENCE

INTRODUCTION
MODERN REASONING
DECLARATIVE KNOWLEDGE
A CRITICAL LOOK AT CURRENT DECLARATIVE KNOWLEDGE

A CLINICAL REASONING MODEL TO INCLUDE PAIN

CLINICAL DECISION MAKING REQUIRES HYPOTHESIS MAKING
PATHOBIOLOGICAL MECHANISMS
DYSFUNCTION/IMPAIRMENT – THE PATIENT'S PROBLEMS
SOURCES
CONTRIBUTING FACTORS
PROGNOSIS
PRECAUTIONS
MANAGEMENT

THE PROCESS OF REASONING

CHAPTER SUMMARY

REFERENCES CHAPTER 6

INTRODUCTION

Neurodynamics, neurobiology, and clinical decision making science are the key elements of this book. They need to be integrated for the best possible clinical use and this is discussed later in the chapter. I want to set the scene first with a broad view of clinical reasoning science and the current state of affairs in manual therapy.

REASONING AND EXPERTS - THE CURRENT STATE OF AFFAIRS

Manual therapists from the various professions usually and sometimes fervently, follow a school of thought or professional name. As Grant (1995) noted there are paradigms of practice where practitioners attach experts' names such as Cyriax, McKenzie or Maitland to an approach. Geographically based therapy systems such as the Norwegian or the Australian approach have existed for many years without real definition. There are anatomically based approaches such as the craniosacral or myofascial approach and there are approaches developed within professions such as chiropractic, physiotherapy, medicine and osteopathy. The development of practice paradigms in this way has meant that each has its own focal points that are often mutually exclusive. We should therefore conclude that there are some myths in all the approaches. Multiple approaches lead to factions and intra-professional politics and are of no real help for patients due to the wide choices on offer (Fig. 6.1). See also figure 1.1.

A more overlapping scenario, based on best evidence and practice would be beneficial. Such a scenario should seek out the common and useful elements of all therapy systems. I have already proposed in this book that a pain report is the most common and consistent feature that our patients present with. A closer look at pain may provide the glue for the merging of concepts.

However before an overlapping scenario is discussed, there are some issues related to evidence based medicine and the current feelings of many clinicians that need discussion.

CLINICIANS, SCIENTISTS AND EVIDENCE

Professionally, we are surrounded by the rapid rise of science in areas such as neurobiology, pain and disability epidemiology, precision of diagnostic tests and pain management. The nineties have been dominated by what Epstein (1990) termed the "outcomes movement", where evidence based medicine (EBM) and practice have come to the fore with willing government support. This has been particularly so in the United States, United Kingdom, Netherlands and Scandinavia. The outcomes movement emerged in the United States due to the obvious need for health cost containment and the competition between Health Maintenance Organisations for the industrial buyer's dollar, with price the basis for competition. It also occurred due to the exposure of great geographical differences in the use of medical procedures (Epstein 1990).

Evidence based medicine (EBM) is best defined by Sackett et al. (1996) as the "conscientious, explicit and judicious use of current best evidence in making decisions about the care of individual patients." Another recent definition from an EBM expert, Silagy (1999) is "...EBM is the integration of the best available scientific evidence with your clinical expertise, your intuition, your wisdom". Perhaps the most practical definition is "... the ability to track down, critically appraise and incorporate evidence into clinical practice (Rosenberg and Sackett 1996). Sackett et al. (1996) go on to say that the practice of EBM means the integration of clinical expertise, such as proficiency and judgement acquired from clinical experience with the best available external evidence from systematic research. External clinical evidence means research from basic sciences, from patient centred trials into the accuracy and precision of diagnostic tests, the power of prognostic markers and the efficacy of management programmes. Most clinicians would be happy if the above description was an accurate portrayal of EBM. However there is palpable unease in the clinic, based mainly on the fact that decision making power is moving more to external bodies.

The outcomes movement has brought another compelling issue for manual therapists. Clinicians who have followed the content of mainstream journals such as Spine and Pain and even a recent issue of Manual Therapy (Vol.4, 1999), will have noted increasing support for the contention that chronic pain development and responses to treatment may have more to do with psychosocial factors than physical factors. These include pain beliefs, movement fears, job satisfaction and childhood experiences. Some clinicians in the musculoskeletal management area may well begin to ponder their worth. We may all go through this, but on the up side, the outcomes movement and the information it brings, combined with the biological revolution is probably providing the most powerful stimulus for change and adaptation of practice ever. It can embellish existing successful management strategies and provide fresh and novel strategies.

CLINICIAN/SCIENTIST RELATIONSHIPS

I believe that there are issues in the clinician/scientist relationship which are stumbling blocks for clinicians integrating science. Mutual attitudes are surely required for the best outcomes. Scientists are often admired if they dabble in the clinic and I would like to push the notion that clinicians in their own way can be considered scientists. Clinician/scientist relationships have often been a bit testy, and some clinicians completely reject scientific evidence that doesn't support their management framework. Some instinctively rebel against science and most clinicians would wonder what a statistician knows about pain and suffering. They also think "it's us, the clinicians, who try and practice EBM not researchers".

It's not that clinicians distrust science. It is the structure of science which may concern them, in particular the advancement of academic careers linked to publication. It is obvious that

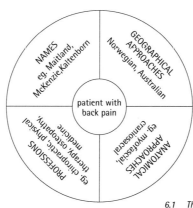

6.1   The patient with back pain has many management paradigms to select from.

research workers want results that validate their choice of subject, their world concept and indeed which validate their choice of career. "Research is like motherhood - there is no such thing as an ugly baby" was an interviewee's comment in Greer (1987). From the clinician's viewpoint, scientists may be seen as professional subscribers to journals - they have a common language and it seems that much is dialogue between researchers. "What does it contribute to the literature?" asks the researcher, whilst the clinician thinks "What does it do for my patients?" Literature is often seen more as a meandering discourse rather than a guide to action. Research conclusions will always be tentative at least initially, yet the practitioner often demands conclusive action. There is a need for clinicians to be able to extrapolate and extract the scientific information into useful clinical material. Many of us may not have these skills, although modern access to databases, informaticians and the enhancement of clinical reasoning skills is available to us all.

Few clinicians will reject the overall legitimacy of the outcomes movement, particularly after the exposure of the huge geographical variations in clinical practice (eg. Wennenberg et al. 1987). However the outcomes movement presents some philosophical difficulties. According to Tanenbaum (1993), the danger is that it may present statistical analysis as superior rather than complementary to other forms of knowledge. The statisticians and those who pay them understandably want neat figures. However uncertainty and subjectivity are at the heart of any clinical encounter. As every clinician knows, good evidence can lead to bad practice if applied in an uncaring way or in an unappealing atmosphere. The clinician wants to know where empathy and the experience of accumulated cases and patterns of clinical responses fits into the equation. Clinicians recognise instinctively that it is a leap of faith to expand the results of a trial to a broad therapeutic principle (Kenny 1997). Many clinicians take quiet umbrage at the randomised clinical trial as it holds all clinicians equal suggesting that the specific clinician does not matter. There are suspicions with trials that test a technique - clinicians realise all the time that a single technique is only a part of the total management package that they provide. The other aspects of the treatment such as associated techniques, explanations with models, empathy, the phone call after the treatment and the friendly healing clinical environment that the clinician carefully constructs seem unnoticed. And, as any good clinician knows from hard earned cumulative experience, there are subgroups of pain patterns and physical features within the diagnosis of neuromusculoskeletal pain on which a certain approach or technique works better than others. However the challenge is now unquestionably on the clinicians to document these groups better, and to realise that intraprofessional research is critical.

There is also suspicion that the outcomes movement is progressing with too much speed and that it could stop development in certain areas (Epstein 1990). Sackett (1996) cautions, reminding us that EBM is a "relatively young discipline whose positive impacts are just beginning to be validated". I would be concerned if meta-analyses had the final say rather than them being tools which expose errors in practice which may be correctable. And after all, isn't science about proving things wrong? For example, exercises may offer little help for acute spinal pain according to Waddell et al. (1996). However, refine the exercise, change the environment in which the exercises are performed, realise that exercise is not just for muscle strength, provide more knowledge and motivation, and specify the group for whom the exercises are given and more efficacy would probably be demonstrated. As Scott and Black (1991) point out, great care should be taken that meta-analyses are not pooling ignorance as much as distilling medicine. The science of neurodynamics is just beginning and there is an existing and growing basic science foundation plus the beginnings of clinical research. It would be sad to see it forced out by an evidence based medicine which hardly considered it, despite its backing in basic sciences. It would be equally sad if it was just taken as dogma and became another concept to fit into figure 6.1.

Black (1998) notes that any movement which encourages self scrutiny and self analysis has to be good so long as it stops short of reducing the self confidence of clinicians. It is this self-confidence after all which enables us to practice while still being aware of the uncertainty in all branches of health care. Self confidence relates to placebo. It's not a bad thing and is the most powerful and consistent pain reliever we have. Hard EBM which denies placebo may destroy confidence.

Despite these differences, which I have presented somewhat one sidedly from my clinically dominated viewpoint, the clinicians and researchers in physiotherapy urgently need to review their relationship with science. Traditional physiotherapeutic approaches must engage a broader science, therefore a shift from traditional experiential based approaches to approaches that critically adopt evidence.

My belief is that a closer look at the phenomenon of pain will take us to that broader science. It will help provide a rational framework in which to embed the neurodynamic concepts. Uncorrupted reasoning science is necessary to address change, particularly if the "grey zones" in which physiotherapists work are contemplated. I urge clinicians to be clinical scientists and take on the responsibility which the word "scientist" endows.

THE GREY ZONES OF MANUAL THERAPY PRACTICE

Most clinicans work in a world of syndromal diagnoses where the underlying pathoanatomy and pathophysiology of the syndrome is not known and neither are the risk/benefit ratios of treatment. This is common in psychiatry (eg. major depression), in neurology (eg. migraine headache) and very frequently in musculoskeletal medicine (eg. thoracic outlet syndrome, myofascial syndrome, fibromyalgia). Most of us work in what has been termed "grey zones of practice" (Naylor 1995) where all is obviously not black and white. Contrast non-specific low back pain, sitting right in the middle of the grey zone with rheumatoid arthritis for example, where the pathophysiology is reasonably well understood.

The grey zone is massive. This is an era of new, chronic and stress related disorders where there is neither vaccine nor cure. And with the grey zone comes an unprecedented growth in new treatments, machines, and professions proclaiming an answer. There will be huge grey areas until the generation of new research (Naylor 1995). Considering that a properly carried out randomised clinical trial may cost 400,000 dollars, this will require a massive financial and social investment and makes clincian/scientist links imperative.

At this stage, best practice clinical reasoning must be applied to traverse the grey zones (Naylor 1995); reasoning which includes, integrates and contributes to relevant evidence based work as it comes about.

CLINICAL REASONING SCIENCE

INTRODUCTION

Many researchers, particularly in physiotherapy, medicine and occupational therapy have studied this science of clinical reasoning. Clinical reasoning has been referred to as "....the thinking and decision making processes which are integral to clinical practice" (Higgs and Jones 1995; 2000). Clinical reasoning is not just judgement of facts, it's a judgement of values, attitudes and expectations as well. Clinical reasoning should actually be EBM carried out by clinical scientists. The opposite of clinical reasoning is "recipe management" where clinicians apply untested similar techniques and principles to all patients. All physiotherapists have routine aspects of their management, particularly when patients have familiar problems. However the more complex a problem becomes, the more decision making skills will be required. This definition of clinical reasoning should not only be considered on a per patient basis, but also for total professional development.

Many clinicians are tempted to say "we do it anyway" in regard to reasoning and evidence based medicine. Maybe. However the most powerful evidence against that is variations in clinical practice. The choices that the patient with back pain has today plus the stark epidemiological data exposing chronic pain levels in society (Crook et al. 1984; Magni et al. 1990) are also evidence that clinicians don't do it that well and need to adapt practice.

Clinical reasoning has been termed many things, such as clinical judgement and clinical decision making. A useful term is "wise action" (Jones 1997). It's more catchy in the clinic and I find more teaching utility in asking a student "is that a wise action" rather than "are you clinically reasoning". I hope that the broader use of available science can be seen as a "wise action".

Reasoning is about uncertainty, but that is what the entire clinical encounter is all about. EBM only makes part of it less uncertain. However this should not be cause for clinical anguish. Rather, there should be a freedom with the knowledge that there is a framework to cope with uncertainty.

MODERN REASONING

Modern clinical reasoning for manual therapists in my view involves a merging of three areas - the best of science, current therapies and the patient/therapist relationship (Fig. 6.2).

THE BEST OF SCIENCE

The best of science means the most current and relevant science related to pathological movement. For manual therapists this includes all that Sackett (1996) outlined - basic sciences, diagnostic tests, prognostic markers, management efficacy - anything related to rehabilitation science. It includes all that is evidence based medicine. However, if we are to take on the paradigm of pain into reasoning, instantly our knowledge deficits are exposed. For example, this may be, depending on where and how you were taught, knowledge of synaptic activity, neurotransmitters, exercise prescription and knowledge of results of randomised clinical trials.

THE BEST OF CURRENT THERAPIES (WITH AN EYE ON THE NEW)

This acknowledges that there are good assessment procedures and management strategies that are either self taught or have been learnt from others. These are particularly beneficial if the right patient for the approach can be selected. For example I would consider that the self management concept of McKenzie, the inherent reasoning strategies of Maitland, the skill in joint management of Kaltenborn/Evjenth and Paris are superb aspects of management that we must never lose, but adapt. There are approaches outside traditional manual therapy which have skills to offer and which could be included, such as counselling. There are also skills which were once commonplace such as relaxation techniques and functional rehabilitation which, to some degree appear to have been lost in the last two decades.

THE BEST OF THE PATIENT/THERAPIST RELATIONSHIP

This implies that a skilled, analytical and defensible physical and subjective examination appropriate to the patient will be undertaken. It also implies that a relationship based on an appropriate amount of empathy is engendered and that the patient is involved in collaborative decision making.

These three aspects of reasoning rely on a basic knowledge common to a profession and are referred to as "declarative knowledge".

DECLARATIVE KNOWLEDGE

"Declarative knowledge" is a term that means to have "knowledge about a topic so that one may declare that knowledge to be theirs" (Biggs and Telfer 1987). This could be considered in a personal sense but also in a professional sense. In the professional sense, it should relate to the knowledge that the profession has which is specific to that profession and it should relate to skills that only that profession has or uses in a particular way. Good clinical reasoning should allow a focus on the uniqueness of a profession - it should make the boundaries clearer.

In some professions the declarative knowledge is quite obvious, for example, dentistry has a near monopoly on the mouth and neonatal cardiologists have few challengers. In the manual therapies it is much more open - there are many professions vying for management rights of painful states. There are many professions with a great interest in the brain.

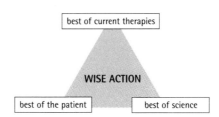

6.2   Clinical reasoning - components of the "wise action" approach.

"Pathokinesiology" (Hislop 1975) has been suggested as the distinguishing central concept in physiotherapy. This is certainly the primary paradigm in physiotherapy, though perhaps "pathological movement" or "movement dysfunction" are more modern terms. Hislop's concept (1975) was also strongly grounded on social and cultural needs and she considered that movement dysfunction could not be considered outside a sociocultural and a scientific framework (Purtilo 1986; Grant 1995).

The mission statements of most national physiotherapy associations are similar. For example, the American Physical Therapy Association mission statement on their website is "to further the profession's role in the prevention, diagnosis and treatment of movement dysfunctions and the enhancement of the physical health and functional abilities of members of the public."

Movement dysfunction is the key, not necessarily the damaged structures which many manual therapy models focus on. What has changed rapidly as part of the outcomes and pain sciences movements is the knowledge of the mechanisms behind the faulty movement and dysfunction, and the best methods to assess it and manage it.

As stated above and discussed in greater detail in chapter 7, the general outcome of the mass of epidemiological data looking at factors related to the development of chronicity of spinal pain points to the importance of psychosocial factors. These include patient beliefs, job satisfaction and educational level (eg. Burton et al. 1995; Kendall et al. 1997; Linton and Hallden 1997). In some cases, they may be more important than the physical health of tissues, although deconditioned tissues and physical dysfunctions are a common feature of patients in a chronic pain state. These more physical factors are still important and addressing them is also a way to address psychological factors.

Manual therapists of all persuasions must become increasingly aware that sensitivity to movement is not only related to tissues but also to changes in ion channel and neurotransmitter activity in the peripheral and central nervous systems and which are driven by biological, psychological and social inputs (chapters 2,3,4). If a patient's pathological movement is negatively influenced by a lack of, or misinformation provided by a health professional, then it is the professional's responsibility to correct this negative input. We should be well placed to contribute here, due to our numbers, time with patients, existing movement improvement strategies, biological and kinaesiological knowledge and the fact that non-surgical rehabilitation costs are low compared with many other services. Indeed we now see repeatedly in the physiotherapy literature the cry that modern physical rehabilitation cannot limit itself to physical methods only (eg Lieberman et al. 1994; Feuerstein and Beattie 1995; Watson 1996; Ford and Gordon 1997; Gifford and Butler 1997; Martinez et al. 1997; Watson 1999). However the critical question arises - is our current declarative knowledge adequate to handle this, not only in technique but in basic sciences?

A CRITICAL LOOK AT CURRENT DECLARATIVE KNOWLEDGE

In the manual therapy approaches, a very dominant tissue or structure based approach still undoubtedly exists, often referred to as a "bottom up" approach. It is a relevant and necessary approach when disease and injury are present in tissues, particularly in acute injury. It also has an important function in chronic pain states where tissues are often unused, unhealthy and unfit. In figure 6.3, this approach is illustrated. The arrows reveal the deeper and deeper search into the tissues for an answer to a patient's pain. In this model the joint is used as an example, but it could equally be fascia, muscle or any tissue. It serves as a reminder that for adequate management of tissue problems we need anatomical and pathoanatomical knowledge of all tissues, including knowledge at a gross anatomical level and down to the molecular level. This approach holds that pain is a passive process beginning at end terminals and relating to impulses going in a straight line to the brain. It appears to neglect current concepts of pain as an endogenous active process and it ignores the role of fear and anxiety, beliefs and the fact that the brain is "on all the time" (McCrone 1997) and thus may not be dependent on peripheral input for activation and output. The phenomenon of pain, particularly in its more chronic modes challenges this approach and calls for a bigger picture. The dominant sources and pain processes may be only partly in the peripheral tissues.

In figure 6.4, which I adapted from Shepherd's classic textbook (Shepherd 1994), a neurobiological approach is presented. I urge the careful and diplomatic integration of this material into current manual therapy practice, ie. expanding our declarative knowledge. Again looking from a macroscopic to a microscopic view, our lack of knowledge is exposed. I believe manual therapists need more knowledge about health related behaviour in general. This includes pain behaviour, illness behaviour and the reasons for it. We need knowledge about neurological centres and pathways. Traditional education has provided us with knowledge about sensory and motor pathways. The more mysterious hypothalamus-pituitary-adrenal axis was left out; we didn't discuss limbic and reticular systems and the autonomic nervous system was never for serious study. Orthodox manual therapy used to stop at the atlanto-occipital joint. We must have knowledge of these centres if we are to understand pathological movement and provide a scientific rationale for management. No one is calling for a great depth of knowledge, even keeping up with lay science journals eg. New Scientist and Science and Medicine and review articles in physiotherapy and mainstream science journals should be adequate for clinicians.

In the model (Fig. 6.4) some knowledge about the function of neurones, synapses, neurone connectivity, receptors and ion channels is also required. Soon we must take more knowledge of genetics into our declarative knowledge. The proteins which constitute ion channels in the axolemma of nerve fibres and ultimately dictate sensitivity are produced by genetic

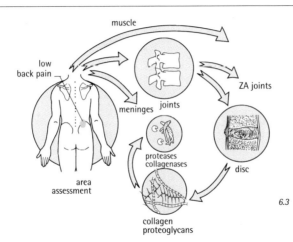

6.3   *The tissue based model. Various tissues could be explored for an answer to the patient's back pain. It is not always successful.*

instruction in response to environmental forces. Perhaps a good example of the need for knowledge down to a genetic/molecular level is recent research (eg. Devor and Seltzer 1999) suggesting that with post peripheral nerve injury, the genetic machinery can alter the expression of receptors at the injury site to make them more responsive to circulating adrenaline (chapter 3). This means that stress may drive a neuropathic pain in a direct way. Clinicians must be professional conduits of this kind of knowledge to patients. I believe that most clinicians would like to take on this new material but just require some assistance with the process.

Utilising a wider declarative knowledge in a clinical reasoning model may assist manual therapists to become more involved with chronic pain professionally. It is well known that most physiotherapists prefer not to work with patients with chronic pain, - all but 4% in a U.S. study (Wolff et al. 1991). As a young therapist I used to dread the "pain everywhere" and the "thick file" patients. It seems that acute injuries and sports injuries are the current preferred options, although it is very likely that clinicians conceptualise recurrent spinal pains as acute rather than the chronic pains they should be framed as. The acute care model predominates in musculoskeletal medicine. The fact that the expression of acute pain depends on peripherally activated central pathways is often forgotten. Not enough is taught about the physiological and cognitive mechanisms in undergraduate training (Wolff et al. 1991). The same problem exists in medicine according to Cherkin (1988). The neurobiological model is as appropriate for acute pain management as it is for chronic pain management.

SO, MANUAL THERAPISTS SHOULD BE PSYCHOLOGISTS THEN?

No. Psychology has its own declarative knowledge, although there will be overlap with many professions. However, the central tenet of manual therapy is faulty movement. If faulty movement comes from a simple fear of movement, fear of reinjury or lack of understanding of the meaning of certain symptoms, then this fear should be dealt with by the managing therapist. Manual therapy approaches for pathological movement should encompass a wider science base which includes stress biology and aspects of psychology. Perhaps two areas, more than any other which have been shown to relate to the development of chronic pain states can be adopted: this is fear of pain and reinjury and lack of understanding of the meaning of pain. Both areas call for a restructuring of basic sciences.

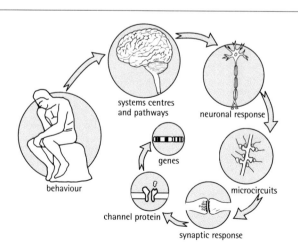

6.4   *The neurobiological model. Knowledge of various processes and structures could be introduced into clinical decision making.*

Professional redefinition points to the awareness of professional limits and boundaries. I believe that the inclusion of the pain paradigm forces this awareness and should create better interprofessional links.

ROLE OF THE CLINICIAN'S EXPERIENCE

Where does experience fit in? Management models that propose new information and the integration of evidence based medicine downplay (or can appear to downplay) the importance of experience. Experience was always the dominant feature of traditional management paradigms (eg. Goldner and Bilsker 1995) and still is, even though EBM has made its mark. The evidence based experts still consider it an important component for current and future management (Sackett et al. 1996). Still, as a recent survey (Tsafrir and Grinberg 1998) showed, physicians relied on review articles and meta-analysis, but for practical patient care purposes they relied more on the opinions of peers and experts.

Experience currently rules supreme in manual therapy as it does in any areas with "grey zones". In this traditional paradigm, clinicians, when faced with a patient, will reflect on experiences with similar presentations, reflect on underlying theory and consult someone who they consider an expert (Jones 1995; Gilroy 1996). We all do this to some degree and most of us reason subconsciously. However, the current underlying theory base needs an injection of pain science and we believe we must be diplomatically critical of who we consider an expert. However there are clinicians who have had 20 years of experience in 20 years of clinical practice, there are others who have 20 years of experience in one year of clinical practice. The latter has reasoned, learned, experimented with management techniques, remained open, been aware of the outcomes movement, and has read widely.

Every clinician has different preprofessional foundations which come into play as part of "experience". These foundations include an outlook on life and a frame of reference or worldview (Hooper 1997). They include culturally mediated beliefs about relationships, the non-organic world, the body, disability and the value and purpose of life. This is the powerful behind the scenes reasoning that has little to do with what was learnt at manual therapy school and which is unique and precious as part of therapy and part of delivery of evidence based medicine.

Medicine and allied practitioners have a firm grasp on pain; people will still visit doctors, physiotherapists, chiropractors, and osteopaths for existential pains, for the sufferring of living in this world, for ailments that no current technology can correct or diagnose (Spiro et al. 1993). I believe that a clinical reasoning approach as defined earlier is necessary for management. There may be non quantifiable differences between patients that an expert may pick up.

Expert opinion is on the lowest scale of the accepted evidential ladder. Clinicians should be aware of this and challenge it. It means that their contribution is less than a poorly conducted trial. It should be clear that there are different kinds of evidence and experience is one kind. Pain management requires flexibility.

While calling for more evidence based practice and a manual therapy contribution to evidence, it is believed that experience is another form of evidence, yet one which is essential for delivering EBM and bridging the gap between knowledge and clinical delivery (for reviews see Tanenbaum 1999; Tonelli 1999).

A CLINICAL REASONING MODEL TO INCLUDE PAIN

There are aspects of decision making in all manual therapy concepts, best articulated for clinicians by Mark Jones and colleagues (eg. Jones 1992; Higgs and Jones 2000). Clinical reasoning provides an evolving framework which easily embraces pain and disability. The inclusion of pain into reasoning strategies was the subject of much discussion and argument with colleagues including Dalton, Gifford, Jones, Shacklock and Slater. See also my combined work with Louis Gifford reflected in the following publications (Butler 1994; Gifford and Butler 1997; Gifford 1997; Butler 1998; Butler 1998; Gifford 1998).

I believe the first step is to consider what pain actually is and what the pain paradigm actually encompasses. I suggest that we seek a broad answer and read widely in pathophysiological areas (eg. Campbell 1996; Melzack and Wall 1996; Raj 1996; Max 1999; Wall and Melzack 1999) but also in sociocultural areas (eg. Scarry 1985; Morris 1991; Delvecchio-Good et al. 1992). Meanwhile, the International Association for the Study of Pain (IASP) definition (Merskey and Bogduk 1994) that "pain is an unpleasant sensory and emotional experience associated with actual or potential tissue damage or described in terms of such damage" is the best starting point.

Ponder on the definition for a moment. "Experience" is the key word. It takes away the usual automatic links which we all have that pain matches injury. It is a reminder that thoughts such as fear and anger can drive a similar pain circuitry that an irritated nerve root can. It encourages a biological, psychological and social assessment.

CLINICAL DECISION MAKING REQUIRES HYPOTHESIS MAKING

Clinical reasoning requires that the practitioner makes educated hypotheses about all kinds of information and processes related to the patient's assessment and management. These can be categorised. A reasoning category is a category or "box" of information collected with the ultimate goal being successful management of the patient (Higgs & Jones 1995). For example, a clinician collects information from a range of sources such as the patient interview, imaging tests, the literature (including EBM), "gut feeling", previous experiences with similar problems and advice from colleagues. This "basket of data" then allows hypothesised identification of a troublesome tissue, hints of disease processes, and guidelines to the kind of physical

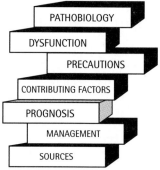

6.5   Clinical reasoning categories. They all relate to each other for stability. The whole reasoning process may topple if information is not collected in each category.

assessment to perform, for example. Although in the following discussion categories are placed in a certain order, the relative importance of each to a particular patient will vary.

The consequences of disease and injury have also been classified by the World Health Organisation (WHO). The organisation published the International Classification of Impairments, Disabilities and Handicaps (ICIDH) in 1980, and updated it in 1999 (ICIDH-2 1999). The recent model allies itself with bio-psycho-social concepts and attempts to capture the variety of experiences which people who live with disabilities have. The classifications in this chapter, especially in regard to dysfunction/impairment, attempt to collect similar information to the ICIDH classifications. The ICIDH classifications are descriptors of health, not really explainers of health (Halbertsma 1995). Medical personnel also require the pathobiology classifications as suggested here and these may help determine the importance and relevance of impairments.

As I have pointed out above, the whole reasoning process may collapse if the clinician cannot provide reasoned information in all categories (Fig. 6.5). On reflection on cases of failed or poor management, it should be easy to see which category was not adequately reasoned. I believe that these categories offer a conceptual design that not only addresses the consequence of injury and disease but also facilitates a management process. These categories are briefly introduced below and elaborated upon in later chapters.

PATHOBIOLOGICAL MECHANISMS

Pathobiology is the physiology of suffering, disease and injury and is obviously a central concept in modern medicine. It is clear that it has not been adequately included in current models of manual therapy. As Loeser (1997) comments, how useful is "sprain" or "strain" as a diagnosis for chronic low back pain? We need to take a closer look at what the "sprain" involves, especially when the diagnosis is still "sprain" 6 months after injury.

Pathobiological mechanisms include biological and pathobiological processes related to all involved systems (eg. motor, endocrine, nervous) in the injury/ disease and responses to the injury/disease. It is in this category that pain can be engaged and our shortcomings in declarative knowledge made evident and corrected. This category can be divided up into **mechanisms related to tissues and mechanisms related to pain.**

We ought to be good at integrating pathobiological mechanisms related to tissue injury or disease. After all, this is where the majority of our training is focussed. This includes making hypotheses about the actual tissue(s) injured, the nature of the injury, the stage of healing, the amount of inflammation and amount of scarring. This is discussed in many textbooks and briefly discussed in chapter 3.

Pathobiological mechanisms related to pain may be a new category for many physiotherapists. Categorising means making a decision on the **class** of pain that a patient has. It is different to the **source** of the pain. It is essentially a biological classification and as such calls for a clinical diagnosis including a categorisation of pain, as well as the traditional diagnosis of tissue. For example, a class of pain could be peripheral neurogenic and the source could be an L4-5 nerve root. Another class of pain could be nociceptive and the sources could be the L2-3 disc and erector spinae muscles. Central sensitivity states will involve multiple central nervous system sources (chapter 2). Management decisions will relate not only to tissues at fault but also to the class of pain the patient has. For example, drugs are not taken for sources of pain, they are taken for processes or classes of pain such as neuropathic pain. Finding the anatomical sources involved in the mechanisms can be invaluable but not always possible. Note that the relative importance of peripheral or central mechanisms cannot yet be judged scientifically. Clinical reasoning is needed to transcend the gap. However, it appears that there has been an error in reasoning in the past with the insistence that all pain should have a dominant tissue source.

A note of caution though. Fordyce (1997) reminds us somewhat cynically that illness expands to fill the diagnostic categories available to fit it. Rigorous attention to basic sciences is needed.

Pain mechanisms can be conveniently divided up into those related to input (eg. nociceptive pain, peripheral neurogenic pain), those related to processing (eg. central nervous system plasticity changes, cognitive influences) and those related to output systems (eg. sympathetic nervous system, immune and endocrine systems). See chapters 3 and 4. Recent reviews and discussions on pain mechanisms include Sidall (1997), Devor (1996) (Gifford 1998) and Markenson (1996). The "Textbook of Pain" divides its introductory chapters into mechanisms of pain (Wall and Melzack 1999).

MECHANISMS RELATED TO INPUT

There are two categories here: **nociceptive** pain and **peripheral neurogenic** pain. Nociceptive pain is pain from the tissues, pain which emerges at the ends of neurones, for example from changes in joint, muscles, dura mater, urethra and skin. The main pain evoking mechanisms will be mechanical and inflammatory. See chapter 3. Note that it also includes the connective tissues of the nervous system such as epineurium and dura mater. The reader may wonder what the difference is between the category of tissue injury and nociceptive pain. The point is that tissue injury does not necessarily have to hurt. To understand pain mechanisms is to understand why an injury may hurt one person but not another.

Peripheral neurogenic pain includes pain generated from peripheral nerves and the cell bodies of peripheral nerve fibres. This includes nerve root injury and nerve entrapment. It also includes injury to cranial nerves and roots. Any injury or disease "outside" of the dorsal horn of the spinal cord in a physiological sense, or the medullary horn in the case of the cranial nerves, could be considered as peripheral neurogenic processes. In peripheral neurogenic pain the split between the tissue approach and the neurobiological approach discussed earlier can be seen. Well known scientists, Devor (1994; Devor and Seltzer 1999) and Lundborg and Dahlin (1996; 1997) have written widely about peripheral nerve injury, but as far as I can see, never mention each other. Devor's group is more interested in the neurobiology of pain, Lundborg's more interested in tissue health issues such as circulation and axoplasmic flow. Both references are highly recommended readings for manual therapists. Peripheral neurogenic mechanisms are discussed in detail in chapter 3.

MECHANISMS RELATED TO PROCESSING

Pain related to input mechanisms is quite understandable. The sprained ankle, the pinched nerve and the aches and pains after unaccustomed exercise make it seem obvious. However, pain is not all like this. If it was all related to input, it would be easy. It would make pain a passive process, a registering of impulse trains in the central nervous system following alterations of input. It is more accurate to consider it as something a person creates or processes actively and highly reliant on endogenous processes (Chapman et al. 1997). The input mechanisms relating to pain are not in use all the time, however the brain is "on all the time". This involves complex processing involving multiple inputs such as feelings and moods, links to existing neural circuitry (memory) which may have been established years previously and biological events including alterations in responsiveness of neurones, receptive field increases, and new neuronal connections (see chapter 2 and 4).

MECHANISMS RELATED TO OUTPUT

The human as a control system will have an output in response to input, processing and feedback. Sometimes these output mechanisms can be considered as pain evoking mechanisms in their own right, mechanisms with powerful influences on tissue health, pain and function. They also function as powerful background homeostatic mechanisms. Muscle spasm or a list are both examples of motor output mechanism responses seen in clinical practice. Clinicians will be familiar with the sympathetic nervous system, but considerations here should also include the parasympathetic system, the sympathetic, endocrine and immune systems. See chapter 4. It might be argued that consciousness could also be seen as an output mechanism.

It is critical that readers realise that all these pathobiological processes will be occurring at one time in both acute and chronic pain, however there may be a clinical dominance of one mechanism over the others. By pattern generation, a reasoned decision about the dominant mechanism(s) in operation may be made. These patterns are discussed in chapter 3 and 4.

DYSFUNCTION/IMPAIRMENT - THE PATIENT'S PROBLEMS

A pathobiological mechanism may result in variable disturbances of function, thus dysfunctions or impairments which hopefully recede as the pathobiological processes get better. Sometimes, due to a wide variety of reasons, members of the public bring these dysfunctions in varying states of recovery to clinicians and then the person becomes a patient. Dysfunctions are what we observe and find in the clinic. They are the clinical manifestations of the pathobiological processes in operation and they represent the patient's main problems at that time.

There are various categories of function/dysfunction which must be understood by clinicians if they are going to integrate pain (Gifford and Butler 1997; Gifford 1997; Butler 1998). All categories should be considered by the clinician.

First is **general physical function/dysfunction**. This is the patient's main problem or problems as outlined by the patient or associates. It may be an inability to walk properly, it could be a limp, poor use of crutches, an inability to perform a particular sporting manoeuvre or creative activities, sleep, use a computer, lack of fitness, etc. Arguably, the rush to find a tissue at fault or apply the favoured manual therapy concept may mean that these general physical dysfunctions, and the fact that they may not need to be associated with unhealthy tissues, may be overlooked. The ICIDH-2 (1999) may classify this under the title of "activity level".

Second is **specific physical function/dysfunction**. This is what clinicians find on examination and what you consider could be a problem. It could be a tight or weak muscle, a loss of reflex, an adherent tight piece of scar, a limited upper limb neurodynamic test, pain on pressure over a certain body part. ICIDH-2 (1999) would refer to this as an "impairment in body function". Manual therapists are usually well skilled at this aspect of examination, especially in joint and muscle evaluation. This is the category where altered neurodynamics could be conceptualised. By themselves, specific physical dysfunctions are only clinical findings. Their relevance must be reasoned. Remember, this is what the therapist finds and it is not necessarily a problem for the patient. The therapist must make a clinical judgement about any links to general physical dysfunction. We all have little bits wrong with us.

Third is **mental or psychological function/dysfunction**. This is what the patient thinks and feels about her injury, you, the treatment and society's ever changing approach to his/her injury and disability. It is best called "distress" (Matthews 2000) and it involves things like mood, anxiety, catastrophising, anger, and enhanced processing of negative stimuli.

MAKING SENSE OUT OF DYSFUNCTION

Obviously all dysfunctions are related. A patient would have to have general dysfunction before a therapist went looking for specific physical dysfunction. General dysfunction is more determined by beliefs, attitudes and motivation as well as physical problems, thus it will often have a significant relationship to mental dysfunction as well as physical problems.

To make more sense in a reasoning approach, dysfunctions have to be seen as **adaptive** or **maladaptive** (Gifford 1997). This can be difficult but a worthy aim. Who are we to say that a certain behaviour is adaptive or maladaptive if the complete picture of the meaning of the pain is not explored. For example, it may be quite adaptive and assist healing for members of certain cultures to exclaim and wail loudly, perhaps seeking as much placebo from society as possible. But in practice, particularly over time, we can usually make decisions when a limp, movement pattern or posture is serving a healing purpose (adaptive) or if there is no benefit in the action (maladaptive). Pathobiological knowledge helps.

We all have dysfunctions. Manual therapists who examine people who are in no distress, even top level athletes, will usually find some specific dysfunction if they want to - perhaps hypomobile joints, limited neurodynamic tests, or muscle imbalance for example. It depends on the particular training or bias of the therapist.

Here is where we need to be careful. These valuable examination skills must be kept but they need to be judged in terms of relevance to the patient's function and outcome, just like the relevance of findings on an X-ray or MRI. We all accumulate dysfunction as we get older, the "kisses of time" in antique seller's language. Taking on the paradigm of pain may help us to determine the relevance of what we find. In a central sensitivity state, minor findings on physical examination may not be that relevant. However, minor findings of tissue ill health may be very relevant in the management of an athlete with minimal problems during a sporting manoeuvre. In the past we have surely found and treated dysfunctions that have no relevance to the patient. We may well have provided a healthy dose of placebo by the ritual of treatment and alleviated a problem which was elsewhere. We should have no troubles admitting this. It has surely happened in all fields of medicine (Spiro and Shapiro 1997).

SOURCES

Sources means the actual anatomical location of the pathobiological mechanisms. It can be invaluable for targeted therapy when this is known. Sources may be graphically explained as "if you had a magic bullet to fix the patient, where would you fire it?" In the case of acute injury and nociceptive pain, you may only need one bullet aimed at tissues and nociceptors supplying the tissues. In the case of a more complex pain presentation, perhaps one magic bullet may not be enough. A "machine gun" approach with careful aim may be more necessary to address the altered tissues - perhaps aiming for the tissues, lamina 11 of the spinal cord, the contralateral cingulate cortex, the pituitary etc.

Clinicians can consider two aspects to sources - **source(s) of the dysfunction** and **sources(s) of the mechanisms**. Patients also have hypotheses about the anatomical location of their problem and this requires respect. Patients may not care much about sources of mechanisms. For a musician who is having difficulty playing an instrument, the source of the mechanisms may be in the peripheral and central nervous system, but the source of the dysfunction could be the hand. The patient's belief here in the importance and reality of structural sources can be extremely powerful. The origin of the belief comes from the same Cartesian based mind-body split which still dominates in the treatment of pain.

CONTRIBUTING FACTORS

This category includes any factor related to the predisposition, development and maintenance of a problem. It includes psychosocial, genetic, anthropometric and ergonomic factors. In understanding this hypothesis category and being aware of the various issues and states which drive a pain state, there should be repercussions for overall management. Sometimes the contributing factors can be treated.

Psychosocial means the interaction between a person and his/her environment and the resultant influences on behaviour. In the last five years the outcomes movement has provided a mass of research in this area. For example, psychosocial factors which have been shown to have a link to the development of pain chronicity include beliefs that all pain is harmful and disabling (Kendall et al. 1997), provision of rational explanations of the problem (Indahl et al. 1995), fear of pain (Klenerman et al. 1995), level of work satisfaction (Bigos et al. 1992) and significant childhood psychological trauma (Goldberg 1994). This reasoning category will provide powerful direction for manual therapy in the future. Knowledge of it, thus creating an awareness of the multiple influences and effects of pain, should emphasise how important it is to include contributing factors into our declarative knowledge. There are more details on contributing factors in the next chapter. It is however, a complex process that turns injury, painful relationships, painful work states, genetic makeup, habits and beliefs into a pain state and a painful world for the patient.

PROGNOSIS

This is perhaps one of the most difficult hypothesis categories to make a decision on. It can be a humbling learning process to make a note on a patient's chart detailing how many treatments she will require and for what result, on her first attendance. This category, like others will draw information from all the other reasoning categories. An example of this for the prognosis category is shown in figure 6.6. In terms of chronic ongoing pain, the prognosis for pain relief may be poor, while that for restoration of functional movement and quality of movement can be excellent. Prognosis should not only be a reasoned judgement of final outcome and duration in relation to goals established by therapist and patient. It should, if possible, provide some guidance as to the course of the disorder, for example exacerbations and remisssions.

Manual therapists can continually reassess the prognosis and attempt to back up their judgement with reasoned hypotheses about pathobiological mechanisms in operation.

PRECAUTIONS

"Do no harm" should be foremost. Or when a manual therapy technique is performed, then the least force for the maximum safe gain should be the ideal. In recent years the terms "red flags" and "yellow flags" have been used (Kendall et al. 1997). Red flags are physical risk factors and often require urgent referral for specialist attention. Many patients come to manual therapists without referral from medical professionals. We must be aware of the red flags and be ever cautious for those who slip through the medical net. An example would be a sudden visual deficit after a neck injury or a rapid loss of weight when there is no obvious reason. Yellow flags refer to psychosocial factors and both red and yellow flags are discussed in chapter 7. Given the phenomenon of pain and the influences upon it there should not only be precautions to what we do, but to what we say and how we act as well.

MANAGEMENT

Management has to be a reasoning category also, as what we actually do can only be a hypothesis. We can be guided by evidence, but the individuality of the patient and the therapist calls for individually tailored and flexible management.

A technique, be it a passive straight leg raise manoeuvre, or education regarding the clicking noise in a patient's back is only a part of overall management. Management also links into the other reasoning categories and it includes knowing when to stop, and when to use other professionals. Given that pain, particularly chronic pain is something that we may never cure, management becomes a critical word. There will always be a place for passively delivered techniques. They are often useful and society demands it. And it is only natural that somatisation is the most common form of expression of pain. However the addition of the paradigm of pain to reasoning makes it obvious that skills including interprofessional work, provision of knowledge, goal setting, activity pacing and rehabilitation of fitness are also critical.

The reasoning categories and subcategories with examples are summarised in table 6.1.

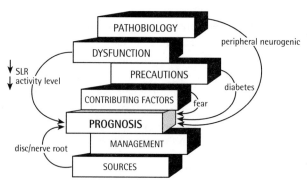

6.6   *Information in one reasoning category is gained from other reasoning categories. Examples of information which may assist prognosis making.*

THE PROCESS OF REASONING

Reasoning is about falsifiable hypotheses. The key is that a hypothesis is not wrong or even fraudulent as the name suggests but one which is subject to being disproven. It can be disproven by response to treatment and various aspects of science. It could be said that hypotheses must be null hypotheses, although in reality few clinicians anywhere operate on the null hypothesis.

Clinical reasoning must be an evolving process. This is perhaps the most critical issue in reasoning (Jones et al. 1995). Clinician and patient knowledge evolves, the patient and his or her injury context evolves, politics evolve, the cultural dimensions of health and illness evolve. For clinicians to keep pace with these evolutions, they must continually look for new patterns, keep up to date with relevant evidence and constantly challenge existing beliefs. The flow diagram below (Fig. 6.7) illustrates the process of reasoning.

I believe the key points are:

• Reasoning is an evolving process throughout the subjective and physical evaluation that continues through subsequent visits.

• All hypothesis categories will be broad at first and then refined, rejected or new hypotheses added.

• Information to formulate hypotheses is gained from two main sources - assessment of the patient and the therapist's knowledge, understanding and previous experiences.

REASONING CATEGORIES	CLINICAL EXAMPLES

Pathobiological mechanisms
• Related to tissues
• Related to pain
  • Input based
  • Processing based
  • Output/homeostatic mechanisms
	tissue healing, inflammation
	
	nociceptive pain
	central sensitisation
	sympathetic maintained pain

Dysfunction/impairment
  • General dysfunction
  • Specific dysfunction
  • Distress
	inability to work, play sport
	hypomobile joint, limited SLR
	fear, catastrophising

Sources	disc, nerve root, spinal cord
Contributing factors	psychosocial, previous injury management, occupation
Prognosis	features will be positive or negative for prognosis
Precautions	cauda equina involvement, tumour,
Management	manipulation, education, graded exercise, passive movement

Table 6.1   Clinical reasoning categories and subcategories with clinical examples.

- the patient must be a part of the reasoning process. They have hypotheses (beliefs) in all the reasoning categories which will alter as the process of assessment and management proceeds.

- Results of an intervention will often effect the evolving concept of the problem.

- Placebo effects could occur anywhere in the process.

- We all reason to varying degrees.

Errors are easily made in reasoning. Two of the most common are adding pragmatic influences and jumping to favourite or trendy hypotheses (Jones 1992), but also read Scott (2000), Sagan (1996) and Sutherland (1994).

If a patient says she has a "pain in the hip", it is easy enough for a therapist to believe her. However this "hip pain" could be arising from a number of structures and be related to various mechanisms. Patients' concepts of where their hips are surely vary. There are often difficulties convincing a patient of your hypothesis that her hip pain is perhaps referred from the spinal tissue or is related to maladaptive central processing. Failure to test the hypothesis in the clinic usually follows.

Because "favourite hypotheses" exist in manual therapy, there are those who will see every problem as a joint, or a nerve, something myofascial or a maladaptive central pain state perhaps. It may relate to the last course they were on or to the most recent successful intervention they may have had. Sometimes it may be the first tissue examined. This also relates to sampling too few hypotheses. We can all be guilty here. Ask yourself why you like

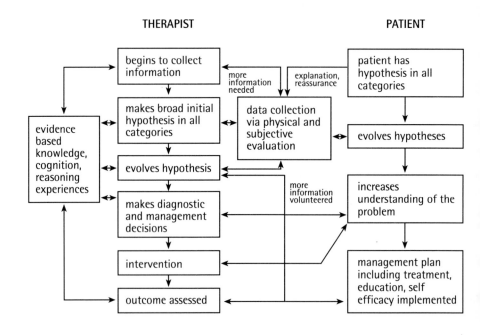

6.7　The clinical reasoning flow model. From: Jones M, Jensen, G and Edwards, I (2000) Clinical reasoning in physiotherapy. In: Higgs, J and Jones M (eds) Clinical Reasoning in the Health Professions, 2nd edn. Butterworth Heinemann, with permission.

the hypothesis and compare it fairly with others. A larger declarative knowledge, particularly one that embraces pain sciences will often be required to make the mistakes obvious.

CHAPTER SUMMARY

Evidence based medicine, the neurobiological revolution, the internet, restless clinicians and patients are all combined and novel forces for adaptation of manual therapy practice. Much current practice exists in the "grey zone" where pathobiology and treatment benefit/risk ratios are not known. Uncorrupted clinical reasoning is seen as necessary to manage "grey zone" patients, and a reasoning framework to include pain and pain behaviours is proposed. Clinical reasoning is not just a judgement of facts, it's a judgement of values, attitudes and expectations as well. Skilled clinical reasoning includes experience. Experience is also seen as a kind of evidence.

CHAPTER 6 REFERENCES

Biggs JB & Telfer R (1987) The Process of Learning, Prentice-Hall, Sydney.

Bigos SJ, Battie MC, Spengler DM, et al. (1992) A longitudinal, prospective study of industrial back injury reporting. Clinical Orthopedics and Related Research 279: 21-34.

Black D (1998) The limitations of evidence. Journal of the Royal College of Physicians of London 32: 23-26.

Burton KA, Tillotson KM, Main CJ, et al. (1995) Psychological predictors of outcome in acute and subchronic low back trouble. Spine 20: 722-728.

Butler DS (1994) The upper limb tension test revisited. In: Grant R (ed.) Physical Therapy of the Cervical and Thoracic Spines, 2nd edn. Churchill Livingstone, New York.

Butler DS (1998) Commentary - Adverse mechanical tension in the nervous system: a model for assessment and treatment. In: Maher C (ed.) "Adverse Neural Tension Reconsidered", Australian Physiotherapy Association, Melbourne.

Butler DS (1998) Integrating pain awareness into physiotherapy - wise action for the future. In: Gifford LS (ed.) Topical Issues in Pain, NOI Press, Falmouth.

Campbell JN ed. (1996) Pain 1996 - An Updated Review. Refresher Course Syllabus, IASP Press, Seattle.

Chapman RC, Oka S & Jacobson RC (1997) Phasic pupil dilation response to noxious stimulation in humans. In: Jensen TS, Turner JA & Wiesenfeld Z (eds.) Proceedings of the 8th World Congress on Pain, IASP Press, Seattle.

Cherkin DC (1988) Commentary. Journal of Family Practice 27: 488.

Crook J, Rideout E & Browne G (1984) The prevalence of pain in a general population. Pain 37: 215-222.

Delvecchio-Good M, Brodwin PE, Good BJ, et al. eds. (1992) Pain as Human Experience, University of California Press, Oxford.

Devor M (1994) The pathophysiology of damaged peripheral nerves. In: Wall PD & Melzack R (eds.) Textbook of Pain, 3rd edn. Churchill Livingstone, Edinburgh.

Devor M (1996) Pain mechanisms and pain syndromes. In: Campbell JN (ed.) Pain 1996- An Updated Review, IASP Press, Seattle.

Devor M & Seltzer Z (1999) Pathophysiology of damaged nerves in relation to chronic pain. In: Wall PD & Melzack R (eds.) Textbook of Pain, 4th edn. Churchill Livingstone, Edinburgh.

Epstein AM (1990) The outcomes movement. Will it get us where we want? New England Journal of Medicine 323: 266-270.

Feuerstein M & Beattie P (1995) Biobehavioural factors affecting pain and disability in low back pain: mechanisms and assessment. Physical Therapy 75: 267-280.

Ford IW & Gordon S (1997) Perspectives of sports physiotherapists on the frequency and significance of psychological factors in professional practice: Implications for curriculum design in professional training. The Australian Journal of Science and Medicine in Sport 29: 34-40.

Fordyce WE (1997) On the nature of illness and disability. Clinical Orthopedics and Related Research 336: 47-51.

Gifford L & Butler D (1997) The integration of pain sciences into clinical practice. The Journal of Hand Therapy 10: 86-95.

Gifford LS (1997) Pain. In: Pitt-Brooke J, Reid H, Lockwood J et al. (eds.) Rehabilitation of Movement, WB Saunders, London.

Gifford LS ed. (1998) Topical Issues in Pain, NOI Press, Falmouth.

Gilroy A (1996) Our own kind of medicine. Inscape 1:52-60.

Goldberg RT (1994) Childhood abuse, depression, and chronic pain. The Clinical Journal of Pain 10: 277-281.

Goldner EM & Bilsker D (1995) Evidence-based practice in Psychiatry. Canadian Journal of Psychiatry 40: 97-101.

Grant R (1995) The pursuit of excellence in the face of constant change. Physiotherapy 81: 338-344.

Greer AL (1987) The two cultures of biomedicine: Can there be consensus. The Journal of the American Medical Association 258: 2739-2740.

Higgs J & Jones M (2000) Clinical Reasoning in the Health Professions, 2nd edn. Butterworth-Heinemann, Oxford.

Higgs J & Jones MA (1995) Clinical Reasoning in the Health Professions, Butterworth-Heinnemann, London.

Hislop HJ (1975) The not-so-impossible dream. Physical Therapy 55: 1069-1080.

Hooper B (1997) The relationship between pretheoretical assumptions and clinical reasoning. American Journal of Occupational Therapy 51: 328-338.

ICIDH-2 (1999) International Classification of Functioning and Disability. Beta-2 draft. Full Version, World Health Organisation, Geneva.

Indahl A, Velund L & Reikeraas O (1995) Good prognosis for low back pain when left untampered: a randomized clinical trial. Spine 20: 473-477.

Jones M (1995) Clinical reasoning and pain. Manual Therapy 1: 17-24.

Jones M, Jensen G & Rothstein J (1995) Clinical reasoning in physiotherapy. In: Higgs J & M. J (eds.) Clinical reasoning in the health professions, Butterworth-Heinemann, Oxford.

Jones MA (1992) Clinical reasoning in manual therapy. Physical Therapy 72: 875-883.

Jones MA (1997) Clinical reasoning: the foundation of clinical practice. Part 1. Australian Journal of Physiotherapy 43: 167-170.

Kendall NAS, Linton SJ & Main CJ (1997) Guide to assessing psychosocial yellow flags in acute low back pain: risk factors for long term disability and work loss, Accident Rehabilitation & Compensation Insurance Corporation of New Zealand and the National Health Committee, Wellington.

Kenny NP (1997) Does good science make good medicine? Canadian Medical Association Journal 157: 33-36.

Klenerman L, Slade PD, Stanley IM, et al. (1995) The prediction of chronicity in patients with an acute attack of low back pain in a general practice setting. Spine 20: 478-484.

Lieberman A, Lieberman MB & Lieberman BR (1994) Psychosocial aspects of physical rehabilitation. In: O'Sullivan SB &

Schmitz TJ (eds.) Physical Rehabilitation, 3rd edn. FA Davis Company, Philadelphia.

Linton SJ & Halldèn K (1997) Risk factors and the natural course of acute and recurrent musculoskeletal pain: developing a screening instrument. 8th World Congress on Pain , IASP Press, Seattle.

Loeser JD & Sullivan M (1997) Doctors, diagnosis and disability. Clinical Orthopedics and Related Research 336: 61-66.

Lundborg G & Dahlin L (1997) Pathophysiology of peripheral nerve trauma. In: Omer GE, Spinner M & Van Beek AL (eds.) Management of Peripheral Nerve Problems, 2nd edn. W.B. Saunders Company, Philadelphia.

Lundborg G & Dahlin LB (1996) Anatomy, function and pathophysiology of peripheral nerves and nerve compression. Hand Clinics 12: 185-193.

Magni G, Caldieron C, Rigatti-Luchini S, et al. (1990) Chronic musculoskeletal pain and depressive symptoms in the general population: an analysis of the first national health and nutrition examination survey data. Pain 43: 299-307.

Markenson JA (1996) Mechanisms of chronic pain. American Journal of Medicine 101 (suppl 1A): 6S-18S.

Martinez A, Simmonds MJ & Novy DM (1997) Physiotherapy for patients with chronic pain: An operant-behavioural approach. Physiotherapy Pactice and Theory 13: 97-108.

Matthews G (2000) Distress. In: Fink G (ed.) Textbook of Stress, Academic Press, San Diego.

Max M ed. (1999) Pain 1999 - An Updated Review, IASP Press, Seattle.

McCrone J (1997) Wild minds. New Scientist 156: 26-30.

Melzack R & Wall PD (1996) The Challenge of Pain, 2nd edn. Penguin, London.

Merskey H & Bogduk N (1994) Classification of Chronic Pain, 2nd edn. IASP Press, Seattle.

Morris D (1991) The Culture of Pain, University of California Press, Berkeley.

Naylor CD (1995) Grey zones of clinical practice: some limits to evidence-based medicine. The Lancet 345: 840-842.

Purtilo RB (1986) Definitional issues in pathokinesiology - A retrospective and a look ahead. Physical Therapy 66: 372-374.

Raj PP (1996) Pain Mechanisms. In: Raj PP (ed.) Pain Medicine, Mosby, St. Louis.

Rosenberg WM & Sackett DL (1996) On the need for evidence-based medicine. Therapie 51: 212-217.

Sackett DL, Rosenberg WMC, Muir JA, et al. (1996) Evidence based medicine: what it is and what it isn't. British Medical Journal 312: 71-72.

Sagan C (1996) The Demon Haunted World, Headline, London.

Scarry E (1985) The Body in Pain, Oxford University Press, New York.

Scott E & Black N (1991) When does consensus exist in expert panels? Journal of Public Health Medicine 13: 344.

Scott I (2000) Teaching clinical reasoning: a case based approach. In: Higgs J & Jones MA (eds.) Clinical Reasoning in the Health Professions, 2nd edn. Butterworth Heinemann, Oxford.

Shepherd GM (1994) Neurobiology, 3rd edn. Oxford University Press, Oxford.

Sidall PJ & Cousins MJ (1997) Spinal update: spinal pain mechanisms. Spine 22: 98-101.

Silagy C (1999) Evidence vs experience. Australian Doctor, April.

Spiro AK & Shapiro E (1997) The Powerful Placebo, The John Hopkins University Press, Baltimore.

Spiro S, McCrea Curnen MG, Peschel E, et al. eds. (1993) Empathy and the Practice of Medicine, Yale University Press, New Haven.

Sutherland S (1994) Irrationality, Penguin, London.

Tanenbaum SJ (1993) What physicians know. The New England Journal of Medicine 329: 1268-1270.

Tanenbaum SJ (1999) Evidence and expertise: the challenge of the outcomes movement to medical professionalism. Academic Medicine 74: 757-763.

Tonelli MR (1999) In defense of expert opinion. Academic Medicine 74: 1187-1192.

Tsafrir J & Grinberg M (1998) Who needs evidence-based care? Bulletin of the Medical Library Association 86: 40-45.

Waddell G, Feder G, McIntosh A, et al. (1996) Low back pain evidence review, Royal College of General Practitioners, London.

Wall PD & Melzack R eds. (1999) Textbook of Pain, 4th edn. Churchill Livingstone, Edinburgh.

Watson G (1996) Neuromusculoskeletal physiotherapy: encouraging self-management. Physiotherapy 82: 352-357.

Watson PJ (1999) Psychosocial assessment: Emergence of a new tool in physiotherapy or a new fad? Physiotherapy 85: 530-535.

Wennenberg JE, Freeman JL & Culp WJ (1987) Are hospital services rationed in New Haven or over-utilised in Boston. Lancet 1: 1185-1189.

Wolff MS, Hoskins Michel T, Krebs DE, et al. (1991) Chronic pain- assessment of orthopedic physical therapist's knowledge and attitudes. Physical Therapy 71: 207-214.

CHAPTER 7

ASSESSMENT, WITH A
PLACE FOR THE NERVOUS SYSTEM

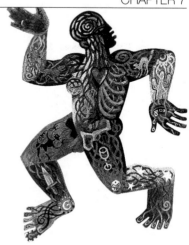

INTRODUCTION

ASSESSMENT AND THE STAKEHOLDERS

BIO-PSYCHO-SOCIAL ASSESSMENT

BIO-PSYCHO-SOCIAL ASSESSMENT IN GENERAL
TALKING ABOUT PAIN AND DISABILITY

COLLECTING INFORMATION AND CATEGORISING IT

PATHOBIOLOGICAL MECHANISMS

TISSUE MECHANISMS/PROCESSES
PAIN MECHANISMS/PROCESSES

DYSFUNCTION

GENERAL PHYSICAL DYSFUNCTION
SPECIFIC PHYSICAL DYSFUNCTION
MENTAL DYSFUNCTION/LEVEL OF DISTRESS
SO WHAT? - CRITICAL DECISIONS ARE NEEDED ABOUT THE RELEVANCE OF DYSFUNCTION

SOURCES

CONTRIBUTING FACTORS

PSYCHOSOCIAL YELLOW FLAGS
PHYSICAL FACTORS

PROGNOSIS

PRECAUTIONS AND CONTRAINDICATIONS

PRECAUTIONS WITH PHYSICAL NEURAL EXAMINATION

MANAGEMENT

GENERAL PHYSICAL ASSESSMENT

REASONS TO PERFORM A PHYSICAL EVALUATION
IT IS ALSO A TIME TO INTRODUCE USEFUL MANAGEMENT PROCEDURES

ASSESSMENT OF PHYSICAL DYSFUNCTION OF THE NERVOUS SYSTEM

PALPATE THE PERIPHERAL NERVOUS SYSTEM
PHYSICAL EXAMINATION OF NERVE CONDUCTION
NEURODYNAMIC TESTS

REFERENCES CHAPTER 7

INTRODUCTION

This central chapter integrates the earlier basic science and clinical decision making chapters with the next five chapters on physical examination of the nervous system. My focus here is on skilled physical assessment of the nervous system. But there is also a focus on placing this essential component of overall physical assessment into a framework which encompasses biological, psychological and societal aspects.

The term "stakeholders" is used. These are people or organisations which have an interest in the patient's outcome. Our aim should be to assess features which are relevant to all stakeholders. Stakeholders will vary from patient to patient.

ASSESSMENT AND THE STAKEHOLDERS

"Whose outcome" is a key question (Grimmer et al. 2000). Those interested in the patient's outcome include the patient, referrer, workplace, insurance company, personnel involved in concurrent management and the therapist. There is often some distrust between stakeholders, particularly when the patient is insured or is being compensated. For example, a physiotherapist usually sides with the patient as does the house doctor. The specialist may go either way but can side with the insurance company and the insurance doctor sides with the insurance company. This is not a healthy situation for the patient. Stakeholders will each have different measures of outcome.

The patient is the major stakeholder. If you were a patient, I suspect that you would probably want to know four things (Butler and Gifford 1997):

1. What's wrong with me?

2. How long will it take to get better?

3. What can you (the patient) do for it?

4. What can you (the therapist) do for it?

These are powerful questions for us to contemplate. We should be prepared to answer them for any patient. Note that therapist technique is last. It's usually number 1 in many clinicians' eyes. To answer questions 1 and 2, some knowledge of neurobiological processes as discussed in chapter 2-5 is required.

The payers are looking for quantifiable outcomes. Return to work and productivity at work are desired. Standard goals of "decrease pain and increase range" are no longer adequate. They are not always related to function and mean little to some of the stakeholders. Some documentation is necessary here and functional disability questionnaires could be considered.

Referring practioners will want to speak on a scientific level and in terms of pathology and outcome. Word of mouth referrals adds another stakeholder. Suggesting a therapist to a friend may end in an unsatisfactory outcome for your friend and you if the referral ends unsuccessfully.

The therapist is often a forgotten stakeholder. There is a financial incentive but it is usually more than that. Happiness, success and growth in a job are important and we all like happy patients via a management construct which supports our own beliefs and training. There are high burnout rates in physiotherapy as there are in all the people orientated professions (eg. Scutter and Goold 1995; Broom and Williams 1996). I believe that one way of countering this is to make the foundations of the movement based therapies wider and stronger.

BIO-PSYCHO-SOCIAL ASSESSMENT

A bio-psycho-social approach (Waddell 1987; Turk 1996; Waddell 1998) is currently seen as the best way to clinically conceptualise and manage neurogenic pain (or any pain for that matter). Although I endorse the concept here, I think we should take great care with this unwieldy word. Many clinicians use it, but with a tendency to use the "bio" or the "psycho" or the "social" component that suits them and their frame of reference. Key parts are often belittled. Bio-psycho-social describes the personal construction of attitudes and beliefs related to injury and nociception and how these interact with social, cultural, linguistic and workplace influences. I prefer to keep the word hyphenated so the components don't get lost.

These three components are intimate, reciprocal and variable in particular presentations (Fig. 7.1). Inputs related to all three components are converted into billions of widely distributed and interrelated action potentials with a dependence on existing neural architecture. My main concern here is that assessment and management processes must deal fairly with all three.

The model presented by Waddell et al. (1984) provides a useful clinical overview. In this "onion skin" model, the components of the pain experience are outlined (Fig. 7.2). I find it helpful in defining roles and considering where a particular profession fits into management. A manual therapist should assess these elements of the clinical presentation or seek help where required. Management could be targeted at any or all of these clinical "levels". Many skilled clinicians have, to varying degrees, thought and performed intuitively like this for a long time. Waddell (1998) warns that the model does not ascribe causes, it represents a cross-sectional look at a particular patient presentation at a particular time. The model closely relates to illness behaviour (Mechanic 1995) where illness is viewed as a mode of coping. It thus includes the variable ways in which humans respond to bodily indications, how they monitor internal states, define and interpret symptoms, take remedial action and ultimately choose care.

The strength of the model is that pain and disability are thought of as responses to the disease/injury and these responses should be the target of management along with the disease process. The bio-psycho-social model also exposes the multiple determinants of the pain

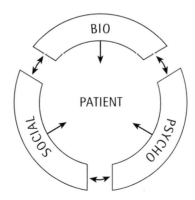

7.1   The bio-psycho-social approach. The components are reciprocally and dynamically interactive.

experience. It is the only way to explain how patients have enormously varying clinical consequences to similar injuries, and why differing clinical patterns occur over time in a particular patient. It also explains why specificity and sensitivity for particular physical tests for particular syndromes are often disappointing. The other strength is that a neurobiological substrate for these components is rapidly emerging (chapters 2-5). In terms of physical dysfunction, combined biological, psychological and sociological models allow a reasoned search and analysis of physical dysfunction.

BIO-PSYCHO-SOCIAL ASSESSMENT IN GENERAL

The movement based therapists currently have a powerful ally - time. Compared to other professions, we have more time with patients and are likely see them a number of times. In patients' eyes, manual therapists are supposed to deal with pain and problems with tissues and function. Allied to this is a professional engagement that involves discussion about many aspects of life, removal of patient's clothes and touch. We even have a licence to provoke a little pain. Manual therapists are therefore in a prime position to expand their routine assessments where needed. Even if your patient's pains are somatised or a result of benign input being maladaptively constructed into a pain experience, the framework for movement and education based therapy is there.

There are two ways to do an assessment. The most common is the face to face subjective enquiry. If you were aware of the various factors that could influence pain and disability and thought them relevant to a particular patient, then you could include them in the interview. Or you could ask your patient to fill out a self report questionnaire, particularly if you had concerns about the development of chronic pain. There are a number of questionnaires available. The "yellow flags" questionnaire (Kendall et al. 1997) is suggested and discussed later in this chapter.

Ideally, you could do an interview and a questionnaire and compare the findings. Questionnaires can be extremely useful, to help identify patients who may develop a chronic pain state. Other stakeholders in the patient's outcome such as their workplace or insurance company are likely to be interested. Be careful though. Precious non-verbal communications are lost if there is a total reliance on questionnaires. The communicator who relies on the

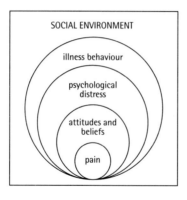

7.2   A bio-psycho-social model of the clinical presentation of a pain state at one point in time. From Waddell G et al. (1984) Symptoms and signs: physical disease or illness behaviour? British Medical Journal 289: 739-741.

slight flush of colour in the face, the tremor, shoulders dropping, voice tonal changes, the precious next question set up to be asked because of the interaction which went on before, will not have access to this while the patient is filling out a form. Life is full of grey areas; it is not black and white. Take care with numerical reflections of life. Hence questionnaires are suggested as a valuable adjunct to a face to face assessment for particular patients.

The assessment categories discussed in the previous chapter and below should be wide open to include bio-psycho-social assessment. Awareness of your limits and the need for other professionals to be involved in the management, especially for chronic pain is most important. When therapists come to testing movements which physically challenge the nervous system and integrate these movements into management, my aim is that they will have assessed all possible contributing inputs to that sensitivity and at the same time, will know the level of importance of the physical dysfunction in the overall clinical picture. Bio-psycho-social concepts facilitate this.

TALKING ABOUT PAIN AND DISABILITY

When a patient comes in for an assessment, they will have selected a set of symptoms and probably movements and postures that they believe are related to their problem. Their central nervous systems have apportioned an importance to these features and will be processing them accordingly. There may be pieces of the story missing, hidden and ultimately irrelevant, but everything which the patient produces is important because it closely reflects the complex thing which has turned that person into a patient. This is his/her model of disease. How this set of symptoms is selected and then prioritised must be extremely complex.

Discussion will invariably focus on pain, at least initially. A constructive use of pain is encouraged (Carmichael 1988). It should be seen as an ally rather than an enemy, or as Sicuteri et al. (1992) comment, view it as "pain the defender not the offender." After all, people who are born without the ability to perceive pain may die from unrecognised injury or disease (Sternbach 1963). The natural response to pain is to express it, however the social response is to suppress pain. Fearing it, distancing it, protecting ourselves from it gives the notion of pain more power, perhaps like a fear of sharks. Your patients need to confront it cleverly, enter into a dialogue with it, and ask it what it is saying to them. This may be particularly so for those patients where the pain has become an "it", something separated from normal inputs and their normal comprehension of what a pain should be. With most acute pains the dialogue is understood. In many chronic pains, the message and purpose of pain is lost.

Some practitioners and therapy systems shy away from pain, preferring to implement a management structure based on function and restoration of tissue health. This is a great start to rehabilitation. Just add the dimensions that a closer look at pain will bring and you will be away! Such an attention to pain must be carried out in the broader context. This will not make a patient focus on his/her pain. Indeed, once pain is understood sufficiently, then in future management interventions the term may disappear, allowing a better focus on goal directed restoration of function. It may be helpful to let the word go and use "back trouble", "neck discomfort", "twinges" or "feelings". There are many words (often colloquial) that describe aches and pains.

Talking about the pain is important for both acute and chronic pain sufferers. The chronic pain sufferer will engage you for much longer in discussion about pain than a person with an acute injury. There are many more biological, sociological and psychological inputs to discuss. Don't feel as though you have to stop and get into the physical examination with chronic pain patients. They have to feel comfortable that they have told their story. Be realistic. You'll never completely get to the core of pain either. It is such a personal, intense, language defying thing. And it's not pain that we are really measuring - what we measure are variables associated with the pain, the behaviours and the suffering associated with it. Pain and these variables may not be directly related. For example, your patient may have back pain, the workplace denies involvement and the patient gets angry at the workplace, not necessarily at the pain. This is where a bio-psycho-social assessment is called for. The value of your physical findings will be diminished while these psychosocial forces are dominant and unrecognised.

SIX KEY AREAS OF PAIN INFORMATION TO COLLECT:

• You'll need to know something of the geography and nature of the pain - where it is and where it travels to. Find out what the links to other symptoms are, check how it progresses over time and find out the aggravating and easing factors, both physical and psychological. Do a body chart and perhaps get the patient to do one as well. A visual analogue scale could be used to help judge pain severity.

• You'll want to know the mechanisms of injury, where and when it started, relation of symptoms now to injury and any aggravating and easing factors. Try to establish the relationship of the pain to various inputs.

• You'll need to explore the patient's classification of severity and her explanatory model. For example, "weak spine", "worn out joints", "nerves compressed". Find out the patient's perception of what brought it on, for example "the car accident" or "began after my baby was born". Ask patients why they think it still persists.

• Try to assess the consequences of the pain and disability state. What are the limitations, how has life changed, what are the effects on work, leisure and creativity, what are the anticipated consequences of activity and what are the thoughts about the future?

• Check what coping styles are used- assess physical and psychological coping methods. For example, is the person "living with it" or "living around it". Does the pain control him/her? For example your patient may say "I work on the computer and then after about 45 minutes I feel a tightness in my neck and I know the pain will come if I continue so I stop".

• Find out what else the pain and the disability does or relates to. For example, anger, blame, sickness. What are the thoughts of the patient's family, work or team mates.

Most patients' goals would include total and permanent relief of pain. Therapists need to be respectful of this. In long term chronic pain states, many patients have been told that total and permanent relief may not be possible. This may be the truth. However it is still a goal for the patient. "Difficult but let's both try and work for a reduction" may be a better response. The future does offer better understanding and pharmacological, physical and psychological management. There should always be hope.

COLLECTING INFORMATION AND CATEGORISING IT

In the clinical reasoning chapter (chapter 6), categories of reasoning were introduced and defined. These are illustrated again in figure 7.3 and in this chapter some practical aspects of information collecting are discussed. Information from all of the categories is necessary to adequately manage patient's needs. You will have your own methods of questioning, but it is worth exploring ways to extract the information or encouraging patients to offer the information. In table 7.1 there are some sample questions and the kind of information they hope to capture. Remember they are sample questions only. The questioning (or listening) necessary for an acute pain state will be different to that for the chronic pain state. I also believe that with more biological knowledge (chapters 2,3,4,5), it will be easier to listen to a patient's story and understand how some of the pain behaviours could be as they are. Better knowledge levels tend to make for better and less biased listening skills. Hadler (1996) authored an article around this topic called "If you have to prove you are sick, you won't get well". Biological knowledge and knowledge of neurodynamics makes it easy to "parallel" while interviewing and the patient may feel they don't have to prove their problem.

Manual therapy models usually include a structured interview method. Just as it should not be difficult to add a neurodynamic evaluation, some of the psychosocial aspects could also be added. These are the categories which Gifford and I have added to existing clinical reasoning models (Jones 1992), in an attempt to introduce pain and neurobiology to manual therapy (Butler 1994; Gifford and Butler 1997; Gifford 1997; Butler 1998; Butler 1998; Gifford 1998).

PATHOBIOLOGICAL MECHANISMS

Clinicians need to make a reasoned attempt at what the underlying processes or mechanisms related to the patient's pain state are. Ask yourself the question, "what is going on here?" and be aware at the same time that there is a growing basic science knowledge to help you construct a reasoned answer.

TISSUE MECHANISMS/PROCESSES

Make a judgement about the tissues involved and the patient's stage of healing. Existing orthopaedic/manual therapy assessment processes are usually good for this. There will be a number of features here to include in decision making. They include severity of injury, tissues injured, age, normal healing rates, coexistent diseases, and the sort of activities that person is still doing. A decision about healing time should be made - given the overall picture has the injury had time to heal, or does it appear that other processes are now contributing?

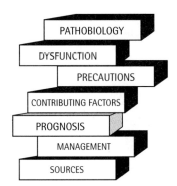

7.3   A reminder of the reasoning categories.
Review text in chapter 6

Remember that pathobiological processes related to the state of the tissues do not necessarily relate to pain perception. I discussed this back in chapter 3.

PAIN MECHANISMS/PROCESSES

This feature of clinical decision making may be new for some. Therapists are asked to make a clinical judgement about the pain mechanisms or processes in operation. This can be easy with the dominant inflammatory nociceptive pain mechanisms associated with acute trauma or rheumatoid arthritis, or the peripheral neurogenic mechanisms of clearly defined nerve root trauma. It becomes more difficult with combined mechanisms, chronic pain and multiple contributing factors. Judgement about the relative contributions of primary hyperalgesia (from peripheral tissues) or secondary hyperalgesia (central nervous system processes) is the initial step to taking on mechanisms. If you can assess a patient under the framework of examining the sensitivity and function rather than a pure "find the structure at fault" thinking, then you are on the way. The patterns which suggest various peripheral and central based mechanisms are presented in detail in chapters 3 and 4. Remember they are not diagnoses, they are states of the nervous system.

DYSFUNCTION

Dysfunctions or impairments are the consequences of the pathobiological processes. Dysfunction is thus a reasoning category in which to include some of the biological,

POSSIBLE QUESTION	KIND OF INFORMATION SOUGHT
What do you do when you get the pain?	Coping styles
Where is the pain and where does it spread to?	Pathobiology
What do you think would happen if you kept working with the pain?	Coping style, catastrophising
Has it changed your life? How?	Activity level, functional level, emotional component
What's it like when you are stressed?	Role of emotions
Does it need something to start it off? What if anything?	Pathobiology, contributing factors
What sort of things can start it off?	Pathobiology, contributing factors
Do some people disbelieve you?	Delegitimisation
Do you think it will get better?	Hope, goals
What do you think is wrong with you?	Explanatory model, beliefs
Have you ever just fought it and kept going?	Coping style, Pathobiology
What treatments do you think are best?	Passive or active coper
How did it start?	Explanatory model, blame
What do you think I can do for you?	Therapist role, passive/active coping

Table 7.1 Some possible questions which could be asked of a chronic pain sufferer and the kind of information sought.

psychological and societal effects of the pathobiological state. There are three categories – general dysfunction, specific dysfunction and distress.

GENERAL PHYSICAL DYSFUNCTION

You'll need answers to the following questions.

• Which are the general activities that aggravate and ease symptoms and distress?

• What is the general level of physical activity? (try to quantify this by time, number or distance)

• Which activities can no longer be done?

• What are the goals regarding the above?

An idea of the general level of work, leisure and creative activity now, compared to before the injury and compared to the short and long term goals will be required. Some idea of environmental restrictions (eg. transport, ability to get to work) will be useful.

Level of fitness, sleep status, and level of socialisation could also be helpful information. Other clinical data conceptualised in this category would include balance, gait, use of appliances and aids. While this reasoning category is important for all patients, it is particularly important for patients in chronic pain.

In more chronic pain states, it may be helpful to draw a diagram of the relationship between pain and activity. This could be useful when setting exercises or activities and demonstrating the level o f control which pain exerts.

Documentation here is important – in particular to state what it is that you are assessing as a gauge of outcome and what your goals should be. This should be something which provides meaningful outcomes to all stakeholders.

For chronic pain sufferers, examples of questionnaires to help with this category are the Oswestry Low Back Pain Disability questionnaire (Fairbanks et al. 1980; McDowell and Newell 1996), the Roland and Morris questionnaire(Roland and Morris 1983) and the Short Form 36 (SF36) (Ware et al. 1993). For a review see Williams (1999).

SPECIFIC PHYSICAL DYSFUNCTION

A good physical evaluation will usually reveal physical findings in every patient. These can be called physical dysfunctions or impairments. Examples of specific dysfunctions include loss of a reflex, a weak or tight muscle, instability at the talocrural joint, SLR limited by 20 degrees compared to the other side, stiffness in the C3-4 zygapophyseal joints, a sensitive trigger point, tightness in a scar and swelling at the ankle. Some of these physical dysfunctions can be helped very quickly, others may never change. As a general comment these are more likely to be a focus of your attention in acute pain states than chronic.

You don't want to miss these findings and your patients will probably want you to check them out. They are, to a varying degree, an expression of the patient's problems. But, their true place in management has yet to be established.

This category is where the neurodynamic evaluation fits in. Tests like the straight leg raise are tests of specific physical dysfunction in the nervous system.

MENTAL DYSFUNCTION/LEVEL OF DISTRESS

Judgements need to be made about the level of distress and the associated thoughts of your patient. These may also be identified in the clinical reasoning category of contributing factors, in particular the risk factors for chronicity. The following are the key categories in which to collect information:

• What is your patient's level of anxiety? Is she catastrophising?

• What is the level of fear and what is she fearful of?

• What coping strategies are being used? Is she an active or passive coper?

• What is the patient's attitude to pain?

• What is the level of anger and to whom is this anger directed.

• What are the influences of others on the patient's thoughts and beliefs.

• What are the patient's beliefs about the pain and injury and healing status.

A useful and recommended strategy here is the yellow flags assessment (Kendall et al. 1997). This can be used in the acute stage and chronic stage. "Yellow flags" are discussed further in the contributing factors section below.

SO WHAT? - CRITICAL DECISIONS ARE NEEDED ABOUT THE RELEVANCE OF DYSFUNCTION

This exercise cannot be a meaningless collection of information. Some key decisions now have to be made. With the information collected so far, the question of "so what?" needs to be answered for all the stakeholders.

To make more sense within a reasoning approach, dysfunctions can be assessed as adaptive or maladaptive (Gifford 1997). This is often difficult, but a judgement can be made about whether, for example, a list, posture, stiffness, mood, thought or behaviour is adaptive (helpful for recovery) or maladaptive (of no help for recovery). This must be made at a particular time. For example, a protective posture may be fine for the early days of a whiplash trauma, but will probably hinder recovery if it is maintained for months after. Some fear of movement can be useful after trauma, but maladaptive if it persists .

Most **general dysfunctions** will need to be addressed in the clinic. After all, these are what the patient and the stakeholders want to improve. This is straightforward in the residual ankle sprain where the patient may want to get back to a particular sport, however in more chronic problems, there may be a number of goals, some short term and some long term.

The decisions regarding the relevance of **specific physical dysfunctions** are tougher. As a very broad guideline, I suggest that specific physical dysfunctions may be more relevant and given priority in management when these circumstances occur:

• when the problem is more acute and related to peripheral sensitisation

• when it stands out glaringly in the overall picture (eg. marked muscle weakness, SLR now 30 degrees whereas prior to injury it was 100 degrees)

• when there is evidence to say that addressing it will help (eg. early movement post trauma, specific muscle stabilising work)

- when it is judged to have links to the general dysfunction (eg. positive slump on the right side and list to the right)

Note that the presence of a physical dysfunction does not necessarily imply that the sole management option is physical.

The relevance of the **distress level** also needs some assessment. You'll need to ask "is this a level of distress which is affecting a healthy outcome?" Most people are upset when they have an injury or disease. A bit of a "downer" could even be beneficial for a short term if it keeps that person from re-injury, but there may be aspects of the distress which could be managed a bit better and help the outcome. Catastrophising and fear of movement are two aspects of distress which are likely to need early intervention.

We all have dysfunctions, even the best athletes. The skill is to ascribe a level of clinical importance to them. In its simplest form, this may mean to forget the dysfunction, keep an eye on it and see if it changes, or deal with it.

THE QUANDARIES OF PHYSICAL DYSFUNCTION

These are the three big quandaries as I see it, ripe for discussion in manual therapy. Let's say our patient has buttock area pain.

- You may have found some unhealthy, sensitive and stiff tissues, say tight muscles and a stiff hip which you announce to the patient. With active and passive mobilisation, the problem could improve considerably. However, it might be the "finding it" (and the examination ritual) which helped her, not only the actual manual effects on soft tissue. She may have thought her buttock pain was something more serious and was very reassured. But then again that's still manual therapy isn't it? Keep your handling skills and try to tap into the cognitions and emotions which may so powerfully contribute to the improvement. For some patients however, this kind of management has side effects - the repeated finding of problems in tissues may in someway diminish their central nervous system's perception of what the tissues are capable of. This can be a problem and is why judgements about relevance of physical findings are so important.

- I may examine the patient and find a limitation in hip movements, say in flexion/adduction. Using this and other clinical data, my judgement of the situation is that there is some physical dysfunction related to neural tissues. A colleague may perform the same examination and his judgement is that it is a myofascial physical dysfunction. Yet another clinician could find that the sacro-iliac joint was the problem. With different techniques we may get the same clinical result. This says many things. Our intra-examinar reliability is not good; our examination protocols were based on limited basic science and if we don't know what was responsible for the improvement then we are missing the opportunity to direct management strategies at those features.

- There may be sensitivity, say on moving the hip into flexion and adduction. It feels a bit stiff so you keep moving it for the patient and it seems to be a very successful part of management. In patient A, her buttock pain could be due to local hip tissue injury and the movement helps tissue healing. In patient B, with a similar presentation, there may be more of a central sensitivity but your movement helps as well. In this case however, it may be a combination of the "finding it", the healing atmosphere of your clinic and the input into the

CNS. This could be processed subconsciously as "if this therapist can do this and reproduce the pain then it can't be too bad after all". We must have been treating secondary hyperalgesia for years. It's now time to try to identify and to target the processes better. Manual therapy can be used for both primary and secondary hyperalgesia.

In summary, I would encourage a multi-tissue and multi-mechanism assessment in a bio-psycho-social framework. Any dysfunctions must be seen as consequences of pathobiological mechanisms.

SOURCES

Most systems of orthopaedic assessments attempt to find the sources of pain - the actual tissues or structure at fault. To identify the structures at fault could be an extremely useful thing. Unfortunately, this is difficult and impractical in many cases. And when you find the source, what do you do with it? It is processes or mechanisms of pain which are treated rather than actual sources. If a source can be recognised or reasoned, then that is an added benefit which may allow delivery of more specific techniques.

The clinician's concept of sources will often differ from the patient's concept. Not only could it be different but the patient's concept of source probably forms a more powerful part of his/her operational diagnosis than the therapist's concept of sources. Patients don't usually think in terms of mechanisms. They frequently need a diagnosis with a structure associated with it to feel satisfied. If you believe that a hand pain has a significant cervical nerve root component, with some elevated central nervous system sensitivity, then this needs to be explained very skillfully and carefully.

Source identification can be useful in peripheral neuropathies. You should be able to identify which nerves are responsible and you may be able to make a reasoned judgement about sites along the nerve where there may be a problem. In particular, identification of whether nerve root or nerve trunk is involved should be possible. This is discussed further in chapter 10.

In nociceptive dominant pain states, reasoned judgements on sources can be made from subjective and physical examination and anaesthetic blocks. There are problems with source identification when there is apparent central sensitisation. Pain is a distributed phenomenon right through the entire nervous system. Still, in the future, certain brain areas and receptors may be targeted accurately.

CONTRIBUTING FACTORS

The presentation of the patient in the clinic represents the tip of an iceberg. Underneath, lurking in the water is the combination of pathobiological processes, damaged structures and contributing factors, all combining to determine the presentation. These contributing factors may be ergonomic, environmental, genetic, physical, social, psychological and cultural.

PSYCHOSOCIAL YELLOW FLAGS

Kendall et al (1997) and the New Zealand government have done us all a favour by sourcing an extensive literature and providing a list of risk factors for chronicity in low back problems. The "yellow flags" (Kendall et al. 1997) document summarises these psychosocial factors. See table 7.2. Refer to the original document and elsewhere for details and useful discussion on its use (Waddell 1998; Kendall and Watson 2000; Watson and Kendall 2000).

ATTITUDES AND BELIEFS ABOUT BACK PAIN

* Belief that pain is harmful or disabling resulting in fear-avoidance behaviour, eg. the development of guarding and fear of movement
* Belief that all pain must be abolished before attempting to return to work or normal activity
* Expectation of increased pain with activity or work, lack of ability to predict capability
* Catastrophising, thinking the worst, misinterpreting bodily symptoms
* Belief that pain is uncontrollable
* Passive attitude to rehabilitation

BEHAVIOURS

* Use of extended rest, disproportionate 'downtime'
* Reduced activity level with significant withdrawal from activities of daily living
* Irregular participation or poor compliance with physical exercise, tendency for activities to be in a 'boom-bust' cycle
* Avoidance of normal activity and progressive substitution of lifestyle away from productive activity
* Report of extremely high intensity of pain, eg. above 10 on a 0-10 Visual Analogue Scale
* Excessive reliance on use of aids or appliances
* Sleep quality reduced since onset of back pain
* High intake of alcohol or other substances (possibly as self-medication), with an increase since onset of back pain
* Smoking

COMPENSATION ISSUES

* Lack of financial incentive to return to work
* Delay in accessing income support and treatment cost, disputes over eligibility
* History of claim(s) due to other injuries or pain problems
* History of extended time off work due to injury or other pain problem (eg. more than 12 weeks)
* History of previous back pain, with a previous claim(s) and time off work
* Previous experience of ineffective case management (eg. absence of interest, perception of being treated punitively)

DIAGNOSIS AND TREATMENT

* Health professional sanctioning disability, not providing interventions that will improve function
* Experience of conflicting diagnoses or explanations for back pain resulting in confusion
* Diagnostic language leading to catastrophising and fear (eg fear of ending up in a wheelchair)
* Dramatisation of back pain by health professional producing dependency on treatments, and continuation of passive treatment
* Number of times visited health professional in last year (excluding the present episode of back pain)
* Expectation of a 'techno-fix' eg requests to treat as if body were a machine
* Lack of satisfaction with previous treatment for back pain
* Advice to withdraw from job

EMOTIONS

* Fear of increased pain with activity or work
* Depression (especially longterm low mood), loss of sense of enjoyment
* More irritable than usual
* Anxiety about heightened awareness of body sensations (includes sympathetic nervous system arousal)
* Feeling under stress and unable to maintain sense of control
* Presence of social anxiety or disinterested in social activity
* Feeling useless and not needed

FAMILY

* Overprotective partner/spouse, emphasising fear of harm or encouraging catastrophising (usually well- intentioned)
* Solicitous behaviours from spouse (eg. taking over tasks
* Socially punitive responses from spouse (eg. ignoring, expressing frustration)
* Extent to which family members support any attempt to return to work
* Lack of support person with whom to talk about problems

WORK

* History of manual work, notably from the following occupational groups
  -fishing, forestry and farming workers
  -construction, including carpenters and builders
  -nurses
  -truck drivers
  -labourers
* Work history, including patterns of frequent job changes, experiencing stress at work, job dissatisfaction, poor relationships with peers or supervisors, lack of vocational direction
* Belief that work is harmful; that it will do damage or be dangerous
* Unsupportive or unhappy current work environment
* Low educational background, low socioeconomic status
* Job involves significant biomechanical demands, such as lifting, manual handling heavy items, extended sitting, extended standing, driving, vibration, maintenance of constrained or sustained postures, inflexible work schedule preventing appropriate breaks
* Job involves shift work or working 'unsociable hours'
* Minimal availability of selected duties and graduated return to work pathways, with unsatisfactory implementation of these
* Negative experience of workplace management of back pain (eg. absence of a reporting system, discouragement to report, punitive response from supervisors and managers)
* Absence of interest from employer

Remember the key question to bear in mind while conducting these clinical assessments is 'What can be done to help this person experience less distress and disability?'

Table 7.2 Clinical assessment of psycho-social yellow flags (Kendall et al 1997)

The yellow flags guide provides a flexible method of screening for psychosocial factors and a systematic approach for assessment (Linton and Hallden 1997). It also suggests better strategies of management for those with acute pain (see chapter 14).

There are a number of points regarding table 7.2.

• Scan the categories and see where your particular job fits in. Addressing the categories of attitudes and beliefs, behaviours and emotions in particular, are categories where movement based therapists could expand their work (Harding and Williams 1995; Harding 1998). If you are part of a multidisciplinary team, or if you worked in an occupational setting, you may have inputs in the other areas.

• This literature is specific for back pain. Given that pain processing only relies partly on the area of input for perception, these features could be extrapolated to the rest of the body.

• There is a possibility that contributing factors are taken in a negative light. There are so many that you may wonder why everyone hasn't got chronic pain. As Mannion et al. (1996) point out, strong associations between psychometric scores and aspects of behaviour related to pain do not prove causation - they are simply two related findings. Depression, litigation, time off work, maladaptive beliefs and antisocial attitudes may be normal human reactions to being upset with medicine, failing treatment and inconsiderate employers. As Kendall et al. stress, these categories are not to label, they are they are to provide an awareness to *prevent* chronicity (Kendall et al. 1997).

• Overall, there is good agreement that the following factors are very important and will consistently predict a poor outcome.

– Presence of a belief that back pain is harmful or potentially severely disabling.

– Fear-avoidance behaviour (avoiding a movement or activity due to misplaced anticipation of pain) and reduced activity levels.

– Tendency to low mood and withdrawal from social interaction.

– An expectancy that passive treatments rather than active participation will help.

– Most guides suggest to screen early. Kendall et al (1997) suggest to note any flags in the initial evaluation and if expected progress in 2-4 weeks is not made, then proceed to a screening questionnaire.

It is an omnipotent viewpoint just to consider the beliefs of the patient. Beliefs of the clinicians and beliefs and worldview of those who provide us with data should be considered. Omnipotence, ego, stress, interactional abilities, behaviours to patients in pain (eg. repeated medicalisation) and prejudices are also part of the pain and disability equation.

PHYSICAL FACTORS

Physical screening of workers was quite commonly done during the 70s and 80s. However there is no evidence that they have prevented the development of work related injuries (eg. Turk 1997) and only a modest correlation between physical signs and disability have been shown (eg. Waddell 1987). We need to create better tests, perform them better and find better categoristion for analysis of tests.

Physical factors which may be predictors of a poorer outcome include:

• signs of nerve root involvement (usually limited SLR and pain below the knee (Bergquist-Ullman and Larson 1977; Roland and Morris 1983; Goertz 1990; Burton and Tillotson 1991; Hellsing et al. 1994; Burton et al. 1995; Cherkin et al. 1996; Selim et al. 1998)). Hellsing et al. (1994) showed that patients with signs of nerve root affection were 8 times more likely to progress to a chronic pain state. This may be due to nerve root involvement.

• where pain is provoked by multiple trunk movements on the initial evaluation (Hellsing et al. 1994). This may well be due to discogenic or an inflammatory problem. It could also be due to widespread secondary hyperalgesia.

• local dysfunction in muscle control. Recent studies support the hypotheses that loss of local muscle support, such as multifidus and transversus abdominis around the injured areas may be a reason for the high reoccurrence rates after low back injury (Rantanen et al. 1993; Sihvonen et al. 1993; Hides et al. 1996; Hodges and Richardson 1996).

• specific risk factors include awkward movements and postures (Riihimaki et al. 1989), vibration and low back pain (Burton and Sandover 1987; Burton et al. 1989) and heavy and repeated lifting.

• higher perceived physical exertion appears to be a risk factor (eg. Josephson et al. 1996; Masset et al. 1998).

• low physical fitness increases the risk of work related low back symptoms (Lindstrom et al. 1994). Physical training is important for the prevention and rehabilitation of musculoskeletal disorders (eg. Biering-Sorenson 1984; Gundewall et al. 1993).

PSYCHOSOCIAL/PHYSICAL CONTRIBUTING FACTORS

The current consensus is that psychosocial features rarely cause acute pain, but are more important than physical features in determining which patients proceed onto chronicity and which patients can be helped (eg. Kulich and Baker 1999; Linton 2000). This has clear repercussions for management strategies

I do not mean to diminish the importance of physical factors. Their current level of predictive power does not lessen their importance in rehabilitation. But what is most important is that readers do not see physical and psychosocial factors as mutually exclusive. This would go against the bio-psycho-social concept and modern concepts of neurobiology. While a physical finding may not be a predictor for an individual, it may still be used as a powerful management tool. For example, if a fear of spinal flexion is conquered by education and physically directed techniques, then anxiety, fears about other movements, and self esteem may be important outcome related factors which change. Psychological and physical measures are abstractions which are really measures of the same underlying process (Graham 1967; Mechanic 1995). It would be an error for clinicians to try to break down the behaviour pattern of the person in pain into distinct psychological and physical compartments. Even range of motion in a test such as a straight leg raise will be influenced by emotions (McCracken et al. 1993).

The "physical deconditioning syndrome" (Mayer and Gatchel 1988) provides a good example of the link. A decrease in strength, cardiovascular fitness and flexibility and an increase in weight often occurs as patients move from acute pain stages into chronicity. This physical deconditioning can lead to a further decrease in emotional well being and self esteem. In addition, the negative emotional reactions "feedback" to physical functioning by decreasing the motivation to exercise, to work and seek recreational activities (Gatchel 1996). Patients may benefit from having this cycle of events pointed out.

Please don't think that an exploration of contributing factors is just for chronic pain. For example, injured athletes who heal faster and have better adherence to rehabilitation programmes, have demonstrated greater use of psychosocial factors than slower healing athletes. Factors included a positive attitude, stress control, social support, goal setting, mental imagery and positive self talk (eg. Fisher et al. 1988; Duda et al. 1989; Ievleva and Orlick 1991; Ford and Gordon 1997).

PROGNOSIS

In order to make a prognosis, clinical data may be collected in other reasoning categories, but can be extracted to allow some form of prognosis based on best evidence available. Making a prognosis is closely associated with goal setting.

You will need to consider what the prognosis is for. Prognosis for pain and prognosis for function may be very different. That is, a person may function much better and yet her pain may remain at or about the same levels. This is probably the most difficult reasoning category to make a decision about. Yet for your own planning and to answer the stakeholders, decisions here can provide valuable information. Conceptualising clinical data into a prognosis category allows reflection on your own decision making processes. For example, a reflection on prognosis in retrospect may come down to analysing your thoughts about "why did I think it a particular good or bad prognosis?"

I believe the best way to address this is to consider a positive and negative column. It's probably what you do intuitively. Information from the other reasoning categories links into this. List the clinical features that point to a good prognosis and then list those that point against it. Information related to contributing factors, pathobiology and dysfunctions will provide most of the information. An example of this is in table 7.3

MORE POSITIVE	MORE NEGATIVE
Young and fit	Whiplash 5 years ago - slow to heal
Has some coping mechanisms	Diabetic
Knows it is in the mind as well as the tissues	Work involves driving
Supportive work place	Husband getting tired of it
Prepared to pace work return	Nerve root involvement
Knows that it could hurt for a while yet	Some spread of pain
No problems with compensation	

Table 7.3   Possible prognostic thoughts for a patient who has sustained a whiplash 6 weeks ago and wished to return to work reasonably painfree.

PRECAUTIONS AND CONTRAINDICATIONS

Manual therapy books have always had a section for precautions and special questions to help identify serious pathology. "Red flags" (AHCPR 1994) is a useful and alerting new term for precautions. These are traumatic, neoplastic, infectious and inflammatory disorders where patients need urgent medical attention. In table 7.4 there is a list of "red flags". From various estimates, 0.8% of patients who visit a doctor with low back pain have a "red flag". The percentage will probably be similar for therapists who work as first contact practitioners. For clinicians who work under referral, a significant number of red flags will be picked up but some will always slip through. Manual therapists have more time with patients than medical practitioners. They may see them more often and they usually undress their patients. There are always more opportunities for reassessment and for picking up subjective clues. It is the subjective clues that should alert clinicians to the presence of a "red flag". For a more detailed account see Waddell (1998) and Deyo et al. (1992). Useful screening texts for manual therapists are Boissonnault (1994) and Goodman and Boissonnault (1998). Roberts (2000) has provided a useful and clinically relevant discussion of red flags.

PRECAUTIONS WITH PHYSICAL NEURAL EXAMINATION

Once patients with suspected "red flags" such as tumours and inflammatory diseases have been identified and managed accordingly, there are other clinical situations where some care and attention is warranted during physical examination. These are clinical thoughts related to physical examination of the nervous system.

TRAUMA, NEOPLASTIC AND INFECTIVE
• Age of presentation, less than 20 years or greater than 55 • Unrelenting, progressive, non-mechanical pain • Night pain • Thoracic pain • Recent weight loss • Cancer history • Drug abuse, HIV • Recent bacterial infections • Persistent severe restriction of lumbar flexion • Structural deformity • Osteoporosis and strenuous activity • Violent trauma, • Widespread neurology
CAUDA EQUINA AND WIDESPREAD NEUROLOGICAL DISORDERS
• Bladder dysfunction (increased frequency, overflow incontinence) • Saddle anaesthesia • Loss of anal sphincter tone • Progressive major motor weakness, gait and balance disorders • Perianal/perineal sensory loss
INFLAMMATORY DISORDERS (RHEUMATOID ARTHRITIS, ANKYLOSING SPONDYLITIS
• Morning stiffness • Gradual onset • Peripheral and spinal joint stiffness in all directions • Skin rashes, colitis • Family history

Table 7.4   *"Red flags" suggestive of serious pathology. Adapted from Waddell (1988) The Back Pain Revolution, Churchill Livingstone, Edinburgh.*

• Take care with elongation and pinching manoeuvres with acute nerve root disorders

• Watch that repeated movements don't aggravate a central sensitivity state.

• Be careful in acute states, when clinical pictures such as disc trauma or compartment syndrome suggests that nerve irritation/compression could occur.

• Remember in chapter 3 there was some discussion on peripheral nerve injuries which could go through a clinically silent period for a few days after injury. Take care with apparent severe nerve injury and wait a few days to see what the clinical expression will be.

• There are some states where peripheral nerves appear tethered and will not move with various physical therapies. Repeated attempts will just worsen the problem. A surgical opinion is necessary.

• Take care with disorders such as diabetes, rheumatoid arthritis, and Guillian Barre. However programmes including graded mobilisation and fitness may be useful for symptomatic relief and to minimise complications.

• When there are hard upper motor neurone signs (chapter 9) as could occur after trauma or with tethered cord syndrome (Pang and Wilberger 1982), seek a specialist medical opinion.

The possibility of aggravating disorders may be reduced if the patient's sensitivity levels can be reduced first before any exercise or passive technique. A positive clinical environment, your good interaction skills, explanations and lessening of blame and anger may facilitate this.

MANAGEMENT

Management will always be a reasoning category. It is trying to make the best use of probability as a representation of uncertainly (Lurie and Sox 1999). A "certain enough" working diagnosis to warrant some management input is necessary. A reasoning model with due attention to all categories should facilitate that. Optimal management for most pain states is not known, particularly spinal pain. Even in well defined pain states where there is good evidence for a particular management protocol, clinical decision making skills are required for best outcomes. For example the treatment technique may have to be timed, varied and different levels of explanation required. Good evidence may not mean good management in the wrong hands.

The information collected in the above categories should lead to a dynamic working clinical diagnosis. Diagnosis is an evocative and proprietal word. It need not be as it belongs to no one. If you don't have a working diagnosis then there is nothing to base management on. It should involve well reasoned hypotheses or known data in each of the reasoning categories. The working diagnosis leads to appropriate physical examination.

GENERAL PHYSICAL ASSESSMENT

Physical assessment of patients is recommended universally although with varying degrees of enthusiasm. It is a time honoured tradition in the manual therapies and medicine to do a physical examination. If possible, a physical evaluation should be valid and reliable. Validity is the degree to which the measurements are a true indication of the phenomenon being measured (Fletcher et al. 1996). This means a test should be performed and researched with the best knowledge of underlying pathobiological processes that are likely to contribute to the finding.

The general research view is that physical examination strategies range from not very reliable (eg. palpation, sacroiliac joint tests and spinal movements) to moderate reliability (eg. nerve compression signs). Many of the suggested tests in the next chapters have not been tested for reliability and validity - they must be taken with other clinical data and kept under the umbrella of big picture management issues discussed in chapter 14.

Therefore, I believe it is important to spell out the reasons why manual therapists should perform a physical examination.

REASONS TO PERFORM A PHYSICAL EVALUATION

MOVEMENT IS THE BASIS OF YOUR ENGAGEMENT WITH PATIENTS

The physical examination is your chance to see how patients move, and how they relate and respond to input. You can view aspects of function and see what they want to show a member of the medical team. How someone gets into a shirt, or takes off shoes is like watching a video which reveals so much. And what an environment it is for patients to talk and unburden and remember and reveal. Movement explorations with the overall goal of better function are a part of management, not necessarily diagnostic tests. A lack of spinal forward flexion may mean little in terms of diagnosis, but it forms a sensitive movement which can be linked to altered function, challenged, moved, discussed and used as something to show mastery over.

Most patients expect and want a physical assessment, particularly the kind of patient who has made his/her way to some form of physical therapy. So often we hear "the doctor (or therapist) didn't even look at my neck - he/she stayed on the other side of the desk all the time" or "he didn't even ask me to take my shirt off". The physical examination may give variable amounts of useful information, but a therapist/patient interaction has been made which will be invaluable for management interventions, especially those requiring compliance.

SUPPORT/REJECTION OF FINDINGS FROM A SUBJECTIVE EVALUATION

Here is your chance to see how physical findings link in to your judgements from the subjective evaluation. For example, if the subjective clinical data points to a moderately severe L5 nerve root disorder, you might expect to find myotomal weakness, a limited SLR or sensitive slump test and perhaps joint stiffness in the lower lumbar spine. If your patient said that she cannot do up her shoe laces, you may expect commensurate physical dysfunction findings in the hip or lumbar spine. If the physical findings are not there, then you may need to take a wider perspective as more psychological and behavioural influences may be in play.

DOCUMENTATION OF PHYSICAL DYSFUNCTION

Some form of documentation of the severity of a physical dysfunction is needed. This will be necessary for a starting point to the programme, enabling outcome evaluation and it could help your patient's motivation.

You could document a range and symptomatic responses to movement, a neurological change, or aspects of a functional activity, for example, walking, going from sit to stand or performing some meaningful work or sports related activity. Documentation should include the current activity level related to what is normal for your patient and her goals. It should also include what you judge to be relevant physical dysfunctions.

General physical dysfunction may be obvious in the person who limps in with a nerve root disorder or sprained medial collateral ligament of the knee. It may need to be quantified in more chronic pain states. For further details on documentation of physical function, with a focus on chronic pain see Simmonds (1997; 1999) Harding et al. (1994) and Williams (1999).

SAFETY ISSUES

A good physical evaluation should make things safer for you and your patients. Findings such as an upgoing Babinski response and multilevel muscle loss may contribute to a "red flag" categorisation.

A physical examination could reveal overt weakness, loss of reflexes, muscle ruptures, skin changes, joint instability, clonus and marked specific physical dysfunctions. These findings could require further investigation or at least a raised index of clinical suspicion and probably care with any physical management. A functional assessment may pick up weakness, balance and coordination problems that would present some dangers for a return to a certain kind of work or sport.

Think widely - you may be the first person for a long time to observe a person's spine and you may spot a malignant melanoma.

MANAGEMENT OF PHYSICAL DYSFUNCTION CAN HELP

Despite the necessity of a wider clinical perspective, we must not lose the specificity of the physical dysfunction/impairment evaluation. Some physical dysfunctions, such as muscle weakness, soft tissue swelling, and "stuck" joints can be quickly helped. Manipulation at the right time has been shown to be beneficial. Appropriate and skilled management of physical dysfunction should have benefits for general dysfunction and psychological dysfunction. Of course there is no use treating physically unless you have examined physically.

IT IS ALSO A TIME TO INTRODUCE USEFUL MANAGEMENT PROCEDURES

Physical examination is also management. Your patient's central nervous system is processing what you are doing and in some cases may be nicely surprised at what can be done. You may have tested movement that had not been performed for some weeks or movement that was expected to hurt. The inputs may provide a useful refreshment for both homonculi and tissues.

I think it is important that the physical evaluation is recognised as part of a management process. It therefore needs to be timed, explained and it will certainly be different for all patients. The entire physical evaluation does not need to be done on the first day and it can be staggered.

Here are opportunities to link physical dysfunction to general dysfunction/disability, to make patients aware of what has to change. Here is a chance to begin to give control to patients. During a reassessment, you might ask "what do you think of that straight leg raise?" An answer may be "a bit better" and your response could be "great, that may be why you can walk further without pain and get less of that tingling feeling. Is there anything else which may have changed?"

Your skill in identifying physical evidence of recovery (such as recovery of a reflex) or evidence of patency of structure (such as stable muscle function in a certain posture) may have beneficial side effects in patient motivation. Now let's turn to a focus on the physical evaluation of the nervous system.

ASSESSMENT OF PHYSICAL DYSFUNCTION OF THE NERVOUS SYSTEM

Physical evaluation routines are well established in many neurological and orthopaedic texts. They might involve observation, a look at functional movement, any painful movements that the patient complains of, active movements, passive movements, resisted movements on testing, palpation and a neurological examination, though not necessarily all and not necessarily in that order. Sometimes specialised testing may be required, for example, tests of autonomic function or a battery of functional tests for patients with chronic pain and disability.

There are three ways, excluding electrodiagnostic testing and scanning, in which an evaluation for physical dysfunction of the nervous system can be carried out. These are palpation, manual tests of conduction and neurodynamic tests.

PALPATE THE PERIPHERAL NERVOUS SYSTEM

Sites of abnormal impulse generation in peripheral nerves will usually be mechanosensitive (chapter 3), and skilled palpation may assist clinical diagnosis. Many nerves are easily palpable, even small ones such as the radial sensory nerve or the infra-patellar branch of the saphenous nerve (chapter 8). Where a nerve is not directly palpable, such as the median nerve in the carpal tunnel, an indirect pressure can be placed upon it to elicit symptoms (eg. Durkan 1991). Once clinicians acquire good neurodynamic test handling skills, they can combine these with palpation.

PHYSICAL EXAMINATION OF NERVE CONDUCTION

A physical assessment of nerve conduction should also be performed. The evaluation will involve an appropriately constructed sensory and motor evaluation of the central and peripheral nervous system. This will add data to an initial diagnosis and is part of a safety net. Unfortunately most clinicians don't do it or limit the testing to the easily performed reflexes. There is a manual handling skill to a neurological examination. The testing doesn't only assist in diagnosis and safety, but is also part of therapy in itself. Explaining findings, for example, "that's strong", or "these nerves are firing well" can be helpful therapy. There are many texts on this aspect of neurological examination including comprehensive texts by the Mayo Clinic (1991) and Nolan (1996). This is what chapter 9 is all about.

NEURODYNAMIC TESTS

The third way, and a major focus of the remainder of this book, is to perform movements which place or presume to place a load onto the nervous system. These are the neurodynamic tests such as the straight leg raise (SLR) and slump test. This is also the focus of chapters 10 to 12. These are not necessarily passive procedures, they can also be performed as active and functional tests.

Read on now to the physical evaluation of the nervous system chapters. There are plenty of useful manual skills to pick up and analyse, with consideration of biological, psychological and social inputs where necessary.

REFERENCES CHAPTER 7

AHCPR (1994) Clinical Practice Guideline Number 14. Acute low back problems in adults. Agency for Health Care Problems and Research. US Department of Health and Human Services. Rockville, MD.

Bergquist-Ullman M & Larson A (1977) Acute low back pain in industry. Acta Orthopaedica Scandinavica 170 (Suppl): 1-117.

Biering-Sorenson F (1984) Physical measurements as risk indicators for low-back trouble over a one year period. Spine 9: 106-119.

Boissonnault WG (1994) Examination in Physical Therapy Practice, Churchill Livingstone, New York.

Broom JP & Williams J (1996) Occupational stress and neurological rehabilitation physiotherapists. Physiotherapy 82: 606-615.

Burton AK & Sandover J (1987) Back pain in grand prix drivers. Applied Ergonomics 18: 3-8.

Burton AK & Tillotson KM (1991) Prediction of the clinical course of low back trouble using multivariate models. Spine 16: 7-14.

Burton AK, Tillotson KM & Troup JDG (1989) Prediction of low back pain frequency in a working population. Spine 14: 939-946.

Burton KA, Tillotson KM, Main CJ, et al. (1995) Psychological predictors of outcome in acute and subchronic low back trouble. Spine 20: 722-728.

Butler DS (1994) The upper limb tension test revisited. In: Grant R (ed.) Physical Therapy of the Cervical and Thoracic Spines, 2nd edn. Churchill Livingstone, New York.

Butler DS (1998) Commentary - Adverse mechanical tension in the nervous system: a model for assessment and treatment. In: Maher C (ed.) "Adverse Neural Tension Reconsidered", Australian Physiotherapy Association, Melbourne.

Butler DS (1998) Integrating pain awareness into physiotherapy - wise action for the future. In: Gifford LS (ed.) Topical Issues in Pain, NOI Press, Falmouth.

Butler DS & Gifford LS (1997) The Dynamic Nervous System: Course Notes, Neuro-Orthopaedic Institute,

Carmichael K (1988) The creative use of pain in society. In: Terrington R (ed.) Towards a Whole Society, Richmond Fellowship Press, London.

Cherkin DC, Deyo RA, Street JH (1996) Predicting poor outcomes for back pain seen in primary care using patient's own criteria. Spine 21: 2900-2907.

Deyo RA, Rainville J & Kent DL (1992) What can the history and physical examination tell us about low back pain? Journal of the American Medical Association 268: 760-765.

Duda JL, Smart AE & Tappe MK (1989) Predictor of adherence in the rehabilitation of athletic injuries. Journal of Sport and Exercise Psychology 11: 367-381.

Durkan JA (1991) A new diagnostic test for carpal tunnel syndrome. Journal of Bone and Joint Surgery 73A: 536-538.

Fairbanks JCT, Davies JB, Couper J, et al. (1980) The Oswestry low-back pain disability questionnaire. Physiotherapy 66: 271-273.

Fisher AC, Domm MA & Wuest DA (1988) Adherence to sports injury rehabilitation programs. The Physician and Sports Medicine 16: 47-51.

Fletcher RH, Fletcher SW & Wagner EH (1996) Clinical Epidemiology, 3rd edn. Williams & Wilkins, Baltimore.

Ford IW & Gordon S (1997) Perspectives of sports physiotherapists on the frequency and significance of psychological factors in professional practice: Implications for curriculum design in professional training. The Australian Journal of Science and Medicine in Sport 29: 34-40.

Gatchel RJ (1996) Psychological disorders and chronic pain. Cause and effect relationships. In: Gatchel RJ & Turk DC (eds.) Psychological Approaches to Pain Managment, Guilford Press, New York.

Gifford L & Butler D (1997) The integration of pain sciences into clinical practice. The Journal of Hand Therapy 10: 86-95.

Gifford LS (1997) Pain. In: Pitt-Brooke J, Reid H, Lockwood J et al. (eds.) Rehabilitation of Movement, WB Saunders, London.

Gifford LS ed. (1998) Topical Issues in Pain, NOI Press, Falmouth.

Goertz M (1990) Prognostic indicators for acute back pain. Spine 15: 1307-1310.

Goodman CC & Boissonnault WG (1998) Pathology: Implications for the Physical Therapist, WB Saunders, Philadelphia.

Graham DT (1967) Health, disease and the mind-body problem: linguistic parallelism. Psychosomatic Medicine 29: 52-72.

Grimmer K, Beard M, Bell A, et al. (2000) On the constructs of quality physiotherapy. Australian Journal of Physiotherapy 46: 3-7.

Gundewall B, Lileqvist M & Hansson T (1993) Primary prevention of back symptoms and absence from work. Spine 18: 587-594.

Hadler N (1996) If you have to prove you are sick, you can't get well. The object lesson of fibromyalgia. Spine 21: 2397-2400.

Harding V (1998) Application of the cognitive-behavioural approach. In: Pitt-Brooke J (ed.) Rehabilitation of Movement, Saunders, London.

Harding V & Williams AC (1995) Extending physiotherapy skills using a psychological approach: cognitive behavioural management of chronic pain. Physiotherapy 81: 681-688.

Harding VR, Williams AC & Richardson PH (1994) The development of a battery of measures for assessing physical functioning of chronic pain patients. Pain 25: 367-375.

Hellsing A, Linton SJ & Kalvemark M (1994) A prospective study of patients with acute back and neck pain in Sweden. Physical Therapy 74: 116-128.

Hides JA, Richardson CA & Jull G (1996) Multifidus muscle recovery is not automatic after resolution of acute first-episode low back pain. Spine 21: 2763-2769.

Hodges PW & Richardson CA (1996) Inefficient muscular stabilization of the lumbar spine associated with low back pain. Spine 21: 2640-2650.

Ievleva L & Orlick T (1991) Mental links to enhanced healing: An exploratory study. The Sport Psychologist 5: 25-40.

Jones MA (1992) Clinical reasoning in manual therapy. Physical Therapy 72: 875-883.

Josephson M, Hagberg M & Hjelm EW (1996) Self-reported physical exertion in geriatric care. Spine 21: 2781-2785.

Kendall N & Watson P (2000) Identifying psychosocial yellow flags and modifying management. In: Gifford LS (ed.) Topical Issues in Pain 2, CNS Press, Falmouth.

Kendall NAS, Linton SJ & Main CJ (1997) Guide to assessing psychosocial yellow flags in acute low back pain: risk factors for long term disability and work loss, Accident Rehabilitation & Compensation Insurance Corporation of New Zealand and the National Health Committee, Wellington.

Kulich RJ & Baker WK (1999) A guide for psychological testing and evaluation for chronic pain. In: Aronoff GM (ed.) Evaluation and Treatment of Chronic Pain, 3rd edn. Williams and Wilkins, Baltimore.

Lindstrom I, Ohlund C & Nachemson A (1994) Validity of patient reporting and predictive value of industrial physical work demands. Spine 19: 888-893.

Linton SJ (2000) A review of psychological risk factors in back and neck pain. Spine 25: 1148-1156.

Linton SJ & Halldèn K (1997) Risk factors and the natural course of acute and recurrent musculoskeletal pain: developing a screening instrument. 8th World Congress on Pain , IASP Press, Seattle.

Lurie JD & Sox HC (1999) Spine Update. Principles of medical decision making. Spine 24: 493-498.

Mannion AF, Dolan P & Adams MA (1996) Psychological questionnaires: Do "abnormal scores precede or follow first time low back pain? Spine 21: 2603-2611.

Masset DF, Piettie AG & Malchaire JB (1998) Relation between functional characteristics of the trunk and the occurrence of low back pain. Spine 23: 359-365.

Mayer TG & Gatchel RJ (1988) Functional restoration for spinal disorders: The sports medicine approach, Lea and Febiger, Philadelphia.

Mayo Clinic (1991) Clinical Examinations in Neurology, 6th edn. Mosby, St. Louis.

McCracken LM, Gross RT, Sorg PJ et al. (1993) Prediction of pain in patients with cronic low back pain: effects of inaccurate prediction and pain-related anxiety. Behavioural Research and Therapy 31: 647-652.

McDowell I & Newell C (1996) Measuring Health. A Guide to Rating Scales and Questionnaires, Oxford University Press, New York.

Mechanic D (1995) Sociological dimensions of illness behaviour. Social Science and Medicine 41: 1207-1216.

Nolan FM (1996) Introduction to the Neurological Examination, F.A. Davis, Philadelphia.

Pang D & Wilberger JE (1982) Tethered cord syndrome in adults. Journal of Neurosurgery 57: 32-47.

Rantanen J, Hurme M, Falck B, et al. (1993) The lumbar multifidus muscle five years after surgery for a lumbar intervertebral disc herniation. Spine 18: 568-574.

Riihimaki H, Tola S, Videman T, et al. (1989) Low-back pain and occupation: a cross-sectional questionnaire study of men in machine operating, dynamic physical work, and sedentary work. Spine: 204-210.

Roberts L (2000) Flagging the danger signs of low back pain. In: Gifford LS (ed.) Topical Issues in Pain 2, CNS Press, Falmouth.

Roland M & Morris M (1983) A study of the natural history of low back pain. Part 1. Development of a reliable and sensitive measure of disability. Spine 8: 141-144.

Scutter S & Goold M (1995) Burnout in recently qualified physiotherapists in South Australia. Australian Journal of Physiotherapy 41: 115-118.

Selim AJ, Xinhua SN, Fincke G, et al. (1998) The importance of radiating leg pain in assessing health outcomes among patients with low back pain. Spine 23: 470-474.

Sicuteri F, Terenius L, Vecchiet L, et al. (1992) Preface. In: Sicuteri F, Terenius L, Vecchiet L et al. (eds.) Pain Versus Man, Raven Press, New York.

Sihvonen T, Herno A, Paljarvi L, et al. (1993) Local denervation atrophy of paraspinal muscles in post-operative failed back syndrome. Spine 18: 575-581.

Simmonds M (1999) Physical function and physical performance in patients with pain: What are the measures and what do they mean. In: Max M (ed.) Pain 1999 - An Updated Review, IASP Press, Seattle.

Simmonds MJ & Claveau Y (1997) Measures of pain and physical function in patients with low back pain. Physiotherapy Theory and Practice 13: 53-65.

Sternbach RA (1963) Congenital insensitivity to pain: a critique. Physiological Bulletin 60: 252-264.

Turk DC (1996) Biopsychosocial perspective on chronic pain. In: Gatchel RJ & Turk DC (eds.) Psychological Approaches to Pain Management, The Guildford Press, New York.

Turk DC (1997) The role of demographic and psychosocial factors in transition from acute to chronic pain. 8th World Congress on Pain , IASP Press, Seattle.

Waddell G (1987) A new clinical model for the treatment of low back pain. Spine 12: 632-641.

Waddell G (1998) The Back Pain Revolution, Churchill Livingstone, Edinburgh.

Waddell G, Bircher M, Finlayson D, et al. (1984) Symptoms and signs: physical disease or illness behaviour. British Medical Journal 289: 739-741.

Ware JE, Snow KK, Kosinski M, et al. (1993) Health Survey: Manual and Interpretation Guide, Health Institute, New England Medical Centre, Boston.

Watson P & Kendall N (2000) Assessing psychosocial yellow flags. In: Gifford LS (ed.) Topical Issues in Pain 2, CNS Press, Falmouth.

Williams AC (1999) Measures of function and psychology. In: Wall PD & Melzack R (eds.) Textbook of Pain, 4th edn. Churchill Livingstone, Edinburgh.

CHAPTER 8

PALPATION AND ORIENTATION OF THE PERIPHERAL NERVOUS SYSTEM

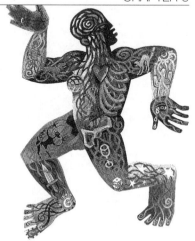

INTRODUCTION

ANATOMY AND PHYSIOLOGY OF PERIPHERAL NERVE PALPATION

NEURONES AND NERVE SHEATH RELATIONSHIPS
PHYSIOLOGICAL RESPONSES TO PALPATION
ANOMALIES
PALPATION AND PERIPHERAL NERVE PATHOBIOLOGY

GENERAL TECHNIQUES OF PALPATION

THE "FEEL" OF A NERVE
GENERAL TECHNIQUES

SPECIFIC AREAS – ORIENTATION AND PALPATION

NERVE ROOTS AND THE SPINAL CORD
THE HEAD AND THE CRANIAL NERVES
THE TRUNK
UPPER LIMB NERVES

INTRODUCTION

We can all physically touch many parts of the nervous system and I encourage clinicians to do this when it is appropriate. Those who inject and place electrodes would also benefit from learning palpation skills. Muscles and joints are quite accessible and for many clinicians, the nervous system may seem hidden and inaccessible to palpation. This is not so. Many peripheral nerves are very easy to palpate. This is a skill worth learning for various reasons.

First, it serves as a rapid, sometimes awe-inspiring way of learning or relearning peripheral neuroanatomy. It should help create a sense of the nervous system as a large, physical and mechanical structure and to some degree, engender a sense of its vulnerability. Undergraduate classes in palpable anatomy have traditionally focused on tendons, muscles and bony protruberances. Many of the mnemonics students learn, for example "Tom, Dick and Harry" to remember the tibialis, digitorum and hallucis tendon arrangements from medial to lateral at the ankle omit adjacent nerves. In this case the easily palpable posterior tibial nerve (Fig. 8.29) has been missed.

Palpation can also serve as a reminder to many clinicians that their training was predominantly based on muscles and joints and that tender structures identified during physical examination could be nerves. For example, when palpating lateral wrist tendons, the radial sensory nerve may be inadvertently palpated, or in the case of manual examination of the medial ankle, the posterior tibial nerve. The spinal segments, particularly in the cervical spine, are also areas where nerves have probably been unwittingly palpated. For example, the greater occipital nerve runs rostrally over the lamina of the C1 vertebrae, an area where many manual therapists try to palpate for assessment and sometimes treatment purposes. In addition, many trigger points may be small cutaneous nerves travelling through muscle or fascia (Maigne and Maigne 1991; Devor and Seltzer 1999).

Sometimes peripheral nerves are visually obvious. The best example here being the cutaneous branch or branches of the superficial peroneal nerve on the dorsum of the foot (Fig. 8.1), particularly when the ankle is plantarflexed and inverted. The sural nerve in the lateral calf and the ulnar nerve at the elbow are also examples of visually obvious nerves. In practical seminars, it is still remarkable how many participants are unaware of the size and accessibility of peripheral nerves or how obvious nerves such as the superficial peroneal nerve at the foot are.

The learning (or relearning) of nerve pathways, neural orientation to other tissues and vulnerable anatomical sites for nerves can be extremely useful in clinical analysis. For example, knowledge of the pathway of the infrapatellar branch of the saphenous nerve may allow its inclusion into the reasoning equation in a patient who has anteromedial knee pain on squatting. The location and vulnerability of the common peroneal nerve at the head of the fibula is always worth a thought when a patient's knee is plastered. An awareness of the orientation of nerves makes the neurodynamic tests much easier to construct. For example, the spiralling around the humerus by the radial nerve (Fig. 8.15) makes shoulder internal rotation a necessary component of testing for radial neuropathy. Similarly, the sural nerve running inferiorly to the lateral malleolus makes ankle dorsiflexion a necessary component of the physical examination for the sural nerve.

A second use of palpation is to assist diagnosis. Most peripheral nerve textbooks such as Mumenthaler (1991), Szabo (1989), Stewart (1993) and Mackinnon and Dellon (1988) suggest it, and there is some experimental support for the contention, (eg. Durkan 1991). I suspect that palpation is rarely used because the skills are not usually taught, nor is there an awareness of the peripheral nervous system as a physical structure with a great potential for the development of abnormal mechanosensitivity. The symptoms evoked by palpation may support or reject a hypothesis of abnormal impulse generation from a segment of peripheral nerve, although more clinical data would be needed to support this assertion. For diagnostic purposes, palpation may be more sensitive if performed in a position where the nervous system is placed on some load, as is the case when palpating the ulnar nerve in the cubital tunnel with the nerve in an upper limb neurodynamic test 3 position (Novak et al. 1994). Remember too, that palpation can still be carried out when great loss of movement prevents a full movement examination.

Peripheral nerve palpation skills are also a part of management. The skills can be used as part of a patient's education about the nature of his/her trouble. For example, the finding that a sensitive infrapatellar branch of the saphenous nerve may be culpable in anteromedial knee pain and that an arthroscopy or re-arthroscopy may not be required should be very reassuring. Patients often ask "what is this tender thing under my fingers?" Knowledge of peripheral nerve anatomy and neuropathic pain behaviour may make the answer simple. In addition, palpation could become a reassessment measure for other management strategies. Massage along or around nerves may well be a treatment technique for selected patients at the appropriate time (eg. Jabre 1994). See chapter 14 for further details.

Palpation skills involve more than an attempt to feel through the skin and find a sensitive structure. It is all part of therapeutic touch. The reasoning process prior to handling, coupled with an awareness of the state of underlying tissues and general body sensitivity makes for educated handling and touch. It should however, be diagnostic while at the same time convey empathy. Professionally, manual therapists are licensed to touch; there usually is a manual handling expectation from the public, therefore the skills should be as refined as possible.

Palpation is of course a primary skill for manual therapists, a part of many routine physical examinations and not performed solely for the purpose of feeling nerves and assisting judgements on the likelihood of peripheral neurogenic pain. This text has a focus on neurogenic pain. There are many patients, particularly those suffering more widespread pain

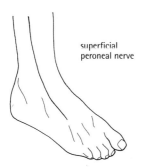

8.1   On the dorsum of the foot, the terminal branches of the superficial peroneal nerve are often obvious, particularly when the ankle is plantarflexed.

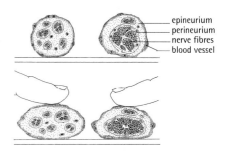

8.2   A varying relationship between connective and conductive tissues can influence the responses to palpation. Where there are more fascicles and more connective tissues, the long fibres are better protected from mechanical forces. From Butler DS (1991) Mobilisation of the Nervous System, Churchill Livingstone, Melbourne, with permission.

states or those with acute trauma where there is no rationale for digging around seeking sensitive peripheral nerves. However in other cases, for example "spot pains", and where there is already a supported hypothesis for peripheral neurogenic pain, then the techniques may be very useful.

There are no texts on detailed palpation of the peripheral nervous system, and nerve palpation usually consists of just a few comments added to muscle and bone palpation in texts such as Field (1994) and Keogh and Ebbs (1984). That makes this chapter somewhat unique. I have also linked my discussion here in with a discussion on the orientation of the nervous system. I hope that this will be useful when applying or constructing neurodynamic tests and analysing painful activities and postures.

ANATOMY AND PHYSIOLOGY OF PERIPHERAL NERVE PALPATION

Hitting the "funny bone", or the ulnar nerve at the elbow is something that you never really get used to. Even for people with normal sensitivity, nerve palpation can be a novel and shocking input into the system. Other than the sensory inconvenience it is not something which usually bothers us, as we understand both the anatomy and physiology of why it occurs. Where patients have sensitive nervous systems, the inputs will probably be enhanced. It's also a rather personal thing to palpate a person's nerves - the responses are likely to be an expression of overall sensitivity, not just local tissue damage. Care needs to be taken.

The physical skill is one aspect. With some knowledge of basic neuroanatomy and neurobiological processes, the foundations for performing palpation in particular groups of patients can be laid and an attempt at analysing responses to palpation can be made.

NEURONES AND NERVE SHEATH RELATIONSHIPS

Part of Sir Sydney Sunderland's enormous contribution to neurology is his knowledge of the internal topography of peripheral nerves (Sunderland 1978). Much peripheral nerve is connective tissue sheath and there are widely varying percentages of conductive and connective tissue between nerves and within the same nerve. Approximately 50% of a nerve is connective tissue with a range of 22% to 88% (Sunderland and Bradley 1949). This is discussed in greater detail in chapter 5. Two simple and broad rules apply. First, where a nerve crosses a joint there is usually more connective tissue, although this doesn't apply to the ulnar nerve. Secondly, the greater the number of nerve fibre bundles (fascicles), the more connective tissue will be present (Sunderland and Bradley 1949) (Fig. 8.2).

Both connective and conductive tissues have the potential to react to mechanical distortion. The connective tissues (epineurium, perineurium and endoneurium) are well innervated by axonal branching (nervi nervorum). The conductive tissues will also react to mechanical distortion, probably due to ischaemia and/or direct effects on mechanosensitive sodium channels in the axolemma. Reactions can occur in normal nerves although responses will be different depending on where the nerve is palpated. One probable reason for this is variations in the cross-sectional connective/conduction tissue relationships. It appears that where a nerve has fewer fascicles and less connective tissue, palpation will more easily evoke a response from the conductive fibres. This is clearly shown in figure 8.2. The most obvious example of this is the ulnar nerve just inferior to the epicondyle at the elbow where palpation will evoke the characteristic shower of paraesthesia towards the ulnar side of the hand. The ulnar nerve here could be up to 80% conductive tissue (Sunderland and Bradley 1949). Similar though less "tingly" responses will also occur if the common peroneal nerve is palpated in the knee crease or the median nerve is palpated in the upper arm.

Thus in some segments of a peripheral nerve, it appears that the higher percentage of connective tissues may protect the nerve and this may be responsible for the more local and less "nervy" response evoked when palpated. This occurs in areas such as the ulnar nerve in Guyon's canal at the wrist or the common peroneal nerve at the head of the fibula. In these areas, a more dull, deep ache is evoked by palpation, these symptoms probably originating from the nervi nervorum (Sunderland, 1989, personal communication), perhaps in combination with responses from surrounding innervated tissues such as fascia and skin. Yet, I believe that there is a quality of pain evoked from peripheral nerve connective tissues which is quite unique and different from our perceptions of muscle or joint pain.

Knowledge of connective and conductive tissue relationships may have some clinical consequences. Post-injury peripheral neurogenic symptoms will be dictated to some degree by internal nerve topography, and will be more neural, eg. paraesthesia, if the site of injury or palpation has less connective tissue. Responses to palpation will also depend on the nerve palpated. Palpation of nerves which have a greater percentage of motor fibres may evoke a deeper ache. The greater the number of sensory fibres in a nerve, the more sensitive the nerve and of course there will be a greater sensory field for responses to be perceived in.

PHYSIOLOGICAL RESPONSES TO PALPATION

People say that nerves do not hurt when palpated. This is usually true. There is no biological advantage of having perpetually tender nerves on pressure. Hence the nervous system has evolved to avoid mechanical forces, particularly external compression. Note how the more sensitive nerves such as the ulnar nerve at the elbow, the median nerve in the upper arm and the posterior tibial nerve at the medial ankle are on the more protected medial body surfaces. In contrast, the more physically tough nerves such as the radial and peroneal nerves are on lateral body surfaces. In addition there are protective behaviours. We have all learnt not to bang our elbows down onto a hard surface. However some areas are normally tender, and these normal responses may be amplified where there is neuropathy.

Normal responses to palpation of a nerve will probably come from mechanical distortion of the nervi nervorum. Physiologically, this is a nociceptive pain. Responses may also come from the conducting tissues. Sensory fibres have mechanosensitive ion channels that will open in response to mechanical forces. If enough of these channels open and the CNS threshold setting allows a significant input, then there may be a painful or dysaesthetic perception. Sustained palpation may be different. Here there is more time for ischaemia and thus metabolically sensitive channels may open. There may even be some physical deformation of the myelin of neurones in outlying fascicles.

ANOMALIES

Clinicians must have some knowledge of anomalies. Neuroanatomy is often not as the textbooks say it should be and anomalies are extremely common, so common that in many cases they could be considered to be variations in anatomy rather than anomalies. There are anomalies in the components of a nerve, the route of a nerve, the innervation fields and in the neighbouring structures with which a nerve must contend during movement. Perhaps the existence of so many neural anomalies is the first clue that the nervous system is not hard wired, not even in a macroscopic sense (see chapter 2).

ANOMALIES OF CONSTRUCTION AND ROUTING

The plexuses are routing mechanisms to assemble neurones with a common function into terminal branches. "Errors" that occur in the nerve assembly, for example, at the brachial plexus are often corrected distally. The best example is the common Martin-Gruber anastomosis, reviewed by Lebovic (1992) and Tountas (1993), where the median nerve communicates with the ulnar nerve in approximately 20% of people, as in figure 8.3A (Sunderland 1978). This anomaly is usually bilateral (Budak and Gonenc 1999). A less common anomaly in the upper limb is the Riche-Cannieu anastomosis which is a communication between the deep branch of the ulnar nerve and the recurrent motor branch of the median nerve (Harness and Sekeles 1971) (Fig. 8.3B). Every nerve has variations and clinicians may need to review literature specific to individual nerves. Tountas and Bergman (1993) have produced a text on anomalies of the upper limb but there is no equivalent for the lower limb.

Not only are they common, but anatomical assemblies can be far from the accepted norm. For example, the spinal accessory nerve may arise from as low as the first thoracic level; the musculocutaneous nerve, like many peripheral nerves can be doubled or absent; and the median nerve can be perforated by the median artery (Tountas and Bergman 1993). The sciatic nerve may divide into the peroneal and tibial branches anywhere between the knee and the sacral plexus. Great variations exist in cutaneous innervations. For example, sometimes the sural nerve may supply the entire dorsum of the foot (Sunderland 1978). Some anomalies in innervation fields are also discussed in the next chapter in the section on sensory testing.

Those who attempt to identify individual nerve or nerve root specificity with the upper limb neurodynamic test should be aware that to date 38 variations of construction of the brachial plexus have been identified (Tountas and Bergman 1993). There are also intradural connections between adjacent cervical (Marzo et al. 1987; Tanaka et al. 2000) and lumbar nerve roots (Mersdorf et al. 1993).

CLINICAL CONSEQUENCES OF ANOMALIES

In some patients, knowledge of anomalies can sometimes help make a little more sense of patient's symptoms. We might realise that a test such as the upper limb neurodynamic test can never be a test solely for a particular nerve trunk or nerve root. However it should also

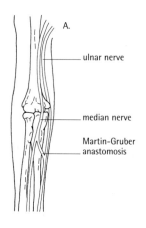

A.

ulnar nerve

median nerve

Martin-Gruber anastomosis

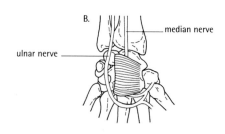

B.

median nerve

ulnar nerve

8.3   Two common anomalies in the upper limb.
A. Martin-Gruber anastomosis.
B. Riche-Cannieu anastomosis. Adapted from Tountas CP and Bergman, RA (1993) Anatomic Variations of the Upper Extremity, Churchill Livingstone, New York.

create more openness when listening to patients' complaints, and anomalies may be just one more reason why patient's symptoms don't always fit with textbook anatomy. Be aware of anomalies when pain reports seem confusing and also be wary of missing a nerve lesion because another nerve may be taking over the role. For example, with the Martin Gruber anastomosis, the ulnar nerve may be severed above the elbow but all hand muscular function may remain intact (Clifton 1948). The radial nerve may provide sensation to the thumb such that a median nerve lesion may not cause an appreciable loss of sensation (Fetrow 1970). Anomalies place some limitations on the analysis of manual muscle testing and electrophysiological studies. A nerve may also be more predisposed to injury due to an anomaly. In support, Werner (1985) demonstrated in nine patients that pronator syndrome (high median nerve compression) was more common when the median nerve pierced the humeral head of the pronator teres muscle instead of its usual passage between the humeral and ulnar heads of the muscle. There are many case studies in the literature of anomalous muscles compressing peripheral nerves.

PALPATION AND PERIPHERAL NERVE PATHOBIOLOGY

In chapter 3, the peripheral and central mechanisms that allowed hyperalgesia on palpation were discussed. Injured nerves often hurt when mechanical forces such as pinch and strain are placed upon them. This must be due to a combination of local changes and the threshold control of the central nervous system. Sensitivity to palpation must be seen as a reflection of total nervous system processes. The molecular targets of palpation are beginning to be understood. The story of abnormal impulse generating sites (AIGS) in nerves is essential to understanding responses to palpation (chapter 3). Once an AIGS is established, contributory inputs to firing could be mechanical, noradrenaline, temperature extremes and metabolic forces. Some may fire spontaneously (Devor and Seltzer 1999).

Take care not to assume that a tender nerve beneath palpating fingers signals the area of damage. Acutely injured nerves will be extremely tender to stimuli such as palpation (Dellon et al. 1983), however this may not always be the case. Nerves can be tender distal to the site of damage, as is frequently observed in radiculopathy. All tissues in a limb or part of a limb may be tender to palpation and movement where there are sensitivity changes in the CNS and thus there may be multiple sensitive sites. There is much potential for false-positive results with nerve palpation.

We do not know the status of the neural connective tissues in injury states. All three components of the sheath are innervated (chapter 4) and thus may be a source of pain, either a nociceptive dominant pain or an ongoing source for a more central pain state. Perhaps there is something special and regulatory in connective tissue so close to neurones. The nervi nervorum characterised in Bove and Light's work (1997) were reactive to stretch and local focal pressure and did not react to normal movement.

Peripheral nerve tumours may arise in any nerve, though fortunately they are rare. Palpation findings may be the first indication of a tumour, particularly where a nerve is superficial. Neurofibromas are a common benign peripheral nerve tumour. These are usually painless, unencapsulated, soft masses often arising from a few cutaneous nerve fibres. They may be associated with neurofibromatosis (Lee and Dick 1998). Schwannomas or neurilemomas are usually benign but can be malignant. They are encapsulated and are more frequently found on the flexor surfaces of the arm and leg, the head and the neck. The ulnar nerve seems to be particularly involved. These are rounded, and may be mobile or fixed. According to Thomas (1984) schwannomas may be rolled over the nerve transversely, but not longitudinally along the nerve. The tumour may be tender to palpation and create problems if it externally compresses a nerve. Most are benign, excision is usually curative, but all suspected tumours require a medical opinion. See chapter 7 for a further discussion on precautions and contraindications. For a review on peripheral nerve tumours see Lee and Dick (1998).

Ganglions are common findings also. These are cysts, often in the peroneal nerve at the knee and in the ulnar and median nerve around the wrist. If they interfere with nerve conduction, surgery is indicated.

GENERAL TECHNIQUES OF PALPATION

THE "FEEL" OF A NERVE

Experienced clinicians have probably acquired the "feel" of a joint and the "feel" of muscle. Peripheral nerve is different. Nerves are pressurised and are hard, harder than tendon, far harder than arteries and have an almost slippery feel as their mesoneurial sheath allows them to slip away from pressure. Due to the internal pressure, they are usually rounded. The "feel" is strongly related to the surrounding anatomy and the depth of the nerve. Probably the best place to start learning nerve palpation skills is on the dorsum of the foot where the terminal branches of the common peroneal nerve are easily available to see and palpate in a high percentage of people, particularly if the foot is placed in plantarflexion and inversion. The tibial and peroneal nerves at the posterior knee are also very easily palpated.

It should go without saying that knowledge of underlying neuroanatomy is the critical basic science underpinning this clinical procedure. A good neuroanatomy text is recommended, in particular those using the Sobotta plates, eg. Clemente (1975) or Netter (1987). Photographic dissection texts such as McMinn and Hutchings (1988) are invaluable.

GENERAL TECHNIQUES

Nerves can be **directly palpated**, meaning the actual nerve structure can be felt, for example, the radial sensory nerve in the forearm or the posterior tibial nerve at the medial ankle. Nerves can also be **indirectly palpated**. This means that although the nerve structure cannot be felt, knowledge of its anatomy means that it is likely that a force which alters its physiology has been placed upon it. Examples where indirect palpation is useful include the sciatic nerve in the buttocks or the median nerve in the carpal tunnel. An indirect palpation must sometimes be used where there is swelling, fat or scar. In some cases however, pathological changes may lead to thickening of nerves and make them easier to identify.

SUGGESTED TECHNIQUES

Palpating the nerve with the tip of your finger or thumb is the easiest technique. Once a nerve is identified, try to palpate the nerve more proximally and distally as well. In some you may be able to follow the nerve to an abnormal impulse generating site.

Maintained pressure as suggested by Durkan (1991) and González del Pino (1997) is another technique that can be used. Durkan suggests a pressure of 150 mmHg over the volar wrist for 30 seconds. This technique has had some research interest (chapter 14). Make sure you are aware of the time it takes for symptoms to be evoked with this test. A technique has been suggested by Goldner and Hall (1997) where "about 10 pounds of pressure is applied at a point 1-2 cm proximal to an area of suspected nerve entrapment", presumably using the examiner's thumb. Distal paraesthesias may be evoked with this technique. Mackinnon and Dellon (1988) also suggest palpation proximal to a site of entrapment.

Where nerves are accessible, I encourage a "twanging" technique using a fingernail or tip of the index finger. Nerves such as the common peroneal nerve on the dorsum of the foot and the infrapatellar branch of the saphenous nerve can be "twanged" rather like a guitar string (Butler 1991). This may sound vigorous but it can be done quite gently. Nerves slip and flick during normal movements and this technique would only be testing their normal physical abilities.

Any of the above techniques can be carried out with the nervous system in more or less tension. For example, the carpal tunnel could be palpated with the fingers extended in an upper limb neurodynamic test position as demonstrated in chapter 15. The ulnar nerve at the cubital tunnel could be palpated with the ulnar nerve loaded as described and tested by Novak and MacKinnon (1994). In most cases, there should be increased mechanosensitivity when the nerve is loaded, unless the movement glides the nerve away from an underlying compressive site. In some patients, a limb can be moved while the palpating fingers are on a nerve. This may provide some information about the physical health of the nerve and its relation to surrounding structures.

When palpating nerves, adjacent tissues should also be assessed and palpated. The skills of surface anatomy and palpation are sometimes forgotten in these days of sophisticated imaging. There are some great surface anatomy books around such as Keogh (1984), Backhouse (1986), Field (1994) and Lumley (1996) among others.

TINEL'S TEST

Tinel's test (Tinel 1915) is the well known tapping of a nerve, universally recommended in peripheral nerve textbooks. Test evoked "tingling" in the distribution of the nerve palpated is indicative of axonal regeneration. The test is limited to superficial nerves or nerves close to the surface such as the median nerve in the carpal tunnel. The nerve should be tapped 4 to 6 times according to Mackinnon and Dellon (1988) and symptoms should be expected while tapping. Overzealous tapping should be avoided as it probably contributes to false-positive signs (Monsivais and Sun 1997).

Take care with analysis of Tinel's test. The incidence of false positives ranges from 6% to 45% (Gellman et al. 1986; Golding et al. 1986; Seror 1987). There has never been any standardisation of the test reported, although a technique and grading scheme has been recently suggested (Spicher et al. 1999). Its best use may be to demonstrate to a patient that the tingling is a good sign of regeneration and recovery.

A CLINICAL DIAGNOSIS FIRST

The basis of this book is best evidence based reasoning. A clinical diagnosis is necessary before physical evaluation. There are many patients whose nerves I would never palpate, in others the refreshed knowledge of nerve orientation points may make some sense of symptoms that arise on movements. In yet others I may well try to place my fingers specifically on a nerve. I am far less likely to palpate the nerves of a patient with a more generalised chronic pain, for example fibromyalgia, than for a patient who has a more focal pain state. Perhaps as an examination technique it is most useful for peripheral neurogenic pain states where the anatomical sources are local segments of peripheral nerve. Nerve palpation should also give some idea of generalised sensitivity.

SPECIFIC AREAS – ORIENTATION AND PALPATION

NERVE ROOTS AND THE SPINAL CORD

The spinal cord starts at the medulla oblongata. If the neck is flexed it will be midway between the external occipital protruberance and the C2 spinous process. The spinal cord is considerably shorter than the spinal canal. The cord ends opposite the space between the L3 and L4 vertebral levels in a child and opposite the upper border of L2 in an adult.

Because the spinal cord is shorter than the spinal canal, the vertebral level will not match the cord level. To emerge from their foramen, the roots of the lower spinal canal have to travel a considerable distance. There are eight nerves which exit the cervical spine, yet only seven vertebrae. They exit above the vertebrae of the same number while the eighth root exits below the seventh cervical vertebrae and above the first thoracic vertebrae.

The thoracic roots emerge from the spinal cord between The T1 and T9 spinal levels and the lumbar, sacral and the coccygeal roots emerge between the spinal cord between the T10 and L1 spines. This cord/vertebral level discrepancy is shown in figure 8.4.

Nerve roots cannot be directly palpated. Most palpation will be an indirect palpation via joint movement. Due to the root/vertebral level mismatch, the more caudal in the spinal canal, the more likely that more than one nerve root may be influenced. The closest palpable nerve roots are the mid to low cervical roots, where anterior palpation of the neck may place some pressure on emerging neural tissues.

THE HEAD AND THE CRANIAL NERVES

GREATER OCCIPITAL NERVE

The greater occipital nerve and its parent C2 dorsal ramus have long been considered candidates for pain at the back of the head (Hunter and Mayfield 1949; Anthony 1992), although cervicogenic referral now appears more likely. It would appear that a local striking

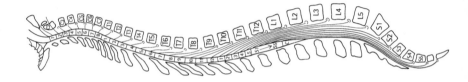

8.4   Nerve root orientation. Adapted from Clemente CD (1975) Anatomy. Urban & Schwarzenberg, Munich.

force may be necessary to cause a painful neuropathy. The nerve runs superiorly over the lamina of C1, deep to the semispinalis and then penetrates the muscle. It enters the subcutaneous tissue on the scalp above a tendinous sling between trapezius and sternocleidomastoid (Bogduk 1981). This emergence onto the scalp, where it may be palpated is between 2.5 and 5 cm from the midline and approximately a centimetre above the intermastoid line (Fig. 8.5) (Bogduk 1981).

THE ACCESSORY NERVE (CRANIAL XI)

The eleventh cranial nerve supplies the upper trapezius. The nerve may be damaged by trauma or, more likely by the surgery involved in the extirpation of a tumour or lymph gland. Persistent tightness in the upper trapezius muscle is probably unhealthy for the nerve. The accessory nerve may be palpable at the root of the neck in the posterior triangle. It will be easier to palpate if the neck is laterally flexed away from the test side and the shoulder depressed a little. The upper trapezius muscle can be pulled posteriorly a little, for better access to the nerve. Occasionally in some individuals it may be visible (Fig. 8.5).

TRIGEMINAL NERVE (CRANIAL V)

The terminal branches of the trigeminal nerve may be palpated to provide an indication of sensitivity in the nerve. The lateral and medial branches of the frontal nerve emerge from the supraorbital foramen and the often sensitive infraorbital nerve emerges from the infraorbital foramen. The terminal branches of the mandibular branch of the trigeminal nerve emerge in

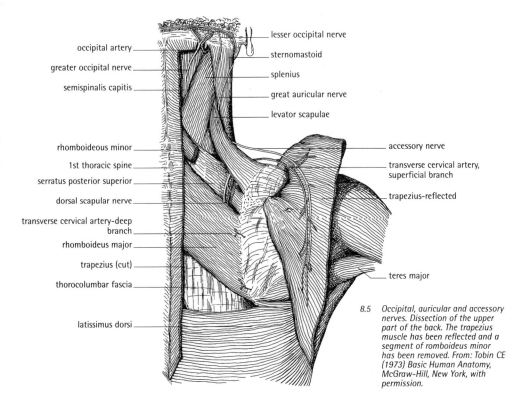

occipital artery —
greater occipital nerve —
semispinalis capitis —

lesser occipital nerve
sternomastoid
splenius
great auricular nerve
levator scapulae

rhomboideous minor —
1st thoracic spine —
serratus posterior superior —
dorsal scapular nerve —
transverse cervical artery-deep branch —
rhomboideus major —
trapezius (cut) —
thorocolumbar fascia —

latissimus dorsi —

accessory nerve
transverse cervical artery, superficial branch
trapezius-reflected

teres major

8.5   Occipital, auricular and accessory nerves. Dissection of the upper part of the back. The trapezius muscle has been reflected and a segment of romboideus minor has been removed. From: Tobin CE (1973) Basic Human Anatomy, McGraw-Hill, New York, with permission.

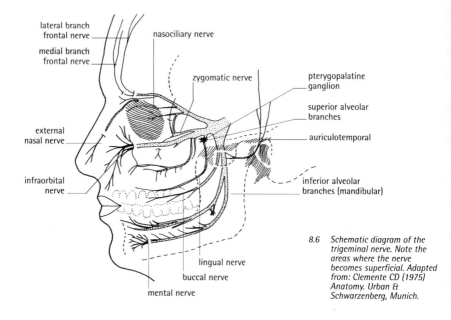

lateral branch
frontal nerve

nasociliary nerve

medial branch
frontal nerve

zygomatic nerve

pterygopalatine
ganglion

superior alveolar
branches

external
nasal nerve

auriculotemporal

infraorbital
nerve

inferior alveolar
branches (mandibular)

lingual nerve

buccal nerve

mental nerve

8.6   Schematic diagram of the
trigeminal nerve. Note the
areas where the nerve
becomes superficial. Adapted
from: Clemente CD (1975)
Anatomy. Urban &
Schwarzenberg, Munich.

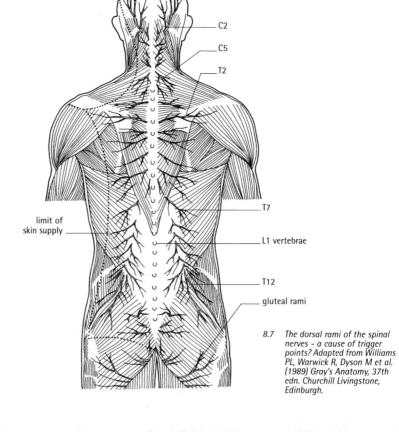

C2

C5

T2

T7

limit of
skin supply

L1 vertebrae

T12

gluteal rami

8.7   The dorsal rami of the spinal
nerves - a cause of trigger
points? Adapted from Williams
PL, Warwick R, Dyson M et al.
(1989) Gray's Anatomy, 37th
edn. Churchill Livingstone,
Edinburgh.

the anterior mandible. The infraorbital branch is easy to palpate just below the orbit and a finger's width from the nose (Fig. 8.6).

THE TRUNK

Nerves of the trunk seem to be infrequently injured, unless further evidence shows that trigger points may involve abnormal impulse generation in small cutaneous nerves.

The cutaneous branches of the posterior primary rami of the thoracic nerves, or at least the emergences of the nerves can be palpated (Fig. 8.7). These small nerves may be relevant in mid-thoracic trigger points. The syndrome involving entrapment of these nerves has been referred to as "notalgia paraesthetica" (Pleet and Massey 1978). This is rare according to some (Narakas 1989), although tender nodules, perhaps precursors to the syndrome are common clinical findings. The palpation site is often more tender if a laterally directed massaging stroke is performed, presumably pulling the nerve out of the fascial opening (see chapter 15). This palpation may also be more tender if the neck is flexed or the thorax is laterally flexed away from the tender side, thus suggesting neurogenic involvement.

Indirect pressures may also be applied to the intercostal nerves between the ribs and may evoke symptoms in intercostal neuralgia. The sympathetic trunk lies approximately 2.5 cm from the midline, attached to the costovertebral joints and would be indirectly palpated when the rib joints are evaluated. Sympathetic neurones will be unavoidably pressured along with motor and sensory fibres during peripheral nerve palpation.

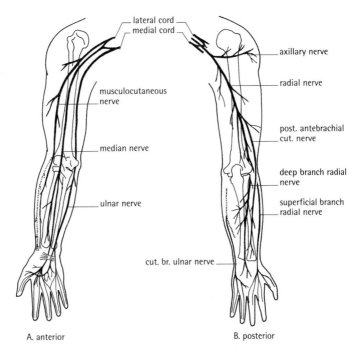

A. anterior   B. posterior

8.8   General overview of innervation of the upper limb.
       A. anterior.
       B. posterior. Adapted from Crouch JE (1972) Functional
       Human Anatomy, Lea & Febiger, Philadelphia.

UPPER LIMB NERVES

The upper limb provides easy access for nerve palpation. This is perhaps reflected in a greater sensitivity here than in the lower limb. There are at least three places along each of the major nerves where they can be palpated. In particular, the ulnar nerve at the elbow and wrist and the radial nerve in the spiral groove are very easy to feel. However the upper limb also offers great chances to palpate indirectly, such as the median nerve in the carpal tunnel. Many small nerves such as the radial sensory nerve can be palpated. A general overview of the upper limb nerves is shown in figure 8.8.

THE BRACHIAL PLEXUS

Clinicians have always palpated the brachial plexus, although I suspect often inadvertently when assessing the first rib and the scalene muscles. Place your hand half way along the clavicle and feel the thickened plexus between the clavicle and the neck. The plexus may be easier to palpate, when the neck is laterally flexed towards the side tested, thus taking tension of the skin and underlying soft tissues. Even better, ask your patient to depress her shoulder girdle. This will often bring the plexus onto your fingers. The brachial plexus and its relationship to arteries and peripheral nerves are shown in figure 8.9.

ULNAR NERVE

Ulnar nerve at the elbow

The ulnar nerve is easily felt in the condylar groove of the humerus and is particularly obvious just proximal to the groove. If palpated with the elbow in extension, the nerve will be looser

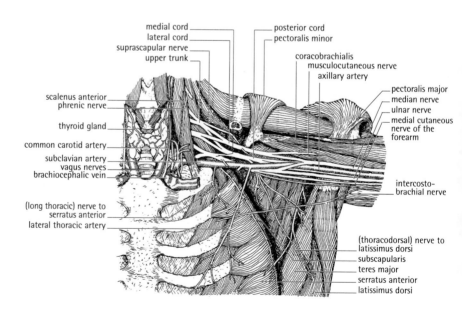

8.9   The brachial plexus. The medial end of the clavicle has been removed and both pectoral muscles reflected. From Tobin CE (1973) Basic Human Anatomy, McGraw-Hill, New York, with permission.

with more side to side migration available. The considerable neurodynamics in this area are discussed in chapter 4. Prolapsing ulnar nerves are quite common, can be easily felt and may be quite alarming for the patient. This is common and has been reported as present in up to 16% of all individuals (Childress 1975), although this figure does seem a little high. Some prolapse more easily if the shoulder girdle is depressed. This movement may physically pull the nerve out of the groove.

From the condylar groove the ulnar nerve can be followed distally to the cubital tunnel where the nerve goes deep into the tissues under the aponeurotic arch of the flexor carpi ulnaris muscle (Fig. 8.10). The entry into the muscle will be on the point of an equilateral triangle, where one point is the olecranon and the other point is the medial epicondyle (Fig. 8.11). Some authors describe the tunnel to include the soft facial sheath which may extend some distance proximally. Palpation can be very specific here, the nerve can be easily felt as it dives into the muscle and then half a centimetre distally it can no longer be felt. Palpating across the nerve at this spot will usually evoke distal paraesthesia. Not only does the ulnar nerve have a small cross-sectional connective tissue sheath content here, the sensory fibres of the nerve are superficial (Sunderland 1945). Try palpating the nerve in flexion also. The distance between the olecranon and the medial epicondyle will be about a centimetre longer in flexion, resulting in a tight aponeurosis, perhaps compressing the nerve (Apfelberg and Larson 1973). In addition, there will be increased forces on the ulnar nerve due to its position behind the flexion/extension axis. There are further details in the neurodynamics chapter (chapter 5), all forming the anatomical basis for palpation in a neurally loaded position. Note that despite its sensitivity, the cubital tunnel is an area where humans frequently rest their arms on tables, or the sides of seats.

Ulnar nerve in the upper arm

The nerve can usually be followed right up to the armpit, straddling the brachial artery for most of the way, closely associated with the median nerve, although the ulnar nerve is a little smaller (Fig. 8.12). The ulnar nerve will also be posterior to the median nerve. It may be easy enough to work out which nerve is palpated. Simply flex the elbow so that the ulnar nerve will tighten up and the median nerve loosens and vice versa. In slim individuals the outline of the nerve running towards the condylar groove can be made out as the elbow is flexed and the wrist extended. The nerve is infrequently injured in the upper arm, compared to the elbow and wrist.

Ulnar nerve at the wrist

The ulnar nerve is quite superficial at the wrist and very easy to palpate in Guyon's canal between the pisiform bone and the hook of the hamate. The floor of Guyon's canal is the pisohamate ligament and the roof of the canal is the palmar fascia and the palmaris brevis muscle. The nerve shares the canal with the ulnar artery which usually runs medial to the nerve (Fig. 8.13). Here, the nerve may be injured by falls onto an outstretched hand or maintained pressure from the demands of various occupations, even manual therapy, or sports such as cycling.

Try palpating this nerve on your own hand. Find the pisiform bone with your thumb. Approximately one thumb width towards the base of the index finger is the hook of hamate bone. The ulnar nerve can be rolled against the hook of hamate where it can create a flicking, almost "thudding" feeling in some. The nerve can then be followed down towards the wrist

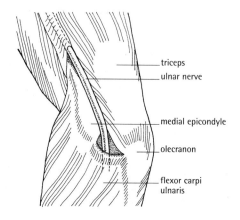

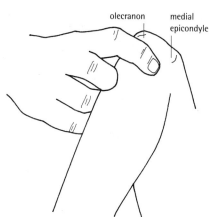

8.10   The ulnar nerve at the elbow, medial aspect.
Adapted from Lundborg G (1988) Nerve
Injury and Repair, Churchill Livingstone,
Edinburgh.

8.11   Palpation of the ulnar nerve at the elbow. The nerve
usually goes into the flexor carpi ulnaris muscle at
one point of an equilateral triangle. The other points
are the olecranon and the medial epicondyle.

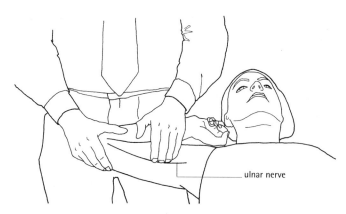

8.12   Palpation of the ulnar nerve in the upper arm. The
nerve becomes more obvious with elbow flexion and
wrist extension.

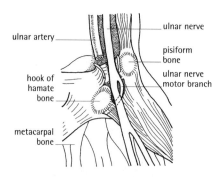

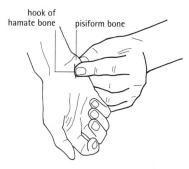

8.13   The ulnar nerve at the wrist in Guyon's canal.
Note the relationship to both the hamate and
the pisiform bone. Adapted from Lundborg G
(1988) Nerve Injury and Repair, Churchill
Livingstone, Edinburgh.

8.14   Palpation of the ulnar nerve at the wrist. Find the
hook of hamate and roll the nerve back towards the
pisiform. The ulnar nerve can also be palpated
proximally to the wrist crease.

crease. Note how the responses are very different to the responses at the elbow. At the wrist, paraesthesia can sometimes be evoked, but it is more likely that the response will be a deep ache, which is perhaps due to firing of the nervi nervorum. You can often follow the nerve for 5 or 6 centimetres proximally in the wrist where the nerve is lateral to the flexor carpi ulnaris muscle.

RADIAL NERVE

Note the general anatomy and nerve orientation in figure 8.8. The radial nerve spirals around the humerus, making it clear that internal rotation of the shoulder is a necessary addition to a radial nerve biased neurodynamic test.

The radial nerve in the upper arm

The nerve can be palpated in the axilla where it lies on the humerus. Here is where the nerve can be damaged in the well known Saturday night palsy, when a person goes to sleep with his/her arm over the back of a hard chair, although the median and ulnar nerves may be injured as well.

The radial nerve should be easy to palpate where it is superficially located in the spiral groove of the humerus where it lies directly on the periosteum. It is easy to strike here too as generations of children have found out. The nerve is approximately 3 finger's width below the insertion of deltoid, and between the lateral and medial heads of triceps. Remember that the nerve runs obliquely across the humerus, thus to feel the nerve it is best to run your fingers perpendicular to the nerve. Palpation creates an uncomfortable sensation and it is obviously not an examination technique for everyone (Fig. 8.15). It is however a reminder of the vulnerability of the nerve.

The radial nerve at the elbow and the sensory radial nerve in the forearm

The deep motor branch (posterior interosseus nerve) winds dorsoradially over the head of the radius as it goes to innervate the wrist extensors (Fig. 8.16). In many systems of manual therapy, techniques for mobilising the head of the radius are employed for lateral elbow pain. The radial nerve may well be palpated during techniques involving anteroposterior pressures on the radius and depending on other clinical information held by the patient, faulty clinical

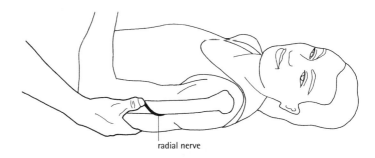

radial nerve

8.15 Palpation of the radial nerve in the spiral groove. The nerve is usually felt as a thick cord. Occasionally the nerve is flattened on the humerus.

diagnoses may emerge. It then enters the arcade of Frohse in the supinator muscle. The nerve can be indirectly palpated as it passes into the muscle. Symptoms evoked by palpation of the nerve here are widely used to assist a diagnosis of an entrapment in the tunnel. The Arcade of Frohse is about one and half finger's width distal to the elbow crease and a thumb width to the medial side of the biceps tendon (Fig. 8.17).

The radial sensory nerve (sometimes referred to as the superficial radial nerve) in the forearm passes over supinator and then deep to brachioradialis and the extensor carpi radialis muscles. In the lower third of the forearm it becomes cutaneous and easily palpable from the point where it emerges between the tendons of brachioradialis and extensor carpi radialis longus, although this emergence site is variable (Mackinnon and Dellon 1988). The nerve runs along the radius making it easy to evoke a Tinel's sign, even in asymptomatic individuals.

Try self palpation here. Place your index finger firmly on the lateral border of the radius about four finger's width distance above the radial styloid. Pronate and supinate the wrist, at the same time feeling the tissues underneath (Fig. 8.18). Don't be confused with the tendon of brachioradialis – it is much softer and thicker than the nerve. Identification is very clear when a shower of paraesthesia is evoked in the thumb and/or anatomical snuff box area. The nerve here sometimes slips away from palpating fingers. This is a good protective measure to avoid impinging forces.

In the anatomical snuff box, when the tendons are relaxed, the terminal branches of the radial sensory nerve can sometimes be palpated. Use a fingernail to rub over the scaphoid bone and you may feel the small nerves like pieces of fine fishing line underneath.

THE MEDIAN NERVE

The median nerve is the largest and most commonly injured nerve in the upper limb. It is not as palpable as the ulnar nerve and techniques of indirect palpation are often necessary.

The median nerve in the upper arm

The median nerve should be easy to palpate in the bicipital furrow, especially when the elbow is extended and the arm is abducted. In slim individuals it becomes obvious that much of the definition of the bicipital furrow is due to the tightness of the median nerve. In the upper furrow the nerve lies anterolateral to the artery, but lies medial to the artery after the insertion of coracobrachialis (Fig. 8.16). Carefully palpate the nerve with the arm in a slightly elevated position (Fig. 8.19). Place your fingers carefully along the nerve and then ask your patient to flex and extend her wrist and fingers or laterally flex her neck. You should feel the nerve sliding on your fingers underneath. Here the median nerve has the ability to slide approximately 2cm in relation to surrounding tissues in movements such as elevating the arm with the elbow extended. It should make you spare a thought for the possible neurological consequences which could occur from lack of movement, oedema and bleeding after breast or shoulder surgery.

At the elbow, the tendon of the biceps makes a good landmark to identify the nerve. Ask the patient to contract against some resistance so that you can find the tendon. If you can't find the biceps tendon you probably shouldn't be reading this text. The median nerve lies medial to the brachial artery and is quite easy to palpate (Fig. 8.16).

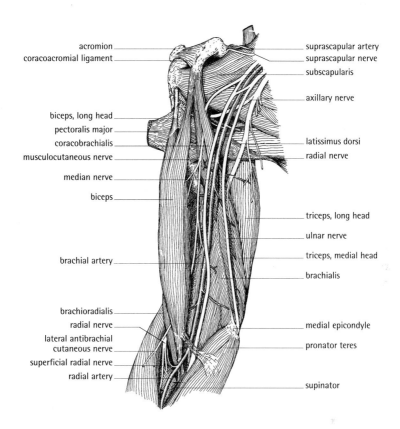

acromion
coracoacromial ligament

suprascapular artery
suprascapular nerve
subscapularis

axillary nerve

biceps, long head
pectoralis major
coracobrachialis
musculocutaneous nerve

latissimus dorsi
radial nerve

median nerve

biceps

triceps, long head

ulnar nerve

triceps, medial head

brachial artery

brachialis

brachioradialis
radial nerve
lateral antibrachial
cutaneous nerve
superficial radial nerve
radial artery

medial epicondyle

pronator teres

supinator

8.16   The nerves, muscles and blood vessels of the forearm. Note also
the radial nerve at the elbow, entering the supinator muscle.
From Tobin CE (1973) Basic Human Anatomy, McGraw-Hill, New
York, with permission.

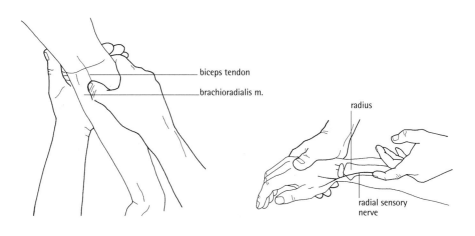

biceps tendon
brachioradialis m.

radius

radial sensory
nerve

8.17   Palpation of the radial nerve at the Arcade
of Frohse.

8.18   Palpation of the radial sensory nerve proximal
to the wrist.

The median nerve at the wrist

The median nerve lies deep in the forearm and cannot be directly palpated. At the wrist the nerve lies deep to palmaris longus between the flexor digitorum superficialis and the ulnar bursa medially and flexor carpi radialis laterally (Fig. 8.20). The nerve cannot be felt directly, however indirect palpation over the carpal tunnel and proximal to the carpal tunnel is a useful test to assist in the diagnosis of carpal tunnel syndrome. This test is now known as the carpal tunnel compression test (eg. Durkan 1991). Note that the carpal tunnel begins at the most distal wrist crease and is approximately one thumb width wide. The technique shown in figure 8.21 involves palpating the tunnel with a web space-to-web space contact. This allows more accurate placement for test-retest, but when a therapist has a small hand and the patient a large hand there will be difficulties and variations needed.

The carpal tunnel and its contents can also be palpated with the nerve and contained tissues on some load. Try with the fingers extended for example. Palpation can be performed with the wrist in flexion (Phalen's test) or extension (reverse Phalen's test), or in combination with an upper limb neurodynamic test. Testing in an upper limb neurodynamic test position would logically be the most provocative way to test the median nerve in the carpal tunnel (chapter 15).

The digital branches of the fingers can only be indirectly palpated. Unless they are swollen they are too small to be palpated.

OTHER UPPER LIMB NERVES

The other long nerve of the upper limb is the musculocutaneous nerve. Check its orientation as shown in figures 8.8 and 8.16. This nerve does not appear to be commonly injured. Tenderness lateral to the biceps tendon may be musculocutanoeous in origin. Frequently, the musculocutaneous nerve anastomoses with the radial sensory nerve at the wrist (Mackinnon and Dellon 1985) and thus may be responsible for symptoms on palpation. Perhaps it could be involved in a syndrome such as de Quervain's tenosynovitis.

Tenderness over the suprascapular notch is regarded as a sign of suprascular nerve entrapment (Vastamaki and Goransson 1993). Horizontal flexion and extension of the shoulder will pull the suprascapular nerve through the notch. See chapter 11 for further details on the suprascapular nerve.

LOWER LIMB SCIATIC TRACT

Lower limb peripheral nerves are larger, yet perhaps not quite as obvious as the nerves in the upper limb. In figure 8.22 the general arrangement and orientation of the nerves in the lower limb are shown.

SCIATIC NERVE AT THE BUTTOCKS

The sciatic nerve is the strongest and thickest nerve in the body. It runs deep to the gluteus maximus in the buttock. The thickness of gluteus maximus makes it difficult to palpate in healthy individuals, but clinicians should know its orientation so that an indirect palpation can be made. In figure 8.23, imagine a line drawn between the ischial tuberosity and the greater trochanter. If this line was divided into three, the nerve would lie on the lower third, towards the medial side. Make this the starting position. Sink your palpating fingers slowly into the tissues, giving the person time to relax and then feel rostrally and caudally from the position described above. The nerve may be more reactive if the patient puts one leg over the side of the bed and is thus in some degree of SLR.

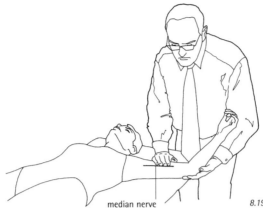

median nerve

8.19 Palpation of the median nerve in the bicipital furrow in the upper arm

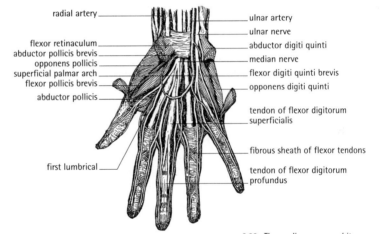

radial artery

flexor retinaculum
abductor pollicis brevis
opponens pollicis
superficial palmar arch
flexor pollicis brevis
abductor pollicis

first lumbrical

ulnar artery
ulnar nerve
abductor digiti quinti
median nerve
flexor digiti quinti brevis
opponens digiti quinti

tendon of flexor digitorum superficialis

fibrous sheath of flexor tendons

tendon of flexor digitorum profundus

8.20 The median nerve and its relationships at the wrist and hand. From Tobin CE (1973) Basic Human Anatomy, McGraw-Hill, New York, with permission.

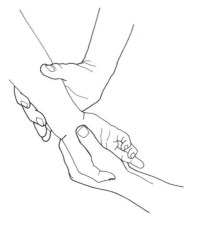

8.21 Indirect palpation of the median nerve in the carpal tunnel.

Mid thigh, the biceps femoris muscle crosses the nerve diagonally. The sciatic nerve branches into posterior tibial and common peroneal nerves, anywhere from mid thigh level to the popliteal fossa, but always superior to the popliteal fossa (Mumenthaler and Schliack 1991).

TIBIAL AND COMMON PERONEAL NERVES POSTERIOR TO THE KNEE

The tibial nerve

It is difficult to palpate the posterior knee region without palpating neural tissue. Note the tibial and peroneal nerves exposed in figure 8.24. The tibial nerve is the larger of the two branches. It can be palpated very easily in the popliteal fossa. It runs between the hamstring tendons of semitendinosis and biceps femoris. The tibial nerve is quite thick here with a diameter of approximately three quarters of a centimetre.

The tibial and peroneal nerves can be easily seen posterior to the knee. Ask your subject to hold her flexed hip and knee and then ask her to extend her knee. Both nerves, but especially the tibial nerve stand out as a thick cord, and can be easily palpated, particularly in a transverse direction through overlying tissues. If the subject dorsiflexes her foot, the tibial nerve will be more easily felt as it tightens up. In this position, even the physical repercussions of dorsiflexion of the great toe may be felt or observed in the tibial nerve.

The peroneal nerve

The smaller branch of the sciatic nerve is the peroneal nerve. It can also be palpated and observed in most individuals in the position described above. The nerve is located towards the lateral side of the posterior knee and medial to the tendon of biceps femoris, the tendon making a good landmark for the nerve and a surface to roll the nerve onto. In the hip flexion/knee extension position described above, if the subject plantarflexes her foot, the nerve will be firmer to palpate and like the tibial nerve, can sometimes be observed tightening up. The common peroneal nerve can also be felt with the subject supine. Just flex her knee a little and then feel under the knee inside the biceps tendon. In some individuals the nerve can be followed out to the head of the fibula where it wraps around before entering the peroneus longus muscle. The nerve can be felt just inferior to the head of the fibula. It is quite firmly attached here and may be quite flattened and will not roll under the fingers as it will at the posterior knee. More than 60 % of the nerve at this point is connective tissue (Sunderland and Bradley 1949), providing some protection in an area well known for nerve trauma from plaster cast compression and trauma to the fibula head and surrounding tissues. There may be tenderness at the tunnel where the common peroneal nerve goes through peroneus longus (Fig. 8.25).

Peroneal nerve branches on the anterior shin and dorsum of the foot

Just past the peroneus longus tunnel, the common peroneal nerve divides into the superficial peroneal branch and deep peroneal nerves. The deep peroneal nerve descends to the foot in the anterior compartment between the tendons of tibialis anterior and the extensor hallucis muscles. If the nerve emerges higher in the shin as in figure 8.1, it can be quite thickened and large and it is not surprising that it is frequently mistaken for a tendon. The superficial peroneal nerve emerges from under the peroneus longus and provides a cutaneous supply to the dorsum of the foot.

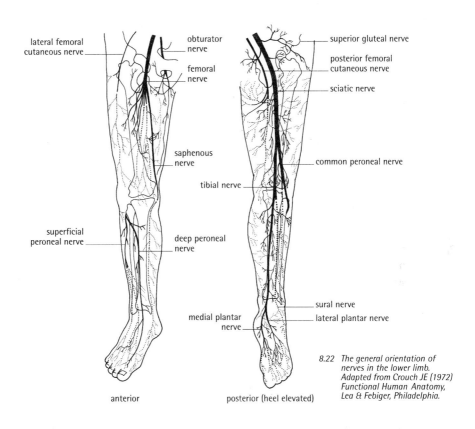

lateral femoral cutaneous nerve

obturator nerve

femoral nerve

saphenous nerve

tibial nerve

superficial peroneal nerve

deep peroneal nerve

superior gluteal nerve

posterior femoral cutaneous nerve

sciatic nerve

common peroneal nerve

sural nerve

lateral plantar nerve

medial plantar nerve

anterior

posterior (heel elevated)

8.22   The general orientation of nerves in the lower limb. Adapted from Crouch JE (1972) Functional Human Anatomy, Lea & Febiger, Philadelphia.

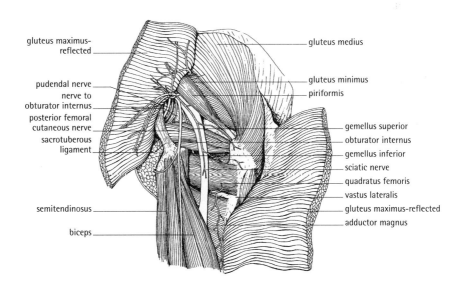

gluteus maximus-reflected

pudendal nerve

nerve to obturator internus

posterior femoral cutaneous nerve

sacrotuberous ligament

semitendinosus

biceps

gluteus medius

gluteus minimus

piriformis

gemellus superior

obturator internus

gemellus inferior

sciatic nerve

quadratus femoris

vastus lateralis

gluteus maximus-reflected

adductor magnus

8.23   The sciatic nerve exposed. Note the sciatic nerve, its relation to the piriformis muscle and its position, one third of the distance between the ischial tuberosity and the greater trochanter. From Tobin CE (1973) Basic Human Anatomy, McGraw-Hill, New York, with permission.

When the foot is inverted and plantarflexed, the dorsal tissues will be stretched. This is quite visible in the fascia, and the veins and in nearly every person the terminal branches of the superficial peroneal nerve can be seen on the dorsum of the foot. The nerve is harder than tendons or blood vessels and the movement will make it stand out more easily. Try "twanging" the nerve(s) here, much like a guitar string. Two branches can often be identified, the more branches, the smaller they will be. If the foot is inverted and everted, the nerve can be seen to slide subcutaneously. Sometimes this movement can be a few centimetres and the nerve may "snap" over the navicular or talus. This is often a useful exercise to appreciate the movement ability of the nervous system. The side to side nerve movement is lessened when the leg is in a straight leg raise position with plantar flexion and inversion of the ankle. Try to trace the nerve back to its emergence from the lateral compartment. Nerve emergence points often appear vulnerable.

The deep peroneal nerve also lies on the dorsum of the foot (Fig. 8.25). It is much smaller than the branches of the superficial peroneal and lies under the retinaculum where it may be a part of an anterior tarsal tunnel syndrome. The nerve can be palpated indirectly at the tunnel just lateral to the tendon of tibialis anterior. Then it runs laterally to the tendon of extensor hallucis longus as it goes to supply the web space. This small, but sometimes problematic nerve can be palpated and twanged with a fingernail moving transversely (Fig. 8.26). It is sometimes easier to find in a symptomatic person because you can go straight to the site of symptoms.

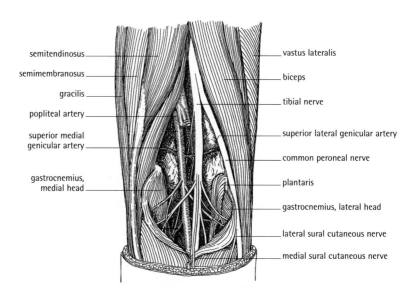

semitendinosus

semimembranosus

gracilis

popliteal artery

superior medial genicular artery

gastrocnemius, medial head

vastus lateralis

biceps

tibial nerve

superior lateral genicular artery

common peroneal nerve

plantaris

gastrocnemius, lateral head

lateral sural cutaneous nerve

medial sural cutaneous nerve

8.24 The tibial and common peroneal nerves posterior to the knee. Note the branches arising from the tibial nerve and also the sural nerve with a branch from the peroneal and the tibial nerves. From Tobin CE (1973) Basic Human Anatomy, McGraw-Hill, New York, with permission.

TIBIAL AND SURAL NERVES AT THE ANKLE AND FOOT

Sural nerve

This little sensory nerve is probably best known because it is often harvested by surgeons and used as an autologous nerve graft. The main sural nerve is a continuation of the tibial nerve and it descends to the foot between the heads of gastrocnemius. It becomes subcutaneous at the lower limit of the gastrocnemius where it is joined by a communicating branch of the common peroneal nerve, called the lateral sural or sural communicating nerve, although this is variable (Ortiguela et al. 1987). The Achilles tendon is medial to the nerve which then runs behind the lateral malleolus (Fig.8.27). The sural nerve then passes along the lateral border of the foot, splitting into medial and lateral branches near the base of the 5th metatarsal. It supplies a considerable amount of the lateral foot including the little toe. Because it is so superficial and so mobile, the sural nerve is one of the easiest to palpate and there are a number of zones where this can be done.

While sitting if you were to reach down and run a fingernail across the lateral side of the Achilles tendon about a hand width above the malleolus, you may feel the nerve. It can be around 3 mm in diameter here. If you "twang" it, there may be a "zinging" down towards the ankle as the nerve probably doesn't have a lot of connective tissue at this point. There is a technique of rolling the fingers from the lateral side of the tendon and then over the tendon, and the nerve will eventually slip under the fingers. In some individuals the nerve can be seen as a line from the mid calf to the inferior lateral malleolus especially in a straight leg raise

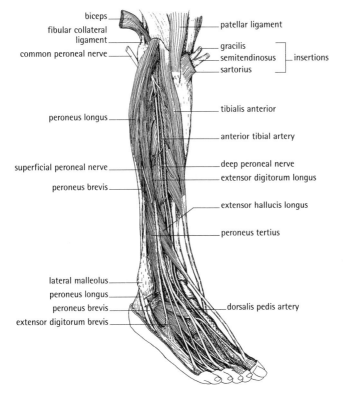

biceps
fibular collateral ligament
common peroneal nerve
patellar ligament
gracilis
semitendinosus — insertions
sartorius
peroneus longus
tibialis anterior
anterior tibial artery
superficial peroneal nerve
deep peroneal nerve
peroneus brevis
extensor digitorum longus
extensor hallucis longus
peroneus tertius
lateral malleolus
peroneus longus
peroneus brevis
extensor digitorum brevis
dorsalis pedis artery

8.25   The anterior shin and dorsum of the foot. Note the deep peroneal nerve. The superficial peroneal nerve has been cut, but would also course onto the dorsum of the foot. From Tobin CE (1973) Basic Human Anatomy, McGraw-Hill, New York, with permission.

position with ankle dorsiflexion. At a point inferior to the lateral malleolus, perhaps a centimetre or so under, the nerve can be easily felt and in patients with lateral ankle pain, this may well be an area of abnormal impulse generation. In some individuals, the nerve can be seen coursing along the lateral aspect of the foot, particularly when the foot is dorsiflexed and inverted (Fig. 8.27).

Having palpated thousands of sural nerves on seminars, it is noticeable that the sural nerve varies in size between individuals. In some the nerve is very large and the superficial peroneal branches are much smaller. It appears that one may partly replace the other (Sunderland 1978). I occasionally notice (perhaps 1 in 20 individuals) that the sural and superficial peroneal nerves or branches of the nerves join on the dorsum of the foot. I don't know whether this makes the nerves more prone to abnormal impulse generation, but it is always a reminder of the great variations in neuroanatomy.

Tibial nerve

In the calf, the tibial nerve remains deep and only becomes superficial and available for palpation for a few centimetres just above the medial malleolus. Here the nerve passes under the very thin fascia of the flexor retinaculum. At this site, the nerve is easily palpable (Figs. 8.28,29). The tibial nerve may divide into medial and lateral plantar nerves here (Fig. 8.30) although this division could occur more proximally or distally. The calcaneal nerve is difficult to palpate and may arise from the level of the retinaculum or more distally.

The tibial nerve is more superficial and is usually more palpable than the tendons. Find the tip of the medial malleolus and approximately two centimetres posteriorly, the tibial nerve can be palpated and rolled against the talus (Fig. 8.29). It is quite thick here, thicker than most clinicians expect, particularly if the nerve hasn't divided into the plantar divisions. This is an important place to palpate the tibial nerve. Injury here could lead to foot disorders such as plantar fasciitis or Morton's metatarsalgia (chapter 15). Palpation of the nerve easily evokes paraesthesia and the feeling can be similar to the palpation of the ulnar nerve at the elbow.

Once past the retinaculum, the tibial nerve has usually split into the medial and lateral plantar nerves. These nerves run deep to the abductor hallucis muscle towards the foot (Fig. 8.30). Once in the foot, direct palpation is not possible.

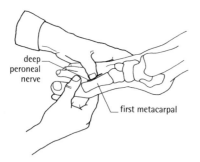

8.26 Palpation of the deep peroneal nerve on the dorsum of the foot.

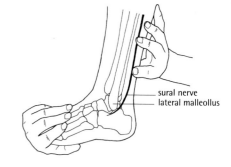

8.27 Palpation of the sural nerve. This nerve becomes more obvious in dorsiflexion and inversion.

THE FEMORAL, SAPHENOUS AND ANTERIOR THIGH NERVES

Note the orientation of the nerves in figure 8.22. Most of these nerves are deep and palpation is difficult, other than the saphenous nerve and branches at the knee. Any inferences of peripheral neurogenic pain from palpation alone would need to be backed up by other clinical data.

Arising from the L 2, 3 and 4 root levels, the femoral nerve descends through the psoas muscles, leaving the lower abdomen about half way along the inguinal ligament between the anterior superior iliac spine and the pubic symphysis (Fig. 8.31). Entrapment is reported as uncommon, although "kinking" during forced flexion such as the lithotomy position or stretch as in some dance movements has been reported (Stewart 1993) (see chapter 14).

The nerve lies lateral, sometimes by a few centimetres to the femoral artery. Thus if the femoral pulse is found a centimetre or so distal to the inguinal ligament, the femoral nerve should also be identified, though this would be best described as an indirect palpation. Approximately 4 cm distal to the inguinal ligament, the nerve divides into its various motor and sensory branches and can no longer be palpated.

THE LATERAL FEMORAL CUTANEOUS NERVE AND OTHER NERVES ANTERIOR TO THE HIP

The lateral femoral cutaneous nerve (LFCN) is reasonably well known because entrapment can cause the syndrome meralgia paraesthetica, which has been widely reported in the literature for over 100 years, sixty years longer than carpal tunnel syndrome. From L 2,3 the LFCN nerve crosses the iliacus muscle and then passes under the lateral end of the inguinal ligament,

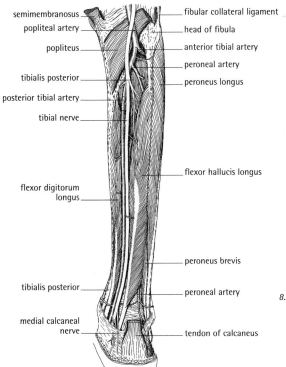

semimembranosus
popliteal artery
popliteus
tibialis posterior
posterior tibial artery
tibial nerve

flexor digitorum longus

tibialis posterior

medial calcaneal nerve

fibular collateral ligament
head of fibula
anterior tibial artery
peroneal artery
peroneus longus

flexor hallucis longus

peroneus brevis

peroneal artery

tendon of calcaneus

8.28   The tibial nerve in the posterior aspect of the leg. Gastocnemius and soleus have been removed. Note the relationship with the tendons and also the emergence of the calcaneal nerve. From Tobin CE (1973) Basic Human Anatomy, McGraw-Hill, New York, with permission.

although many variations to this route are reported. Note that the nerve is lateral to the axis of abduction and adduction and thus for testing, adduction of the hip could be a useful inclusion in a neurodynamic test for the nerve.

The lateral femoral cutaneous nerve can sometimes be palpated, though it will primarily be an indirect palpation, particularly when it runs through or deep to the inguinal ligaments. Find the anterior superior iliac spine and then the nerve should be approximately one finger's width, sometimes a little more, medially and inferiorly (Fig. 8.32). Occasionally a nerve can be felt rolling under the fingers. This may be a variation where the nerve is superficial to the inguinal ligament. This area is often reported as tender to palpation in meralgia paraesthetica. In chapter 11, a technique for examining and treating the nerve in a sidelying/slump/knee flexion position is described.

The other anterior groin nerves, the iliohypogastric, ilioinguinal and genitofemoral nerves are not palpable. The iliohypogastric and ilioinguinal nerves both originate from L1 and L2 roots and proceed to run parallel to each other in the groin (Fig. 8.33). No direct palpation is possible although in suspected neuropathy, a tender point just medial to the anterior superior iliac spine may be noted in ilioinguinal nerve neuropathy according to Kopell and Thompson (1963). The ilioinguinal continues down to the pubic tubercle. The iliohypogastric has a small lateral cutaneous branch, sometimes irritated by belts. Hip adduction and medial rotation will place some strain upon the nerves.

The genitofemoral nerve is not palpable, but its course along the line of the psoas major muscle should be remembered when psoas testing is performed. Perhaps the psoas test is also a test of the mechanosensitivity of a number of nerves. Note also the obturator nerve. It is not palpable however its location suggests that activities such as abduction of the hip will load the nerve (Fig. 8.33)

SAPHENOUS NERVE

The saphenous nerve can be a forgotten nerve. Students often think that the femoral nerve somehow ends at the knee, but it continues to the medial ankle as the saphenous nerve. An indirect palpation can be performed at the subsartorial or Hunter's canal where the nerve changes its name from femoral to saphenous (Figs. 8.31,34). Remember that the femoral vessels and the motor nerve to vastus medialis are also in the canal.

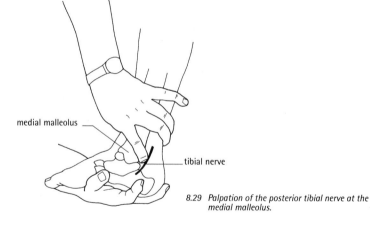

medial malleolus

tibial nerve

8.29 Palpation of the posterior tibial nerve at the medial malleolus.

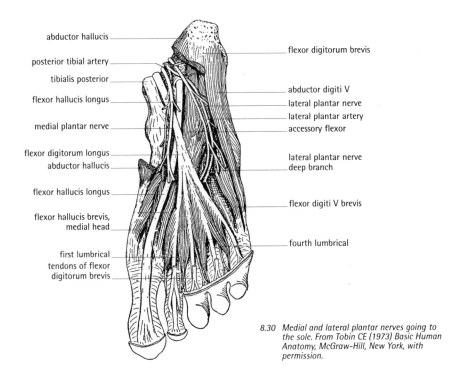

abductor hallucis

posterior tibial artery

tibialis posterior

flexor hallucis longus

medial plantar nerve

flexor digitorum longus
abductor hallucis

flexor hallucis longus

flexor hallucis brevis,
medial head

first lumbrical
tendons of flexor
digitorum brevis

flexor digitorum brevis

abductor digiti V
lateral plantar nerve
lateral plantar artery
accessory flexor

lateral plantar nerve
deep branch

flexor digiti V brevis

fourth lumbrical

8.30 Medial and lateral plantar nerves going to
the sole. From Tobin CE (1973) Basic Human
Anatomy, McGraw-Hill, New York, with
permission.

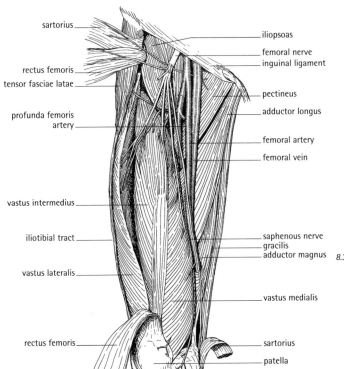

sartorius

rectus femoris
tensor fasciae latae

profunda femoris
artery

vastus intermedius

iliotibial tract

vastus lateralis

rectus femoris

iliopsoas
femoral nerve
inguinal ligament

pectineus
adductor longus

femoral artery
femoral vein

saphenous nerve
gracilis
adductor magnus

vastus medialis

sartorius
patella

8.31 The femoral nerve
at the inguinal
ligament. Note
that it is lateral
to the artery and
divides into
numerous branches
just past the
inguinal ligament.
From Tobin CE
(1973) Basic Human
Anatomy, McGraw-
Hill, New York, with
permission.

Note in the medial view (Fig. 8.34) that the main trunk of the nerve is posterior to the axis of flexion and extension at the knee. This means that a prone knee bend test will actually slacken the nerve, however knee flexion will tighten up the infrapatellar branches. Because of this, an alternate test is suggested in chapter 11.

The saphenous nerve can also be palpated on the medial side of the knee, where it may be injured in knee trauma, particularly that which involves the medial collateral ligament (Fig. 8.34). The nerve is usually found between the sartorius and gracilis muscles. Sometimes there is a slight depression or "pouch" between the two muscles here where it can be palpated. The nerve at this spot is probably 2-3 mm in diameter. It can also be felt posteromedially just below the head of the tibia. With the knee flexed as in sitting it is quite mobile and will flick under the finger. Although rare, ankle arthroscopy may injure a terminal branch of the saphenous nerve (Ferkel et al. 1996) and a thumbnail may activate a mechanosensitive abnormal impulse generating site at the ankle.

INFRAPATELLAR BRANCHES OF THE SAPHENOUS NERVE

The infrapatellar branches of the saphenous nerve are often easier to palpate than the main branch of the saphenous nerve. Two or three branches may be palpable. The nerve(s) emerges from the main nerve at the inferior pole of the patella and then runs obliquely towards and across the patella tendon (Tennent et al. 1998) (Fig. 8.34). Injury to the nerve could occur during meniscectomy or arthroscopy, or trauma ranging from dashboard injury to surfers gripping the sides of the board as they wait for a wave. The nerve is quite mobile and is best palpated in knee extension when it runs obliquely 45 degrees to the articular surface of the tibia. In knee flexion of 90 degrees, the nerve will run almost parallel and horizontal to the joint line (Mochida and Kikuchi 1995).

Try palpating the nerve by running a fingernail or thumbnail across the nerves on either the femur or the tibia. They feel like pieces of fishing line and will flick under the nail. Sometimes there may be one large branch. There is usually no paraesthesia evoked. If there is an arthroscopy incision which is causing persistent pain, palpate on either side of it. You may well reproduce the pain. Remember that the saphenous nerve goes to the ankle though it doesn't go much past the medial malleolus (Williams and Sugars 1998). It might be a good time to do a quick review of the cutaneous nerve innervation fields of the foot. This can be done in the next chapter.

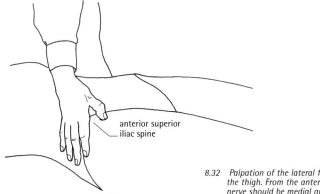

anterior superior
iliac spine

8.32   Palpation of the lateral femoral cutaneous nerve of
the thigh. From the anterior superior iliac spine, the
nerve should be medial and distal.

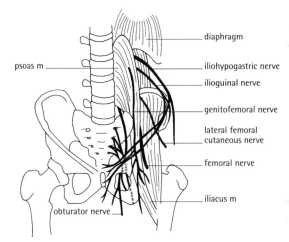

diaphragm

psoas m

iliohypogastric nerve

ilioguinal nerve

genitofemoral nerve

lateral femoral
cutaneous nerve

femoral nerve

iliacus m

obturator nerve

8.33   The anterior nerves of the groin. Adapted from
Stewart JD (1993) Focal Peripheral Neuropathies,
2nd edn. Raven Press, New York.

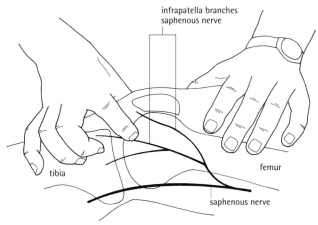

infrapatella branches
saphenous nerve

tibia

femur

saphenous nerve

8.34   Palpation of the saphenous and infrapatellar
branches of the saphenous nerves at the knee.

CHAPTER 8 REFERENCES

Anthony M (1992) Headache and the greater occipital nerve. Clinical Neurology and Neurosurgery 94: 297-301.

Apfelberg DB & Larson SJ (1973) Dynamic anatomy of the ulnar nerve at the elbow. Plastic and Reconstructive Surgery 51: 76-81.

Backhouse KM & Hutchings RT (1986) A Colour Atlas of Surface Anatomy, Wolfe Medical Publications, London.

Bogduk N (1981) The anatomy of occipital neuralgia. Clinical and Experimental Neurology 17: 167-184.

Bove GM & Light AR (1997) The nervi nervorum. Pain Forum 6: 181-190.

Budak F & Gonenc Z (1999) Innervation anomalies in upper and lower extremities (an electrophysiological study). Electromyography and Clinical Neurophysiology 39: 231-234.

Butler DS (1991) Mobilisation of the Nervous System, Churchill Livingstone, Melbourne.

Childress HM (1975) Recurrent ulnar-nerve dislocation at the elbow. Journal of Bone and Joint Surgery 38A: 978-984.

Clemente CD (1975) Anatomy. A Regional Atlas of the Human Body, Urban & Schwarzenberg, Munich.

Clifton EE (1948) Unusual innervation of the intrinsic muscles of the hand by the median and ulnar nerves. Surgery 23: 12-19.

Dellon AL, Schneider R & Burke R (1983) Effect of acute compartmental changes upon response to vibratory stimuli. Plastic and Reconstructive Surgery 72: 208-216.

Devor M & Seltzer Z (1999) Pathophysiology of damaged nerves in relation to chronic pain. In: Wall PD & Melzack R (eds.) Textbook of Pain, 4th edn. Churchill Livingstone, Edinburgh.

Durkan JA (1991) A new diagnostic test for carpal tunnel syndrome. Journal of Bone and Joint Surgery 73A: 536-538.

Ferkel RD, Heath DD & Guhl JF (1996) Neurological complications of ankle arthroscopy. Arthroscopy 12: 200-208.

Fetrow KO (1970) Practical and important variations in the sensory supply to the hand. Hand 2: 178-186.

Field D (1994) Anatomy: Palpation and Surface Markings, Butterworth-Heinemann Ltd., Oxford.

Gellman H, Gelberman RH, Tan AM, et al. (1986) Carpal tunnel syndrome. An evaluation of the provocative diagnostic tests. Journal of Bone and Joint Surgery 68A: 735-737.

Golding DN, Rose DM & Selvarajah K (1986) Clinical tests for carpal tunnel syndrome: an evaluation. British Journal of Rheumatology 25: 388-390.

Goldner JL & Hall RL (1997) Nerve entrapment syndromes of the lower back and lower extremities. In: Omer GE, Spinner M & Van Beek AL (eds.) Management of Peripheral Nerve Problems, 2nd edn. W.B. Saunders, Philadelphia.

Gonzalez del Pino JG, Delgado-Martìnez AD, Gonzalez-Gonzalez I, et al. (1997) Value of the carpal compression test in the diagnosis of carpal tunnel syndrome. Journal of Hand Surgery 22B: 38-41.

Harness D & Sekeles E (1971) The double anastomotic innervation of thenar muscles. Journal of Anatomy 109: 461-466.

Hunter CR & Mayfield FH (1949) Role of the upper cervical roots in the production of pain in the head. American Journal of Surgery 78: 734-749.

Jabre JF (1994) "Nerve rubbing" in the symptomatic treatment of ulnar nerve paraesthesiae. Muscle & Nerve 17: 1237.

Keogh B & Ebbs S (1984) Normal Surface Anatomy, William Heinemann, London.

Kopell HP & Thompson WAL (1963) Peripheral Entrapment Neuropathies, Williams and Wilkins, Baltimore.

Lebovic SJ & Hastings H (1992) Martin-Gruber revisited. Journal of Hand Surgery 17A: 47-53.

Lee DH & Dick HM (1998) Management of peripheral nerve tumors. In: Omer GE, Spinner M & Van Beek AL (eds.) Management of Peripheral Nerve Problems, 2nd edn. W.B. Saunders, Philadelphia.

Lumley JSP & 1996 (1996) Surface Anatomy: The Anatomical Basis of Clinical Examination, Butterworth-Heinemann, London.

Mackinnon SE & Dellon AL (1985) The overlap pattern of the lateral antebrachial cutaneous nerve and the superficial branch of the radial nerve. Journal of Hand Surgery 11A: 522-526.

Mackinnon SE & Dellon AL (1988) Surgery of the Peripheral Nerve, Thieme, New York.

Maigne JY & Maigne R (1991) Trigger point of the posterior iliac crest: painful iliolumbar ligament insertion or cutaneous dorsal ramus pain? An anatomic study. Archives of Physical Medicine and Rehabilitation 72: 734-737.

Marzo JM, Simmons EH & Kallen F (1987) Intradural connections between adjacent cervical spinal roots. Spine 12: 964-968.

McMinn RMH & Hutchings RT (1988) A Colour Atlas of Human Anatomy, 2nd edn. Wolfe Medical, London.

Mersdorf A, Schmidt RA & Tanagho EA (1993) Topographic-anatomical basis of sacral neurostimulation: neuroanatomical variations. Journal of Urology 149: 345-349.

Mochida H & Kikuchi S (1995) Injury to the infrapatellar branch of the saphenous nerve in arthroscopic knee surgery. Clinical Orthopaedics and Related Research 320: 88-94.

Monsivais JJ & Sun Y (1997) Tinel's sign or percussion test? Developing a better method of evoking a Tinel's sign. Journal of the Southern Orthopedic Association 6: 186-189.

Mumenthaler M & Schliack H (1991) Peripheral Nerve Lesions, Thieme, New York.

Narakas A (1989) Compression syndromes about the shoulder including brachial plexus. In: Szabo RM (ed.) Nerve Compression Syndromes, Slack, Thorofare.

Netter FH (1987) The CIBA Collection of Medical Illustrations, CIBA-Geigy Corporation, Summit, New Jersey.

Novak CB, Lee GW, Mackinnon SE, et al. (1994) Provocative testing for cubital tunnel syndrome. Journal of Hand Surgery 19A: 817-820.

Ortiguela ME, Wood MD & Cahill DR (1987) Anatomy of the sural nerve. Journal of Hand Surgery 12A: 1119-1123.

Pleet AB & Massey EW (1978) Notalgia paresthetica. Neurology 28: 1310-1313.

Seror P (1987) Tinel's sign in the diagnosis of carpal tunnel syndrome. Journal of Hand Surgery 12B: 364-365.

Spicher C, Kohut G & Miauton J (1999) At which stage of sensory recovery can a tingling sign be expected? Journal of Hand Therapy 12: 298-308.

Stewart JD (1993) Focal Peripheral Neuropathies, 2nd edn. Raven Press, New York.

Sunderland S (1945) The internal topography of the radial, median and ulnar nerves. Brain 68: 243-250.

Sunderland S (1978) Nerves and Nerve Injuries, 3rd edn. Churchill Livingstone, Melbourne.

Sunderland S & Bradley KC (1949) The cross sectional area of peripheral nerve trunks devoted to nerve fibres. Brain 72: 428-439.

Szabo RM (1989) Nerve Compression Syndromes, Slack, Thorofare NJ.

Tanaka N, Fujimoto Y, An HS, et al. (2000) The anatomic relation among the nerve roots, intervertebral foramina, and the intervertebral discs of the cervical spine. Spine 25: 286-291.

Tennent TD, Birch NC, Holmes MJ, et al. (1998) Knee pain and the infrapatellar branch of the saphenous nerve. Journal of the Royal Society of Medicine 91: 573-575.

Thomas PK (1984) Clinical features and differential diagnosis. In: Dyck PJ, Thomas PK, Lambert EH et al. (eds.) Peripheral Neuropathy, 2nd edn. Saunders, Philadelphia.

Tinel J (1915) Le signe du "fourmillement" dans les lesions des nerfs peripheriques. Presse Medicale 47: 388-389.

Tountas CP & Bergman RA (1993) Anatomic Variations of the Upper Extremity, Churchill Livingstone, New York.

Vastamaki M & Goransson H (1993) Suprascapular nerve entrapment. Clinical Orthopaedics and Related Research 297: 135-143.

Werner CO, Rosen I & Thorngren KT (1985) Clinical and neurophysical characteristics of the pronator syndrome. Clinical Orthopaedics and Related Research 197: 231-236.

Williams RP & Sugars W (1998) Lumbar root innervation of the medial foot and ankle region. Australian and New Zealand Journal of Surgery 68: 565-567.

CHAPTER 9

MANUAL ASSESSMENT
OF NERVE CONDUCTION

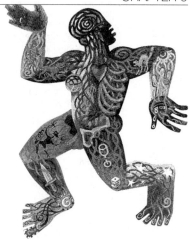

INTRODUCTION

THE VALUE OF A NEUROLOGICAL EXAMINATION

MENTAL STATUS

SENSORY EXAMINATION

INTRODUCTION
LANGUAGE OF THE SENSORY EXAMINATION
USE OF DERMATOMES AND PERIPHERAL NERVE INNERVATION FIELDS

SENSORY EXAMINATION PERFORMANCE

SKIN SENSATIONS – LIGHT TOUCH
SKIN SENSATIONS – SUPERFICIAL PAIN
SKIN SENSATIONS – HOT AND COLD
DEEP SENSATIONS – PAIN
DEEP SENSATIONS – PROPRIOCEPTION
DEEP SENSATION – VIBRATION SENSE
CORTICAL SENSORY FUNCTION

MANUAL TESTS OF MOTOR FUNCTION

MUSCLE WASTING
TREMOR AND FASCICULATION
MUSCLE POWER – GENERAL COMMENTS ON TECHNIQUE
COMMONLY PERFORMED TESTS OF MUSCLE POWER
UPPER LIMB
LOWER LIMB
QUICK/FUNCTIONAL MUSCLE TESTS
USE THE MUSCLE INNERVATION MAP

REFLEXES

THE SKILL OF MUSCLE-STRETCH REFLEX TESTING
SPECIFIC MUSCLE-STRETCH REFLEXES
ANALYSIS AND RECORDING OF REFLEX BEHAVIOURS
OTHER REFLEXES

THE CRANIAL NERVES

TESTS OF AUTONOMIC FUNCTION

THE EYE AND HORNER'S SYNDROME
OBSERVATION AND PALPATION OF THE SKIN

APPENDIX 9.1

REFERENCES CHAPTER 9

MANUAL ASSESSMENT OF NERVE CONDUCTION

Well known author and patient, Robert Murphy (1987) wrote about his medical experiences with a progressive tumour in his spinal column. He was hospitalised many times and neurologists frequently used him as a model for students. Murphy wrote:

"A recently retired clinical neurologist asked if he could use my body to demonstrate a standard workup to a young resident. He went though the entire process for an hour, explaining to his student the purpose of each test and the meaning of my responses, both verbal and reflexive. By the end I knew a lot more about my malady and I knew that he could have diagnosed my illness without a CT or even a myelogram."

INTRODUCTION

The series of largely reductionist tests described in this chapter are only a part of a neurological evaluation of conduction. From the moment a patient is met to the time of discharge, a neurological examination really never ceases. In particular, there will be situational effects on conduction. For example, unguarded movements, certain moods, familiar testing patterns and even a subjective interview could influence nerve firing.

The rapid advances in nervous system imaging techniques such as magnetic resonance imaging (MRI) and nerve conduction studies may have raised the notion that manual tests of nerve conduction are no longer essential. I disagree. Imaging and conduction studies are not foolproof nor are they universally available. They are expensive and in many cases may not be required. Pathological changes such as disc degeneration are frequently demonstrated by tests such as X-ray and MRI tests but may have no link to the patient's pain state (eg. Jensen et al. 1994). They are no replacement for a manual examination; they are an additional form of evaluation, and more useful in severe cases or where there are hints of "red flags" (chapter 7).

There is an art to a good manual neurological examination. Adept handling and patient communication skills plus an interlinked knowledge of neuroanatomy, neurophysiology and neuropathology are the basic critical skills. A neurological examination should not be performed unless an adequate subjective examination has been done and analysed. Thus the examination should be a clinically reasoned event. The examiner then performs the neurological tests, expecting certain findings which either support or reject hypotheses made in the various reasoning categories as defined and discussed in chapters 6 and 7, and represented in figure 9.1. The physical neurological examination can provide much knowledge to both patient and therapist if it is performed under this empowering reasoning framework, rather than a series of isolated and protocol driven tests.

I regularly note that tests of conduction are poorly performed by many clinicians. Some clinicians fail to perform the tests and others may perform a recipe style neurological examination without any reasoning base. For example, there is no use performing a detailed examination of light touch trying to find a dermatomal loss when the patient has pain everywhere and it appears that there may be maladaptive central influences on sensitivity. Equally, with a clear L3 nerve root compromise, testing of muscles innervated by the S2 root could be eliminated or quickly tested. The tests may aggravate the patient's symptoms anyway. However, spending time on a careful sensory examination for what appears to be an entrapment of the lateral femoral cutaneous nerve (meralgia paraesthetica) may be appropriate to help clarify a diagnosis. It is all about having a reasoned diagnosis first. In my experience, patients who have been told they have no reflex, often have a reflex, particularly in the case of the ankle reflex (S1-2) and the triceps reflex (C8-T1). Other clinical data collected may point to the fact that there should be a reflex and therefore it is worth spending some time testing. The technique may have just been performed badly and it can be of great encouragement to a patient to be told and shown that her nerve impulses are functioning well. Equally, many minor changes in nerve conduction can be missed because of poor testing and analytical technique (Impallomini et al. 1984).

The terms sensory and motor examination (although used here and elsewhere) are dated. Motor responses must always be sought and should be expected if there are sensory symptoms. Tests of proprioceptive abilities for example, involve combined input (deep sense) and output (motor) related components. Most of the tests rely on the patient's subjective responses. Examiners should also remember that the sensory and motor examination does not only reflect a tissue injury. It also reflects the response of the uninjured pathways to that injury. In addition, concepts of searching for a discrete lesion may be limiting. It is impossible to have a focal lesion in the nervous system, such are the multiple response systems and inherent neuroplasticity.

I therefore emphasise the handling and analytical skills in the neurological examination and encourage clinicians to practice the examination techniques. While it is clear that a manual neurological examination alone is inadequate for research purposes (Sunderland 1978), there are many reasons and uses of a manual nerve conduction examination that are worth stating.

THE VALUE OF A NEUROLOGICAL EXAMINATION

The neurological examination is a series of inputs that presumes to test particular normal and altered tissues, pathways and processing systems of the patient. In reply to the inputs, the responses in output systems such as the motor system, sympathetic system and patient's perceptions, (which could be called consciousness) are measured clinically. Deficits and changes found on a neurological examination may originate from a number of anatomical sites and pathobiological mechanisms. For example, a depressed quadriceps reflex may relate to the health of the muscle, related afferent and efferent neurones and central nervous system

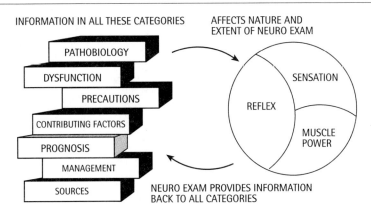

9.1   A neurological examination is a clinically reasoned event and the responses may contribute to further clinical reasoning involving all categories.

IMPAIRMENT STUDIED	AUTHOR(S)	POPULATION STUDIED	N	SENSITIVITY %	SPECIFICITY %	COMMENTS
Ankle dorsiflexor weakness	(Spangfort 1972)	HNP Surgery	2504	49	54	70-90% of patients with dorsiflexor weakness had HNP L4/5
	(Hakelius 1970)	HNP Surgery	1986	20	82	
Great toe extensor weakness	(Hakelius 1970)	HNP Surgery	1986	37	71	
	(Knuttson 1961)	HNP Surgery	206	63	52	
	(Spangfort 1972)	HNP Surgery	2504	30	68	
	(Kerr et al. 1988)	Patients with sciatica	136	54	89	
	(Kortelainen et al. 1985)	HNP Surgery	403	57		In 57% of cases with extensor weakness, HNP was at L5-S1, 32% at L4-5
Ankle reflex	(Spangfort 1972)	HNP Surgery	2504	31	80	HNP at L5-S1 level in 80-90% for ages 20-45, and 60% after age 50
	(Hakelius 1970)	HNP Surgery	1986	52	63	Absence of reflex has higher specificity than decreased reflex
	(Kerr et al. 1988)	Patients with sciatica	136	48	89	
	(Knuttson 1961)	HNP Surgery	206	56	57	
Patella reflex	(Spangfort 1972)	HNP Surgery	2504	.04	96	Sensitivity of 50% in L3-L4 HNP. In 67% of cases of impairment, HNP is at L4-5 and L5-S1 levels
	(Hakelius 1970)	HNP Surgery	1986	7	93	If this is an isolated finding then the sensitivity is worse
	(Kortelainen et al. 1985)	HNP Surgery	403	7		In 85% of impairments, HNP is at L4-L5 and L5-S1 levels
	(Aronson 1963)	Upper Lumbar HNP	73	50		
Quads weakness	(Hakelius 1970)	HNP Surgery	1986	<1	99	
Ankle plantar flexion weakness	(Hakelius 1970)	HNP Surgery	1986	6	95	
Lower limb sensory testing	(Peeters et al. 1998)	Lumbar nerve root disorders		Low	High	Positive predictive values 75%
	(Knuttson 1961)	HNP surgery	206	29	67	
	(Kerr et al. 1988)	Patients with sciatica	136	16	80	

Table 9.1 Studies of manual neurological examination for the lumbar spine. Adapted from Andersson and Deyo (1997) and van den Hoogen et al. (1995).

processing including the involvement of other tissues such as the knee joint. It may also involve events not directly associated with the knee reflex such as the patient's cognitions and environment of testing. The fact that most clinicians think that they are going to sample the nervous system may be restrictive. In fact the patient's nervous system is going to sample you the clinician, and your performance.

A manual neurological examination can only provide a moderately accurate diagnosis at best. One sign by itself may not offer much diagnostic strength but in combination there may be more power (van den Hoogen et al. 1995). For example, weakness of ankle dorsiflexion and extension of the 4 lateral toes plus disturbed sensation in the L5 dermatome gave positive predictive values of approximately 75% and negative predictive values of around 50% for an L4 disc lesion verified by operative findings (Jensen 1987). In this study however, similar findings could not be repeated for L5. A summary of experimental findings for the neurological examination related to herniated lumbar discs is in table 9.1. Chapter 12 provides information on the meaning of sensitivity, specificity and the value of various physical tests of the nervous system. Future research directions will be to evaluate the validity of the complete diagnostic process and then to study the added value of the different tests (Deville et al. 2000).

The information gained from a neurological examination adds to clinical decision making in all of the clinical reasoning categories endorsed by this book and defined in chapter 6. Some examples follow, linking the neurological examination to clinical reasoning categories.

PATHOBIOLOGY

The neurological examination can provide supportive information to operant pain mechanisms. For example, hyperreflexia may be suggestive of increased central sensitivity. A simple light touch examination might alert the clinician to the presence of tactile allodynia, and the clinician would then hopefully make an educated decision as to whether this was a primary or secondary allodynia (see chapter 3). Diminished sensitivity in a peripheral nerve innervation field should point to some conduction change in that peripheral nerve. Marked sweating increases after minimal examination may alert the therapist to a labile sympathetic system and the presence of fear or uncertainly with the examination processes. Information can be provided to both clinician and patient about the state of healing of neural and adjacent tissues (eg. reflex changes, muscle strength changes).

DYSFUNCTION

Many of the changes frequently found on a neurological examination, such as loss of a reflex or weakness in a specific muscle could be considered as specific dysfunctions or impairments. Some of these findings may not be relevant to the diagnosis and management. Their relevance will have to be reasoned, based on other clinical data or in retrospect. For example, a tendon reflex may not return, but your patient may report no pain and be able to function very well. Loss of proprioception or balance may be part of a general dysfunction. A neurological examination will provide clues as to the presence of adaptive or maladaptive distress. For example, the examination may reveal that there is really no somatic reason for a patient to continue to limp. Review the descriptions of dysfunction and impairments in chapters 6 and 7 if you wish.

SOURCES

Neurological examinations can be particularly helpful with localisation of anatomical sources of problems. The symptom patterns may suggest neurogenic involvement and then the tests can provide assistance in defining the actual sources of the problem. With nerve root problems, this may be identifying the nerve root level and perhaps associated discogenic pathology. In the case of a nerve trunk, the tests may provide information identifying which nerve is injured and also the site of injury along the nerve trunk. For example, loss or preservation of muscle power may help identify the site of the lesion. In other cases, tests and observations might provide evidence of a central nervous system lesion. It should be clear that in order to make diagnostic decisions, the information gained from a neurological examination must also be allied with information from a subjective history and other aspects of the physical examination.

CONTRIBUTING FACTORS

This may be the category under which clinicians like to conceptualise a variety of findings. For example, weakness and sensitivity to input may be contributing factors to function and outcome and be identified on a neurological examination. Altered function is often linked to sensory changes or perceptions of sensory changes.

PROGNOSIS

Results from a neurological examination may impact upon the prognosis. In many situations, the long term loss of a reflex may not be a good sign, particularly if coupled with the knowledge that there was significant damage at the root level in the spinal canal. Rapid return of strength and reflexes following surgery or injury is clearly an encouraging sign. The patient and the therapist will only know if this is so, if they perform the tests properly, if they repeat the examinations over time and have good handling skills that allow reproduceability of tests.

PRECAUTIONS

Some findings from neurological examination could be considered as "red flags" (chapter 7). This could include findings of multilevel sensory and motor loss, rapid neurological loss, or an upgoing Babinski response. These are indicators that may limit a form of treatment or act as strong indicators that a referral to a specialist medical practitioner is warranted.

MANAGEMENT

In addition to the diagnostic aspects impacting on a working clinical diagnosis, neurological examinations may sometimes be used as part of the reassessment of any therapy. They can also assist in the education of patients about the status of their nervous system and thus powerfully direct therapy. Findings may be a part of validating the pain experience for the patient. Some tests, such as muscle strength tests can be used for patient self assessment and thus allow greater inclusion of the patient on the management team. There are many places for cognitive behavioural inputs during neurological examinations. It could just be a simple "wow, that reflex is looking good." Physical assessment should always be considered a part of management.

MENTAL STATUS

The patient's mental status can be evaluated during all parts of the physical examination. Symptoms suggestive of excessive alcohol intake, drug use, delusions, orientation problems and suicidal intention, all require medical assessment and possible attention. Memory and general cognitive function can be assessed via self report from the patient and sometimes from family members. The important aspect here for movement based therapists such as physiotherapists, is to consider what cognitive functions may influence movement. Two very common ones will be lack of understanding of the pain and its nature, and also fear of movement because of possible re-injury.

A higher index of suspicion of altered cognitive functioning may be present in a patient who has sustained trauma, particularly whiplash. Vagueness may be a symptom, not a part of a particular patient's personality, concentration difficulties may not be necessarily related to pain, but to the trauma. For greater details, consult Mayo Clinic (1991), Nolan (1996) and Haddox (1999). Even though this text focuses on typical patients seen by manual therapists, the content of an examination of mental status is the same as for the seriously injured patient. The list by Nolan (1996) covers the major aspects of mental function.

1. level of consciousness

2. attention

3. orientation

4. language function

5. learning and memory

6. cortical and cognitive functions

7. mood and affect

8. thought content

Cognitive and emotional aspects related to the manual therapy based management of pain and disability states is discussed in chapter 7.

SENSORY EXAMINATION

INTRODUCTION

There are two basic methods of sensory evaluation - bedside sensory evaluation and quantitative sensory testing (QST). QST requires specialised equipment, trained staff, and time to analyse data. For reviews see Bovie (1994) and Omer and Bell-Krotoski (1997). This chapter is about bedside testing. However, it is recognised that manual bedside testing is often a crude procedure; examiners have variable skills, patients have different levels of reporting, the stimuli are variable and we still have some ignorance regarding mechanisms of perception of sensory stimuli.

There is no critical order for performing a neurological examination. During a typical assessment most patients will go from sitting for the subjective examination to standing for active movements, to sitting again, then to supine. It is best to fit an examination into this, meaning that parts of the sensory and motor examination may be performed in sitting, parts of the motor examination may be performed in standing, then a sensory examination and the rest of the motor examination is in supine. My preference and habit is to perform the majority of the sensory examination in supine.

As suggested by the title, a sensory examination is an examination of the sensitivity of the patient in response to various stimuli. The bedside examination essentially involves stimuli to the skin, although the tests involve peripheral and central discriminatory abilities.

LANGUAGE OF THE SENSORY EXAMINATION

The International Association for the Study of Pain (IASP) has developed terminology for use in clinical practice (Merskey and Bogduk 1994). These terms are defined primarily in relation to the skin and exclude the special senses, but may be adapted to other somatic stimulation. The physiological bases for these pain and sensitivity states are described in chapter 3 and 4.

Confusion often abounds with these terms and few clinicians outside of pain units actually use them. The IASP taxonomy committee acknowledges that the use of individual terms varies widely in medicine and simply suggests that authors make it clear precisely how they employ the words (Merskey and Bogduk 1994). I think it is important that all clinicians begin to utilise these terms and that we contribute to the ongoing discussions about pain terminology (eg. Chaplan and Sorkin 1997).

Allodynia is pain due to a stimulus that does not normally provoke pain. For example, if gently stroking the arm evokes pain, this could be referred to as tactile allodynia.

Hyperalgesia is an increased response to a stimulus that is normally painful. For example, pinprick may evoke more pain than usual or more pain in one limb than another. An Upper Limb Neurodynamic Test may be more sensitive on one side than the other and thus be hyperalgesic.

Analgesia is the absence of pain in response to a stimulus that would normally be painful. Patients frequently call this "numbness" although the term is often used with an absence of sensation to light touch.

Hyperpathia is a painful syndrome characterised by an abnormally painful reaction to a repetitive stimulus. Hyperpathic states often include allodynia and hyperalgesia. Clinicians may note hyperpathia during some of the repetitious testing during a sensory examination.

Hypoalgesia is diminished pain in response to stimulation that would normally be painful.

Hypoesthesia is diminished sensitivity to stimulation, excluding the special senses. The stimulus and site of the stimulation should be specified.

Hyperesthesia is increased sensitivity to stimulation. The stimulus and site of stimulation should be specified. There will often be obvious overlap with allodynia and hyperalgesia.

Dysesthesia is an unpleasant but not painful sensation.

The differences between "esthesia" and "algesia" becomes easier if their Greek roots are remembered - esthesia pertaining to the senses and algesia pertaining to pain.

Movement based clinicians will instantly recognise most of these sensitivity states because movement is an extremely common stimulus. The pathobiological states related to these definitions often overlap.

Hyperalgesia is the key sensory state and a good place for clinicians to begin integrating the terms. To begin utilising the terminology, I encourage therapists to consider that their physical examination is mainly an examination of hyperalgesia, that is, increased sensitivity. Primary hyperalgesia (source from tissues) and secondary hyperalgesia (source from central nervous system) have been dealt with in chapters 3 and 4. Be aware that hyperalgesia has become something of an umbrella term in the literature and it often encompasses the term allodynia.

USE OF DERMATOMES AND PERIPHERAL NERVE INNERVATION FIELDS

Well known maps of dermatomes exist and are presented in most orthopaedic and neurological textbooks including this one (Figs. 9.2, 9.3). A dermatome is the area of skin innervated by a single dorsal nerve root. A myotome is an area of muscle and a sclerotome is an area of bone innervated by a single dorsal root. Although myotomal and sclerotomal maps are available they are rarely used as it is difficult to stimulate the deeper structures.

A SHORT HISTORY OF DERMATOMES

Clinicians may have noted that in different texts the dermatomal maps are slightly different, particularly around the sacrum, cervicothoracic and sometimes the foot area. This has occurred because the original researchers had different ways of determining where a particular dermatome was. They also had different theories of how a dermatome came to be. The maps shown here (Figs. 9.2, 9.3) are from the original work by Foerster (1933) and popularised by Haymaker and Woodhall (1953).

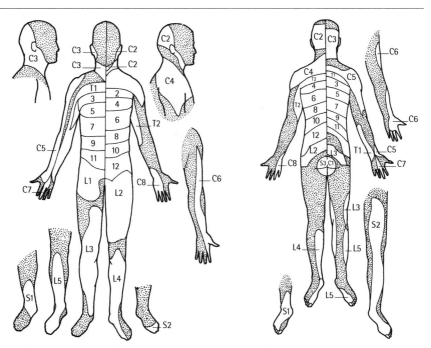

9.2   Dermatomes anterior view. The degree of overlap is shown by the alternating dermatomes on the right and left halves. Based on Foerster (1933). Adapted from: Gardner E, Gray DJ, O'Rahilly, R et al. (1975) (eds.) Anatomy, 4th edn. WB Saunders, Philadelphia, with permission.

9.3   Dermatomes posterior view. Based on Foerster (1933). Adapted from: Gardner E, Gray DJ, O'Rahilly, R et al. (1975) (eds.) Anatomy, 4th edn. WB Saunders, Philadelphia, with permission.

Foerster revised early dermatome descriptions by Head (1900) by examining a series of patients after he had severed various nerve roots. Unfortunately what Foerster did not know then, was that cutting a nerve involves a massive change of input into the central nervous system which is very likely to increase a patient's pain. To confirm his findings, Foerster also electrically stimulated the distal end of the divided root causing vasodilation in the area of the dermatome. You have to suspect that many of Foerster's patients may have ended their days in pain. At the same time we can be grateful for modern day university ethics committees.

The other dermatomal model used is the more strip-like dermatome style of Keegan and Garrett (1943) which often adorn clinic walls. The Foerster based dermatomes have been used here because I feel they are less ordered, focus more on overlap, are more accurate for the low back and seem more appropriate in the clinic.

There is very little recent research into dermatomes and, as Nitta et al. (1993) comment, it is probably not worth the effort. There have been some recent revisions. The L4 dermatome does not go onto the foot as it does in most dermatome maps including the map in figure 9.2. Williams and Sugars (1998) showed that the saphenous nerve terminated at or about the medial malleolus. This finding was also shown electrophysiologically by Liguori et al. (1992). The Keegan style dermatomes show L5 and S1 across the lateral aspect of the buttock. This has been disputed, as Maigne et al. (1989) have shown that the lateral buttock/iliac crest area is usually innervated by the dorsal rami of T12 and L1, and occasionally L3. Also it is possible for the S2 dermatome to go onto the dorsolateral aspect of the foot and to the posterolateral aspect of the ankle (Liguori et al. 1992).

USE OF DERMATOMAL MAPS

Some caution is needed when using dermatomal and cutaneous nerve maps:

• As discussed above, the various maps reproduced in texts are different, depending on the method used to construct them (Nitta et al. 1993; Dubuisson 1994).

• Anatomical variations to nerve distributions are very common.

• Symptoms of nerve injury are often represented in only part of the innervation field. The dermatome shows the whole field of the dorsal nerve root.

It is equally important to recognise that patients may have a neuropathic pain state and their symptoms may not resemble these maps at all. These fields relate primarily to peripheral neurogenic pain. Many patients, particularly those with maladaptive central processing, present with pain and symptoms which defy these territories even though an initial injury could have been manifest in one nerve field. The main message for clinicians is that sensory changes in dermatomes are just one part of information collecting.

Cutaneous nerve innervation fields and dermatomes are different, except in the thorax where the lack of plexus formations means that the nerve root continues as the peripheral nerve. In compressive lesions by tumour in the thoracic spine, dermatomal involvement is often the only indication of anatomical level of the tumour (Hirabayashi et al. 1995). It is worth noting here that the anatomical level of the tumour may be above the level indicated by the dermatomal change.

"SIGNATURE ZONES"

There are zones in the body which are autonomous to a particular nerve or root. These have been called "signature zones" (Stewart 1993), or "distinctive regions" (Nitta et al. 1993). These zones, in relation to nerve roots are demonstrated in figure 9.4. Most textbooks announce them without stating the research backing it, nor the variations possible, although the zones demonstrated seem clinically reasonable. However, the L4, 5 and S1 zones are accurate in about 85% of patients (Nitta et al. 1993). This group defined "distinctive regions" of spinal nerves as the region most involved after nerve blockade and least involved after blockade of adjacent roots.

CUTANEOUS ZONES

Dermatomes are routinely learnt by clinicians, however knowledge of the areas of skin innervated by post plexus peripheral nerves can also be useful clinical knowledge. Like dermatomes, cutaneous nerve distributions are approximate also. Overlap and variations are a feature of the nervous system. In figures 9.5 and 9.6, the cutaneous fields are demonstrated.

CLINICAL REASONING AND THE USE OF SENSORY TESTING.

Experienced clinicians will comment that a level of nerve root involvement can frequently be approximated from dermatomal involvement, and there is some research support for this, particularly in the lower lumbar spine (Kortelainen et al. 1985). However this clinical finding must be reasoned along with other information collected (eg. reflex tests, kind of injury, gross

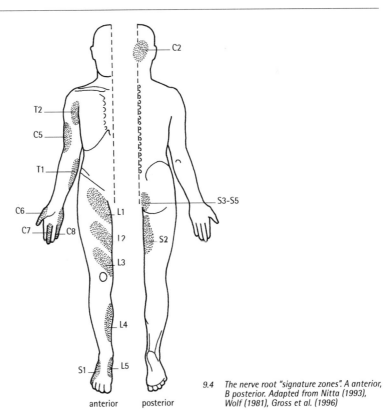

9.4   The nerve root "signature zones". A anterior, B posterior. Adapted from Nitta (1993), Wolf (1981), Gross et al. (1996)

anterior   posterior

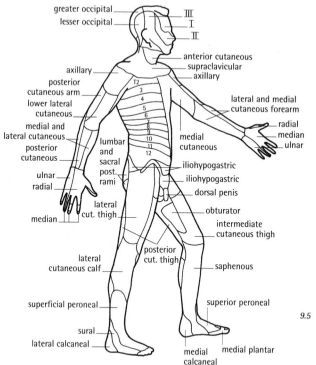

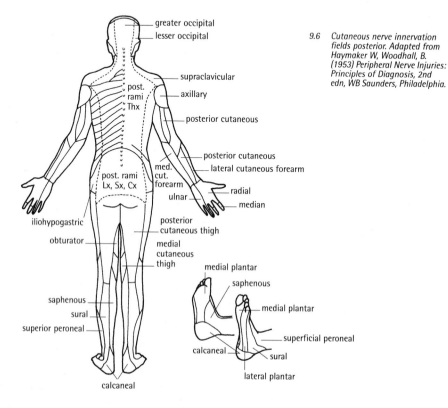

9.5   *Cutaneous innervation fields side view. Adapted from Haymaker W, Woodhall, B. (1953) Peripheral Nerve Injuries: Principles of Diagnosis, 2nd edn, WB Saunders, Philadelphia.*

9.6   *Cutaneous nerve innervation fields posterior. Adapted from Haymaker W, Woodhall, B. (1953) Peripheral Nerve Injuries: Principles of Diagnosis, 2nd edn, WB Saunders, Philadelphia.*

presentation, absence of other dermatomal involvement) and linked with the clinician's previous patterns of nerve root involvement collected over the past.

Similarly, symptoms in the signature zones do not announce a nerve root disorder. It provides information, which in the presence of other information strengthens a clinical diagnosis that a nerve root disorder is a part of the patients clinical picture.

SENSORY EXAMINATION PERFORMANCE

There are a number of components to the sensory and motor examination. These are summarised in table 9.2.

SKIN SENSATIONS - LIGHT TOUCH

The impulses conveying light touch (and proprioception and vibration) travel predominately in the large myelinated fibres (A alpha and beta), whose cell bodies are in the dorsal root ganglia or the ganglia of the cranial nerves. Dendrites enter the spinal cord via the dorsal roots. Considerable convergence occurs here as numerous primary afferent fibres link onto one spinal cord neurone. They ascend in the dorsal columns on the same side, in a somatotopic organisation (chapter 2). The dorsal column nuclei are at the foramen magnum. From this synapse, axons decussate and form the medial lemniscus which then projects to the thalamus. All the time the dorsal columns and the medial lemniscus collect incoming neurones from the arm and face. Somatotopic organisation is preserved all the way to the cortex (see discussion in chapter 2). The thalamus then projects to the somatosensory cortex, where due to the decussation, the contralateral body surface is represented in numerous somatosensory homonculi. This is essentially a serial processing of information.

TECHNIQUE

The guidelines for the examination of light touch sensitivity also applies for sensitivity tests using other stimuli. A sensory examination can be performed in sitting or lying supine or both. My habit is to perform the tests in supine.

The basic approach for sensory (and motor) conduction testing is to compare the responses to the stimuli from side to side and from distal to proximal, appreciating the possibilities of bilateral involvement. The patient must have the parts to be tested uncovered. Neurological

SENSORY	MOTOR
Skin sensation	**Observation**
light touch	Muscle wasting, tremor, fasciculation
superficial pain	Muscle strength tests
hot and cold	Quick/functional tests
Deep sensations	**Reflexes**
Pain	Specific muscle stretch reflexes
Proprioception	Superficial skin reflexes
Vibration	Central nervous system reflexes
Cortical sensory function	**Tests of autonomic function**

Table 9.2 Components of the standard neurological examination.

examinations cannot be done through socks. A tissue, piece of cotton wool, camel hair brush or Semmes-Weinstein filaments should be used. Semmes-Weinstein filaments are nylon monofilaments rather like thick fishing line that when placed perpendicular to skin will bend but maintain a constant force (Bell 1978; Omer and Bell-Krotoski 1997) (Fig. 9.7). These articles allow a more consistent stimulus to be applied than if the examiner's hands or an object like a cotton swab was used. The skin should not be depressed and this is why compliant objects should be used.

TECHNIQUE GUIDELINES - 8 KEY POINTS

1. Ask your patient to outline the area of sensory changes.

2. Describe what you are going to do to your patient and why you are going to do it. Establish a clear means of communication such as "yes" when sensation is considered normal or "no" when it is deficient. Ask your patient to say "don't know", if that is the case. Also, your level of interest in change should be made obvious to your patient. For example, small changes in a finely delineated peripheral nerve entrapment can be of interest; minor changes in a patient with widespread sensitivity changes may not.

3. Ask your patient to close her eyes.

4. A base sensation response is needed so that the responses can be compared. This may be extracted from the opposite limb or the abdomen. Where possible, when seeking a comparison, the tested parts should be matched to similarly sensitive areas. For example, the ventral aspect of the forearm is much more sensitive than the dorsal aspect, therefore a comparison is difficult.

5. The testing method is dependent on sources and mechanisms of neural deficit. For example, skirt around a peripheral nerve and dermatomal deficits (Fig. 9.8). Start distally and work proximally where there is a long strip of change or a total limb change. In the extremities, don't forget to test between digits and along digits

6. Traverse as many innervation fields and dermatomes as is necessary.

7. Always record findings on a body chart and in the neurological examination section of notes. "Tactile allodynia," or "hypoesthesia in the L2 dermatome" would be example of the

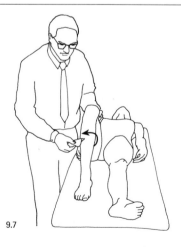

9.7

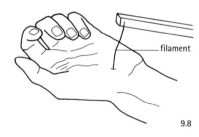

filament

9.8

9.7   *Test around the limb to include a number of dermatomes and cutaneous fields. From: Butler DS (1991) Mobilisation of the Nervous System, Churchill Livingstone, Melbourne (with permission).*

9.8   *Sensory testing, using a monofilament. The filament should be perpendicular to the surface of the skin. Increase pressure until the filament bends.*

terminology that could be used with appropriate findings. It is best not to do this on a bodychart which has the dermatomes marked on it. The urge to fit the patient's complaint into the therapist's construct of the problem may be too great.

8. All neurological dysfunctions, like any biological process, include a function of time. This means that they are likely to require repeat testing.

SENSORY EXAMINATION HINTS

These hints may be applicable to all sensory stimuli tests.

1. With patients who have very hairy skin, touching the hair could be a way of testing.

2. Repetitive touch or pressure may be needed to assist with a diagnosis of hyperpathia.

3. The processing of the sensory inputs may be distorted by the patient in severe pain. Do it at another time.

4. Always aim to decrease the patient's fear and anxiety before and during a neurological examination. Results may be different on the second visit.

5. It is important to have a "don't know" category of response for the patient. Patients may not be able to formulate a response in the categories the therapist has given them for a number of reasons. They may say "yes" or "no" when really they do not know.

SKIN SENSATIONS - SUPERFICIAL PAIN

Impulses which may be interpreted as pain are usually initiated in A delta and C fibres, the high threshold fibres to the spinal cord. Stimuli interpreted as superficial and deep pain run primarily in the lateral spinothalamic tracts. These tracts are not bundles as represented in texts but have considerable diffusion. In some pain states activation of A beta fibres may cause pain. Higher central nervous system pathways related to pain are discussed in chapter 2, 3 and 4. There is much more complexity processing a pain stimulus than a sensory stimulus.

TECHNIQUE

1. Superficial pain should be tested after light touch.

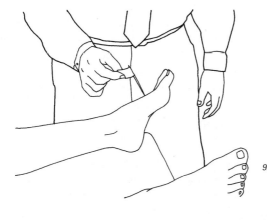

9.9   The flagged pin. Holding the flag and tapping the pin on the skin should give a repeatable stimulus. From Butler DS 1991 Mobilisation of the Nervous System, Churchill Livingstone, Melbourne with permission.

2. Use a new pin, or the sharp point of a new broken wooden tongue-blade for each patient. Get the patient to answer "nothing", "dull", or "sharp" or "don't know".

3. A flagged pin is also suggested. This can be easily constructed by placing a piece of sticking plaster around the end of a large pin (Fig. 9.9). It is possible to touch or tap the skin, while holding onto the plaster. This should allow a more repeatable stimuli.

4. The same general guidelines discussed above for the examination of light touch can be followed.

5. Be aware that some patients may have delays in pain appreciation and others may demonstrate summation, where repeated testing evokes an increasing pain response.

6. Allow a few seconds between each stimulus.

SKIN SENSATIONS - HOT AND COLD

Thermal sensitivity is not tested routinely and is not required if superficial pain sensation is intact. Thermoreceptors utilise A delta and C fibres and the anterolateral tracts as do impulses related to superficial pain. However, for patients who complain of symptoms related to temperature, thermal sensitivity should be tested. Following the suggestions of the Mayo Clinic (1991) test tubes should be filled with the hottest and coldest water available from free flowing taps, ensuring that the exterior of the tubes are dry to prevent evaporation and cooling of the subject's skin. Follow the same guidelines as described above for the testing of light touch.

DEEP SENSATIONS - PAIN

In the context of the sensory examination, deep pain refers to pain from somatic tissues such as muscle and bone, in fact any tissue other than skin. This is not tested routinely. However in the movement examination, where muscles and joints are moved, deep pain sensations are automatically tested.

Deep pain sensation is rarely performed as a passive test and is only routinely performed with comatose patients. In these patients the Achilles tendon can be squeezed.

DEEP SENSATIONS - PROPRIOCEPTION

Impulses related to proprioception (the sense of position and passive movement) pass along fibres in the posterior columns and medial lemniscus system, and then are distributed primarily to the thalamus and sensory cortex. Along with vibration sense, altered proprioception is a good indicator of problems in the columns (Mayo Clinic 1991), although the dorsal spinocerebellar tract is also likely to be involved (Ross et al. 1979). Clinicians may become aware of proprioceptive loss and thus the need for specific examination during a general examination. For example, while performing functional examinations such as getting out of a chair, performing balance tests or during a routine physical examination the loss may be noted. Remember that many aspects of nervous system function, such as cerebellar and basal ganglia function will be also tested during these movements.

A person's precision of proprioceptive recognition is the opposite to light touch; less than one degree of movement can be recognised in the shoulder, whereas an interphalangeal joint requires 5-10 degrees of movement for recognition (Cohen 1958). It makes you realise how important shoulder stability is for good hand function.

SPECIFIC TECHNIQUES FOR PROPRIOCEPTION

1. Ask your patient to close her eyes.

2. In the case of the foot, grasp a toe at the sides and then with a mimimum of pressure, gently move the digit in an up or down direction and ask her to specify which direction the digit is being moved.

3. Test slowly for a more refined test and ask her to comment as soon as she can feel the toe moving. Minute deflections can usually be appreciated. When a whole digit is moved, tendon and muscle stretch receptors along the muscle are activated, meaning that distal proprioceptive peripheral nerve involvement might be missed. To refine testing, place the joints in the mid position.

GENERAL TECHNIQUES FOR PROPRIOCEPTION

For the upper body, ask your patient to touch her nose with her index finger. Remember that this test gets easier to do with practice (try performing it yourself). The difficulty of this test can be increased by asking her to alternately touch her nose and your index finger, while the location of the finger is changed during the test. Seidel (1995) suggests asking the seated patient to pat both knees, alternately with front and back of both hands, increasing the rate gradually, while observing for stiff, slow, non-rhythmic movements. For the lower limb, test her ability to slide her heel down the shin of the opposite leg. This should be easy to do without any irregular deviations.

Ask yourself how long it has been since someone performed a neurological examination on you. It may be a worthwhile experience that takes you closer to understanding how your patient may feel.

DEEP SENSATION - VIBRATION SENSE

The sense of vibration (pallesthesia) is often altered with disease and/or injury in the nervous system. A tuning fork that vibrates at 128 Hz or 256 Hz should be used (Fig. 9.10). Nolan (1996) notes that although vibratory sensation is often regarded as a deep sensation, the stimulus will also activate low threshold rapidly adapting Pacinnian corpuscles in the skin. The Mayo Clinic manual (1991) indicates that a sharp gradient of vibration loss with a marked

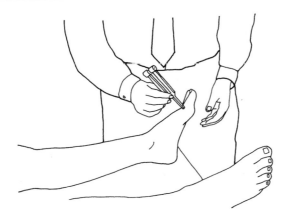

9.10 The tuning fork. From Butler DS 1991 Mobilisation o f the Nervous System, Churchill Livingstone, Melbourne with permission.

deficit peripherally and little proximally, suggests a peripheral nerve lesion. A cord lesion is more likely when there is no such gradient. Loss of vibration sense in peripheral nerve injuries may be seen more when associated with disease. The use of vibration sensation via a tuning fork to detect diabetic patients at risk of foot ulceration has been demonstrated by Thivolet (1990). Vibration presents quite a barrage of input into the nervous system. In some patients with chronic pain vibration testing may cause symptoms elsewhere in the body. However, its main use is in peripheral neuropathies.

TECHNIQUE

1. The best areas to test are the bony surfaces such as the clavicle, sternum, patella and extremities. A prong of the fork is struck on a firm object and the single pronged end is placed on the area to be tested.

2. Place the vibrating fork on your patient's sternum, foot or forehead and let her feel the buzzing sensation. Stop the fork buzzing by holding it and let them feel the sensation when the fork does not buzz. A very clear verbal relationship must exist. Have her say "yes" or "no," or "buzzing" or "not buzzing" or "don't know."

3. Once the prongs are struck, the fork slowly loses amplitude, hence double testing is required to allow for this (ie. test left side first then right side first). Another way of checking when testing the vibration sense of a digit is to place your finger under the digit and feel the sense of vibration to see if it is similar to that experienced by the patient.

CORTICAL SENSORY FUNCTION

All tests are of course tests of various aspects of cortical function. Some sensory tests can involve higher perceptual abilities, often referred to as cortical sensations. Inability to perform them should evoke suspicions of lesions in the sensory cortex, parietal lobe or posterior columns (Mayo Clinic 1991; Nolan 1996), although clearly intact input and output systems are required. These tests may not need to be routinely performed. They may be useful for a functional examination and should be evaluated in any movement dystonia.

Some of these sensory discriminatory activities are also suggested as exercises for cortical retraining (Byl and Melnick 1997). All tests are performed with the patient blindfolded.

GRAPHAESTHESIA

This is the ability to recognise and identify numbers or letters written on the skin. Use a blunt stick or pen. Let the patient watch one or two demonstrations first and then test her with her eyes closed. Make sure that the numbers and letters are written with the clinician facing the same way as the patient so that they are not presented as "upside down".

FINGER IDENTIFICATION

One of the subject's fingers is touched by the examiner and the subject uses her other hand to identify the touched finger.

STEREOGNOSIS

This is the ability to recognise and identify an object by handling it. Keys, coins and paper clips are commonly used. The objects or forms could then be identified in a picture.

TWO-POINT DISCRIMINATION

This is an innervation density test, requiring considerable cortical abilities. The ability of the nervous system to discriminate two points of sensory input depends on the part of the body tested. As a guideline, the approximate distances where two points of stimulation can be correctly identified are: fingertips 2-7mm; palms 8-15mm; dorsum of the hands 20-30mm; dorsum of the feet 30-40mm; and 40-80mm on the back (Mayo Clinic 1991; Barkauskas 1994). As with all tests, explain the procedure to the patient and then ask her to respond to your testing by saying "one", "two" or "don't know". A paper clip opened out could provide an adequate stimulus although commercial "two-point discriminators" are available (Mackinnon and Dellon 1988).

MANUAL TESTS OF MOTOR FUNCTION

Many clinicians will perform reflex testing - it's easy and quick, but muscle testing and a sensory examination are often omitted (Little et al. 1996). Time is often a problem. I also believe that many manual therapists tend to neglect these aspects of the examination or perform them with routine non-analytical monotony because that is what they were taught to do. This is unfortunate because the tests can provide much valuable information. In particular, some neurological lesions can be localised and their severity judged. Manual muscle testing is a skill that must be based on a sound knowledge of anatomy and tissue relationships. It is also a skill that takes time to learn and which must be enhanced by experiences with strong, weak and injured patients. The descriptions in texts are easy - the integration into clinical examination and analysis are sometimes not.

MUSCLE WASTING

Wasting is an objective change which can be measured by a tape measure. It is a finding that can relate to treatment goals and it is something that the patient can relate to. Often patients will be unaware of wasting, especially in the calf, gluteals and around the scapula and may be quite shocked when they are made aware of it. The word "wasting" is quite evocative so be careful using it. Wasting may be due to previous muscular or neurological injuries and some clarification will be needed to ascertain this. Be aware that swelling can sometimes mask the extent of wasting and that easily observable asymmetries are a possibility, particular in sportspeople with dominant use of one side, such as a tennis player. Kerr at al. (1988) showed in 136 patients with sciatica, that calf muscle wasting had a low sensitivity (.29) but very high specificity (.94) for diagnosing disc disease. Calves are worth observing in sciatica. They can also by easily measured with a tape measure.

The muscle power examination is very important for motor nerves, such as the suprascapular nerve on the basis that there is no sensory field to assist diagnosis. In this case, atrophy of the supraspinatus and infraspinatus may be observed (Vastamaki and Goransson 1993). A wasted muscle should also be palpated. The texture may be different from the muscle on the contralateral side. It may not even be palpable. Kirkpatrick (1982) demonstrated in 100 patients that if the extensor digitorum brevis muscle could not be palpated, it was a likely predictor of neuropathy in the peroneal nerve.

TREMOR AND FASCICULATION

Tremor and fasciculation are common, particularly where patients have long standing chronic pain or Parkinson's disease. Tremor is an involuntary rhythmic contraction of muscles, producing the appearance of trembling or quivering. Fasciculations are spontaneous visible or palpable contractions of muscle fibres associated with a single motor unit (Nolan 1996). Many tremors are physiological. Nearly everyone would have experienced tremor from fatigue, fright, hunger and certainly from the cold. The tremors seen in many chronic pain patients may result from emotional stress or fatigue.

Fasciculations are usually benign, but may result from peripheral nerve and nerve root disorders, poliomyelitis and spinal cord disease (Mayo Clinic 1991). The stress of worrying about the meaning of fasciculations is what is usually harmful, particularly if people know it may represent motor neurone disease.

MUSCLE POWER – GENERAL COMMENTS ON TECHNIQUE

1. Muscle power evaluation may not be necessary in some patients. In some there may be no diagnostic value, in others the testing may aggravate symptoms. In some patients, a more general examination of movement and functional movement may be more important than a focused examination of specific muscles or movements. Individual muscle testing is usually performed for the localisation of sources of damaged muscles, nerve roots or peripheral nerves.

2. A maximal contraction is required if possible, and then you apply a counterforce until the muscle "gives".

3. Some muscles require careful positioning prior to testing. For example, for most patients, calf strength may need to be tested in its outer range thus requiring the test to be performed in standing. The biceps should be tested in its outer range as it can be too powerful for the examiner if tested in its inner range.

4. I prefer to do most muscle testing with the patient in supine as this offers good stabilisation for the rest of her body and should offer better re-test accuracy.

5. As in sensory testing, reasoned hypotheses in all categories (chapter 6) (Fig. 9.1), should be made prior to examination. The muscle power examination simply allows strengthening or rejection of hypotheses already made. Surprising findings may significantly change your reasoning.

0	no contraction
1	flicker or trace of contraction
2	active movement with gravity eliminated
3	active movement against gravity
4	active movement against gravity and some resistance
5	normal power

Table 9.3 Grading of muscle function
From: Medical Research Council (1976) Aids to the Examination of the Peripheral Nervous System.
Memorandum No. 45, H.M.S.O., London.

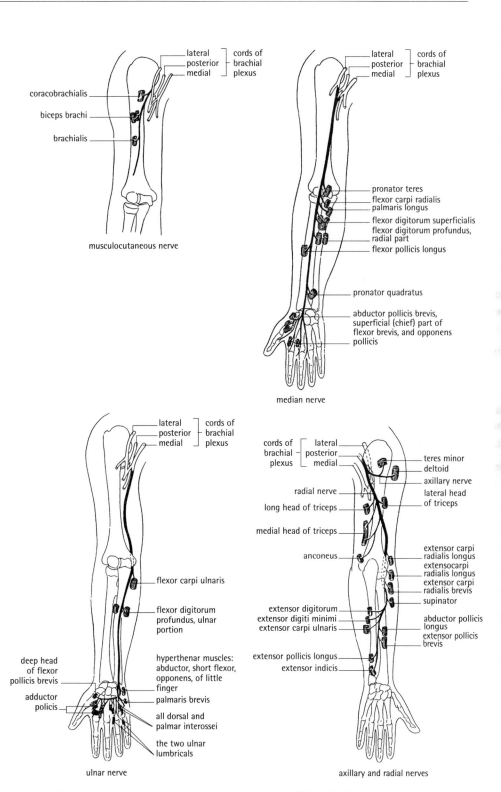

lateral ⎤ cords of
posterior ⎬ brachial
medial ⎦ plexus

coracobrachialis

biceps brachi

brachialis

musculocutaneous nerve

lateral ⎤ cords of
posterior ⎬ brachial
medial ⎦ plexus

pronator teres
flexor carpi radialis
palmaris longus
flexor digitorum superficialis
flexor digitorum profundus,
radial part
flexor pollicis longus

pronator quadratus

abductor pollicis brevis,
superficial (chief) part of
flexor brevis, and opponens
pollicis

median nerve

lateral ⎤ cords of
posterior ⎬ brachial
medial ⎦ plexus

flexor carpi ulnaris

flexor digitorum
profundus, ulnar
portion

deep head
of flexor
pollicis brevis

adductor
policis

hyperthenar muscles:
abductor, short flexor,
opponens, of little
finger

palmaris brevis

all dorsal and
palmar interossei

the two ulnar
lumbricals

ulnar nerve

cords of ⎡ lateral
brachial ⎬ posterior
plexus ⎣ medial

teres minor
deltoid
axillary nerve

radial nerve

long head of triceps

lateral head
of triceps

medial head of triceps

anconeus

extensor carpi
radialis longus
extensocarpi
radialis longus
extensor carpi
radialis brevis
supinator

extensor digitorum
extensor digiti minimi
extensor carpi ulnaris

abductor pollicis
longus
extensor pollicis
brevis

extensor pollicis longus
extensor indicis

axillary and radial nerves

9.11   *The motor distribution of nerves in the upper limbs. From Jenkins DB (1991) Hollinshead's Functional Anatomy of the Limbs and Back, 6th edn. WB Saunders, Philadelphia, with permission*

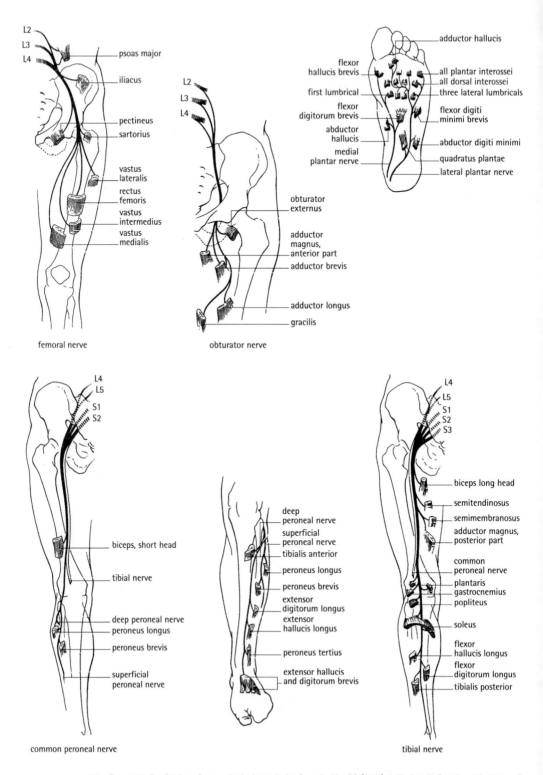

9.11   The motor distribution of nerves in the lower limbs. From Jenkins DB (1991) Hollinshead's Functional Anatomy of the Limbs and Back, 6th edn. WB Saunders, Philadelphia, with permission

6. Comparisons are made with the other side and you will need to draw on previous experiences with muscle testing.

7. Where possible, palpate the tendons of the muscle being tested. Feel for the "springiness" in the tendon and compare this with the other side. This is particularly useful for testing muscles such as tibialis anterior and the extensors of the toes, or the tendons which make up the anatomical snuff box.

8. Documentation is important. The grading suggested by the Medical Research Council (1976) is an easy to use grading system in the clinic (Table. 9.3).

Rather than list particular muscles for testing I have listed the examination techniques by movement and have included the most commonly tested movements. For further details of individual muscle testing, there are a number of useful texts (Kendall et al. 1971; Daniels and Worthingham 1972; Hoppenfeld 1976; Smorto and Basmajian 1980; Mayo Clinic 1991). In figures 9.11A and B, individual muscle innervations and in particular the site of innervation along the main nerve trunk are shown.

COMMONLY PERFORMED TESTS OF MUSCLE POWER

In this section, the movement to be tested is listed, followed by the principal and usual innervating motor roots, the peripheral nerve and the major muscle/muscles involved. Any variations to testing are also noted and common muscle tests for peripheral nerve trunks are also discussed. It is hoped that the system where movement is tested rather than specific anatomy will facilitate easier use in the clinic.

UPPER LIMB

SCAPULAR RETRACTION: C4-5, DORSAL SCAPULAR NERVE, RHOMBOIDS AND LEVATOR SCAPULAE

The muscles innervated by the dorsal scapular nerve attach the medial border of the scapula to the thoracic and cervical spines. They have an important scapula stabilising function during arm movement and act to adduct, elevate and rotate the scapula. Lay your patient prone, flex her elbows and ask her to take her flexed elbows away from her body as in figure 9.12A. Encourage her not to elevate her shoulder girdle. The examiner's hand on the shoulder can prevent this. Make sure she lifts hands and elbows off the bed. The scapula will abduct away from the spine if the muscles are weak and this should be easily seen.

SHOULDER ELEVATION: C4, SPINAL ACCESSORY NERVE, UPPER TRAPEZIUS ASSISTED BY LEVATOR SCAPULAE

This is best performed with the patient in sitting. Stand behind her and place your hands on her shoulders as in figure 9.12B. Ask her to shrug her shoulders as high as possible and then apply an increasing downward pressure. The scapular elevators can be particularly powerful in some patients and they may not be able to be "broken".

SHOULDER ABDUCTION: C5-6, AXILLARY NERVE, DELTOIDS AND SUPRASPINATUS

Test both sides at once. Stand behind your patient. Guide her arms with flexed elbows out to approximately 30 degrees of abduction. Then ask her to hold against you while you gradually increase the inwards pressure on her arms (Fig. 9.12C).

By altering your hand position and thus moving the direction of resistance, shoulder internal and external rotation can also be tested conveniently in this position and so can shoulder adduction (C6-7-8).

During shoulder abduction, the muscles can be palpated. Palpate the supraspinatus muscle while the patient abducts the shoulder. If the overlying trapezius muscle is relaxed by lateral flexion to the sided tested and then rotated away from the side tested, this should allow for a better quality palpation of the supraspinatus.

ELBOW FLEXION: C5-6, MUSCULOCUTANEOUS NERVE, BICEPS, BRACHIALIS

The elbow flexors are best tested in greater than 100 degrees of extension, otherwise they are usually too powerful to test adequately. Note in figure 9.12D that the examiner has positioned himself so that the body weight is behind the movement. Remember when retesting, that the same starting range should be used. It is best to test in supination as this will exclude some of the automatic contribution from the radial nerve innervated brachioradialis muscle. Remember to retest with the same degree of supination each time.

The musculocutaneous nerve also innervates the coracobrachialis muscle. To test this muscle, test shoulder flexion with the arm in external rotation, elbow flexed and the forearm supinated.

ELBOW EXTENSION: C6-7-8, RADIAL NERVE, TRICEPS

A very similar position to the test for the elbow flexors can be used as shown in figure 9.12E. Triceps is best tested with the elbow more flexed, say to 70 or 80 degrees. Scrutinise the contraction as well as feel the action when the muscle is particularly weak.

Resisted elbow extension will test for any proximal injuries of the radial nerve, although high radial nerve lesions will leave the triceps intact. Brachioradialis should be tested in mid range supination/pronation, that is with the "thumb up", and then elbow flexion resisted. The muscle can be observed and palpated.

THUMB TIP EXTENSION: C7-8, POSTERIOR INTEROSSEUS NERVE, EXTENSOR POLLICIS LONGUS

Note in figure 9.12F, the examiner has grasped and stabilised the patient's whole thumb complex, leaving only the interphalangeal joint free. The subject is asked to extend her thumb. The examiner can use an index finger to test the muscle. Flexor pollicis longus can also be tested in this position, if required.

TIPS OF FINGERS FLEXION: C7-8-T1, ANTERIOR INTEROSSEUS NERVE, FLEXOR DIGITORUM PROFUNDUS (DIGITS 4 AND 5 ARE INNERVATED BY THE ULNAR NERVE).

This test is shown in figure 9.12G. The patient is asked to fold her fingers in and then the therapist places his fingers on the tips of the patient's fingers and tries to straighten them. Note in the figure that the wrist is carefully stabilised.

For the median nerve, test the first or second distal interphalangeal joint flexion (functional muscle tests are described below).

FINGER ABDUCTION AND ADDUCTION: C8-T1, ULNAR NERVE, INTEROSSEI AND LUMBRICALS.

These muscles are best tested as in figure 9.12H. The patient is asked to "make a platform" with her flexed metacarpophalangeal joints. This position is stabilised, then the examiner

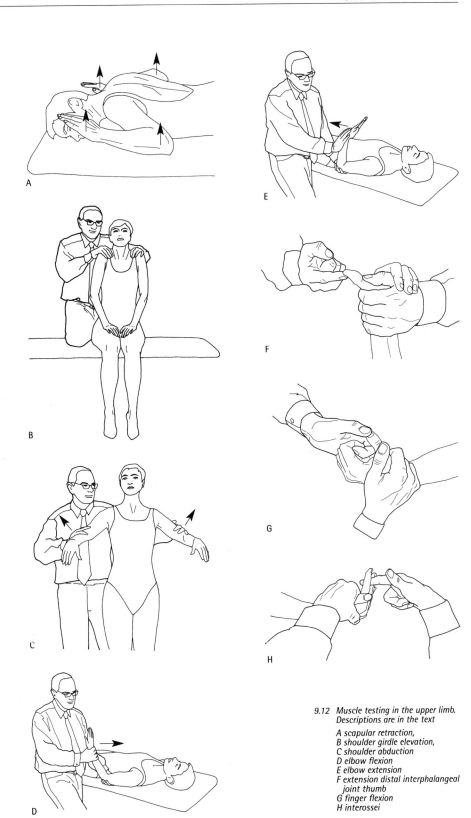

9.12 *Muscle testing in the upper limb.*
Descriptions are in the text

A scapular retraction,
B shoulder girdle elevation,
C shoulder abduction
D elbow flexion
E elbow extension
F extension distal interphalangeal
* joint thumb*
G finger flexion
H interossei

places a finger individually in each of the web spaces and asks the patient to "hold on as hard a possible" as the examiner tries to draw the finger out. Some patients may be helped by saying "pretend my finger is a cigarette" and hold onto it as hard as you can". Make sure your patients don't "cheat" by flexing their fingers.

Injury to the ulnar nerve at the elbow may affect all ulnar motor and sensory function. Refer to figure 9.11 for the levels of motor supply. If the wrist is stabilised, the health of motor fibres in the ulnar nerve can be tested by resisted flexion of the distal interphalangeal joints of the little and ring fingers. See functional muscle tests below for further muscle tests of ulnar nerve function.

LOWER LIMB

HIP FLEXION: L2-3-4, LUMBAR PLEXUS, FEMORAL NERVE, ILIACUS AND PSOAS MAJOR

The test can be performed with the patient in sitting and in supine. In supine (Fig. 9.13A), place your hands around the patient's thigh, flexed to 90 degrees, and then ask her to hold against your increasing pressure until she is using all her strength. The test in sitting may well be a more functional test, although variations are more likely with the changes in body position For the test in the sitting position, ask her to lift her leg against gravity and then against increasing resistance. While the sitting position is useful for a strong patient, the supine position may be better to identify weak muscle action.

Resisted hip adduction (L2-3-4, obturator nerve, adductor longus, brevis, magnus, and gracilis and pectineus) could also be tested in the position described above.

HIP EXTENSION: L5-S1, INFERIOR GLUTEAL NERVE, GLUTEUS MAXIMUS

This is tested with the patient prone. Ask your patient to extend her leg, keeping her knee flexed. Increasing resistance can be given as needed. This can be an important test to differentiate a site of neuropathy as the nerve supply to the gluteals arises proximally to the L5, S1 innervated muscles around the ankle (figure 9.11).

KNEE EXTENSION: L2-3-4, FEMORAL NERVE, QUADRICEPS

There are a number of ways to test knee extension. With your patient in supine, place her knee over yours and then encourage her to straighten her knee as far as possible. (Fig. 9.13B). You then try to resist the knee extension until it gives. This can be difficult with a strong patient and in this case, testing in sitting can be appropriate. More power is generated in the last 30 degrees of extension, so it may be necessary to test in 90 degrees of flexion in the sitting position.

KNEE FLEXION: L5-S1, SCIATIC NERVE, HAMSTRINGS

Knee flexion is best tested in prone. Place the knee in maximal extension and ask the patient to flex against resistance. Be careful as the hamstrings may cramp in this position. Consider also that the hip extension as described above will also test the same nerve roots. Remember that biceps femoris is more an S1 innervated muscle and the semimembranosus and semitendinosus are more L5 root innervated.

ANKLE DORSIFLEXION, L4-5-S1, DEEP PERONEAL NERVE, TIBIALIS ANTERIOR

There are no muscle-stretch reflex tests for the L4 and L5 nerve roots so muscle testing is particularly important. The patient is asked to dorsiflex both her ankles as much as possible. The examiner then tries to pull the ankles towards plantarflexion as in figure 9.13C. This position also allows you to apply some resistance against inversion. Where there is more weakness, the patient can hold her feet dorsiflexed, while the tendon of tibialis anterior can be palpated for firmness. As in all tests, a comparison must be made with the other side.

GREAT TOE EXTENSION: L4-5-1, DEEP PERONEAL NERVE, EXTENSOR HALLUCIS LONGUS

The patient is asked to maximally dorsiflex her ankles and then her great toes. The examiner places the tips of his index fingers on the toenails and then asks the patient to "hold against me" while pulling them towards flexion (Fig. 9.13D). It is advisable to swap hands and perform the test using the opposite hand to eliminate any left and right side strength and perception bias. The tendon of extensor hallucis longus can also be palpated for alterations in tension. Extension of the other 4 toes can also be tested (Fig. 9.13E). These have the same innervation and the tendons are easily palpable. The extensor digitorum brevis assists in extension of all toes, except the little one. It can be palpated for firmness on the lateral aspect of the foot during toe extension.

Drooping of the big toe at rest has been noted in patients with L5 root dysfunction (Madden and Lazaro 1997), suggesting involvement of the motor components of the nerve.

ANKLE EVERSION: L5-S1, COMMON PERONEAL NERVE, PERONEUS LONGUS AND BREVIS

Ask your patient to place her heels together as in figure 9.13F. You then place your hands on the lateral borders of her feet and ask her to "turn your feet out", as you apply pressure against the movement. This test can be difficult for some patients to perform as they tend to plantar flex the feet. Careful hand placement as exhibited in the figure, and verbal encouragement can overcome this. The peroneal tendons can also be palpated.

ANKLE PLANTARFLEXION: L5, S1-2, TIBIAL NERVE, GASTROCNEMIUS AND SOLEUS

The leverage of the powerful calf muscles makes them difficult to test in the manner of other muscles. Therefore the weight of the patient's body is usually necessary. If you are organised, you will have realised from the subjective examination that a muscle test will need to be done and performed the test before the patient lies down. Have the patient standing on one foot, hands on a wall for balance. Ask her to go up on her toes as far as possible (Fig. 9.13G). The patient will need to be encouraged to get ankle plantarflexion. The test should be carried out at least six times. With suspicion of injury to the innervation of the muscle, continue testing for longer if required. Note the time or number of repetitions to tire for each calf.

TOE FLEXION L5-S1: POSTERIOR TIBIAL NERVE, FLEXOR HALLUCIS LONGUS, FLEXOR DIGITORUM LONGUS

The foot is kept in the neutral position. Place your fingers under the patient's toes and then ask her to curl her toes. Ask her to hold the toes curled as you try to straighten them out (Fig. 9.13H).

DORSIFLEXION OF THE METATARSOPHALANGEAL JOINTS: L5-S1-2, POSTERIOR TIBIAL NERVE, INTRINSIC MUSCLES OF THE FOOT

The tibial nerve innervates all the intrinsic muscles on the plantar aspect of the foot, via the medical and lateral plantar nerves. The test is similar to the one described above for the flexor digitorum longus. Get your patient to plantarflex their toes against resistance and then attempt to dorsiflex the metatarsophalangeal joints. Ask them to try and "cup the sole of the foot".

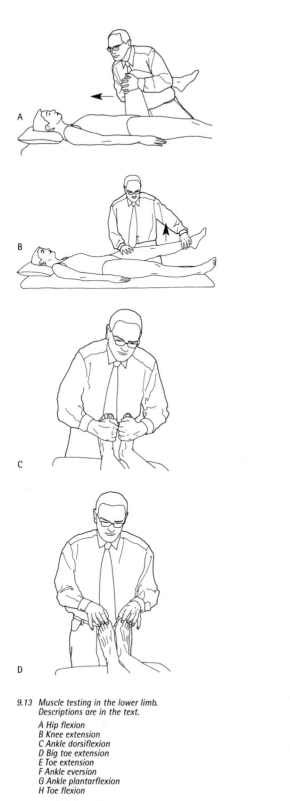

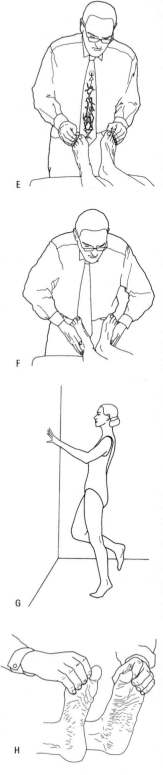

9.13 Muscle testing in the lower limb.
Descriptions are in the text.

A Hip flexion
B Knee extension
C Ankle dorsiflexion
D Big toe extension
E Toe extension
F Ankle eversion
G Ankle plantarflexion
H Toe flexion

QUICK/FUNCTIONAL MUSCLE TESTS

Tests that patients can do themselves have a special place. They create an awareness of the nature of the problem, they may form part of an exercise or a goal for the patient, and for the clinician they can be regarded as quick tests.

UPPER LIMB

For the **median nerve**, the patient tries to make a circle with the thumb and index finger. With weakness of the flexor digitorum longus, the patient will only be able to make a pear shape (Fig. 9.14A). Encourage them to turn the "pear" into a nice rounded orange and then test this action repeatedly. There may be fatigue.

The lateral key pinch test or the similar Froment's test (Fig. 9.14B) are good tests of the **ulnar** innervated first dorsal interrosseus muscle. For Froment's test, ask the patient to grasp a piece of cardboard between thumb and index finger as in the figure. Make sure she has an extended distal interphalangeal joint of the thumb. As she pulls on the cardboard, a difference in right/left strength can be easily seen as the interphalangeal joint of the thumb flexes on the weak side. (I have never been able to find out who Froment is or was.) Make sure you take a close look at the hand. Wasting in the first dorsal interrosseus muscle can easily be observed.

Another useful test for the ulnar nerve, particularly when there is minor weakness, is the ulnar border test. Note this in figure 9.14C. Try it on yourself first. It may take a little practice. Supinate your forearms and place your palms at eye level, ulnar borders together, fingers

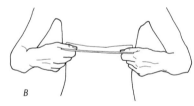

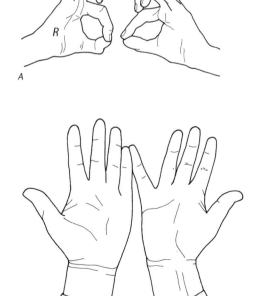

9.14 *Quick functional tests for the upper limb*

A *Median nerve. The right hand (R) flexor digitorum pollicis is strong and the left is weak*
B *Froment's test. The interphalangeal joint of the thumb on the weak side will flex.*
C *Ulnar border test. The weak side will quickly collapse*

extended. Keep the tips of the little fingers together and carefully tap the ulnar borders together. The weak side will collapse very quickly. Note that all these signs have never been experimentally validated and they need to be used with other data. However, their validation would make useful research projects.

LOWER LIMB

Walking on heels is a quick test for the ankle and toe dorsiflexors, and walking on the toes is a test of calf strength. Observe and also ask your patient which one feels weaker. The extensor hallucis longus and extensor digitorum longus can be quick tested by asking your patient to stand with equal weight on both feet and then to lift their toes up and down.

In sitting, flexing the hip is a quick test for the hip flexors. Minimally affected muscle power may be noticed from the squat to stand position.

USE THE MUSCLE INNERVATION MAP

In figure 9.11A and 9.11B the sites of branching of nerves to innervate muscles are clearly shown. Use of the maps is simple. Branches above a nerve lesion will continue to innervate, branches below will have altered innervation. For example, if the deep radial (posterior interrosseus) nerve is damaged at the radial head, wrist extension may remain intact because the innervation of extensor carpi radialis brevis may arise proximal to the lesion. In this case there will be weakness in finger and thumb extension because the innervation to extensor digitorum longus arises below the radial head.

REFLEXES

There are two kinds of reflexes that can be tested - the skin reflexes and the muscle-stretch reflexes. The latter are of major interest to clinicians. Sudden stretch of a skeletal muscle will result in a reflex contraction of that muscle. This contraction is dependent on monosynaptic connections between primary afferent fibres from muscle spindles and spinal cord motor neurones which innervate that muscle (Sherrington 1906). This is a simple reflex, the only known monosynaptic reflex in the mammalian nervous system. The term muscle-stretch reflex is used in preference to other terms such as deep tendon reflex and myotatic reflex as it imparts more physiological meaning (Brazis et al. 1990; Mayo Clinic 1991).

Reflexes are motor behaviours activated by sensory input or descending input from higher motor centres. This descending input is a balance of excitatory and inhibitory currents which provide a sensitivity adjustment. Therefore reflexes can be used to assess the integrity of both afferent and motor connections as well as the general sensitivity of the central nervous system. Note that muscle strength and tendon response do not necessarily correlate. For example an anterior cruciate ligament reconstruction will frequently result in a strength deficit in the quadriceps but will not alter reflex behaviour (Tsuruike and Koceja 1999).

THE SKILL OF MUSCLE-STRETCH REFLEX TESTING

Even the simple stretch reflex is not entirely stereotyped. The reflex behavior in normal and injured people can be altered by body position, gravity, load on the muscle and will be dependent on inhibitory and excitatory currents acting in the central nervous system. These are all possible reasons for the considerable inter-observer disagreement in testing (Stam and van Crevel 1990). Various techniques of eliciting reflex behavior have been described and are used clinically, however there are some common features to testing.

1. For all reflex testing, the major requirements are a relaxed patient, the muscle to be tested on slight stretch, an adequate stimulus and some reinforcement if required.

2. It is well worth taking some time to achieve relaxation. A pain free position if possible, an adequate explanation of the test and careful handling are necessary. Tests can be done in various positions and clinicians are encouraged to explore other test positions when necessary, especially for the Achilles tendon reflex. All reflexes can be performed with the patient in sitting or in supine. It is difficult or impossible to elicit a reflex when the patient is actively contracting the muscle to be tested, although sometimes a slight contraction may enhance the reflex (see below).

3. If the muscle to be examined is on too little or too much stretch, it may be difficult to elicit a reflex. Appropriate amounts of muscle stretch are shown in the following drawings (Figs. 9.15A,B,C,D).

4. Although reflexes can be elicited by the examiner's hand, a tendon hammer should be used. Beware the hard rubber tendon hammers - they can hurt if you strike your own thumb, the softer rubber ones are far better. Remember that rubber hardens with age. The tendon should be struck a few times, letting the hammer fall onto the tendon, allowing an even distribution of weight. The lightest percussion necessary to elicit a reflex should be used. In some cases, such as the biceps reflex testing, (Fig. 9.15A) use of indirect percussion via the examiner's thumb is suggested. This allows accurate localisation of the tendon to be tested and also allows some determination of the amount of tendon tension prior to the test. In addition, indirect percussion probably relaxes the patient in that she realise thats the examiner is hitting his own thumb before he hits hers.

5. Careful scrutiny of the muscle being tested is also needed. Sometimes a flicker of reflex muscle activity can be a valuable sign of pathological changes and a very positive sign of recovery for a particular patient. Always tell the patient what you are finding.

REINFORCEMENT TECHNIQUES

When a tendon jerk is hard to realise, reinforcement via muscular exertion remote from the test site can be used. Clenching the teeth will improve the triceps reflex as will turning the head to the side being tested (Tarkka and Hayes 1983). Other examples are clenching the jaw or the fists for lower limb reflexes, and tightening the quadriceps or the buttocks for upper body reflexes. As a general comment, reflex behaviour will be facilitated by contraction of muscles in remote parts of the body, and this applies to both upper and lower limbs (Delwaide and Toulouse 1981). Reinforcement can also be provided by asking the patient to think hard about making the movement related to the muscle tested (Stam et al. 1989). Make sure you test the reflex immediately after the reinforcement stimulus as the effect is only brief. Often, if your patient looks at what you are doing, the reflex response will be stronger.

The reinforcement techniques have become known as Jendrassik manoeuvres (Jendrassik 1883; Jendrassik 1885). Jendrassik tested the knee jerks of 1,000 subjects. Fifteen were missing knee jerks but all could be restored using the Jendrassik manoeuvre. A recent study showed that the manoeuvres improved reflex latencies of the knee jerk, but not the ankle jerk in normal subjects (Zabelis et al. 1998).

Perhaps muscle stretch reflexes can be enhanced if the muscle to be tested is contracted slightly, as was shown recently (Toft et al. 1991; Uysal et al. 1999). The results of Uysal et al.

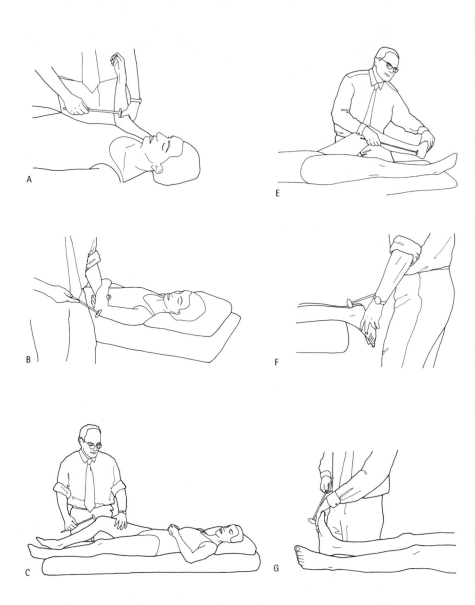

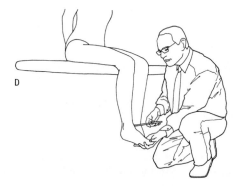

9.15 Muscle-stretch reflex testing

A Biceps reflex
B Triceps reflex
C Quadriceps reflex
D Gastrocnemius reflex in sitting
E Gastrocnemius reflex in supine
F Gastrocnemius reflex in prone or
  kneeling
G Gastrocnemius reflex, plantar strike
  technique

(1999) suggests that around 10-20% of full contraction is worthwhile. Experiment with this in the clinic by asking patients to contract the test muscle a little, by taking a little bit (say 10%) of the weight of the limb prior to the test. Altering the test posture may also assist in achieving a reflex. See the discussion below on testing the ankle jerk in various postures.

I firmly believe that all aspects of a neurological examination can be improved. Reflex testing has always been considered the easy part of the neurological examination and sometimes may be the only part of a neurological examination that some clinicians perform. The study by Impallomini et al. (1984) demonstrates the need for good handling skills. These authors reviewed the literature and found that the incidence of missing ankle jerks in the elderly had been reported as being between 27% and 50% in persons over the age of 65 and between 38% and 80% over the age of 80. Impallomini et al. (1984) examined 200 consecutive elderly patients admitted to hospital and by using Jendrassik manoeuvres, testing on the second day of admission, and using a plantar technique (Fig. 9.15G), found that only 6% of the patients had a missing ankle jerk and only 1.5% of these could be attributed to old age. The skill is in the testing and the patient-clinician relationship. Benassi et al. (1990) also showed that absence of muscle-stretch reflexes rarely occurred in the 67-87 year age group. The myth of missing reflexes in older people should be put to sleep.

SPECIFIC MUSCLE-STRETCH REFLEXES

Numerous reflexes have been described in texts. The most commonly used tests are described below.

BICEPS REFLEX (C5-6)

The test can be performed with the patient in supine as in figure 9.15A or in sitting. Find the biceps tendon at the elbow crease by asking the patient to flex her elbow against your resistance. Her forearm rests relaxed and pronated against your forearm. Your thumb is on the biceps tendon. To elicit the reflex, the tendon hammer is dropped carefully onto your thumbnail. This is an excellent reason to use a soft rubber hammer. Others may prefer to perform the test with the patient in sitting, with her forearm resting on her thigh.

TRICEPS REFLEX (C7-C8)

This reflex may be more difficult to elicit than the biceps reflex in normal subjects. See figure 9.15B for positioning. Note the patient's relaxed arm resting on her stomach and the gentle grasp of the examiner so that a contraction can be readily identified. The examiner's aim will need to be good. A good place to percuss the tendon is about 3cm proximal to the olecranon and central in the limb. Watch for a contraction in both the lateral and long heads of the triceps. The only difficulty with this technique is that in testing the opposite side, the examiner will need to turn around and face the opposite direction. With a little practice, this should be no difficulty.

QUADRICEPS REFLEX (L2-L3)

This test can be performed with the subject sitting with her legs dangling or in supine as shown in figure 9.15C. In the supine position, her knee should be flexed approximately 20 to 30 degrees and can be rested on the your knee. While some reflex behaviours here can be quite dramatic, in others, careful attention to flickers in the quadriceps muscle will be necessary. Because asymmetry is a key clinical indicator, it is worth testing both knees together. Try to have both of her knees resting on your knee so that both quadriceps reflexes can be tested with a minimal alteration of position. This test can also be performed with the patient in sitting and dangling her knees over the side of the bed.

CALF REFLEX (S1-S2)

In figure 9.15D, the test has been performed with the subject sitting and the examiner kneeling and resting her foot on his hand. There are a number of postures in which the Achilles tendon can be struck and it may be worth experimenting (Postacchini and Perugia 1992). The test can also be performed in a similar position as the quadriceps reflex, (Fig. 9.15E) with the leg externally rotated, the foot held in some dorsiflexion and then the tendon tapped or it can be quite adequately performed in prone (Fig. 9.15F) or in the kneeling position. In this test, she may need to be reminded to "let go" and relax her foot prior to testing. Some gentle passive movements from the examiner may facilitate this. The calf reflex has been researched in regard to posture. Two hundred and ten patients with a unilateral S1 radicular syndrome were tested (Postacchini and Perugia 1992). The calf reflex was normal in 58 patients, absent in 77 and varied depending on the test posture in 65. In this group of 65, the diminished calf reflex was best detected in prone, followed by testing in sitting, supine and in the kneeling positions. Relaxed calf muscles and decreased reflex activity in prone were given as reasons for this finding in the study.

Striking the tendon is the traditional method, but it is worth testing calf reflexes by striking your own fingers placed over the plantar surface of the passively dorsiflexed foot (Fig. 9.15G). This is likely to be a more appropriate test for elderly and bed bound patients and was the technique used by Impallomini et al. (1984). In one study, this technique was shown to have better intra and inter-observer agreement than the tendon strike method (O'Keefe et al. 1994). If a reflex is absent with one technique, then try the other.

THE PROBLEM OF MUSCLE-STRETCH REFLEXES FOR THE L5 RADICULOPATHY

There are no standard reflexes for the common L5 radiculopathy, although there have been some trials. The extensor digitorum brevis (EDB) reflex was described by Marin et al. (1995). The technique involved tapping the tendons of EDB just distal to the muscle belly. In Marin et al's study, sensitivities were low and specificities were high. The medial hamstring test has also been described (Felsenthal and Reischer 1982) and Jensen (1987) demonstrated a positive predictive value of 85-89% and a negative predictive value of 51-61% for L5 radiculopathy. These tests are not regarded as standard tests, but my suggestion is to try them.

LESS FREQUENTLY USED MUSCLE-STRETCH REFLEXES

If you strike any muscle there is likely to be a reflex reaction in that muscle, and textbooks often have long lists of reflexes. The four reflexes listed above are the most useful and have had some experimental attention. There are others which may be useful. For the **brachioradialis reflex**, positioning is similar for the biceps reflex, although the forearm is held in mid pronation and supination and the distal end of the radius is percussed. There may be little reason to perform this test given that the biceps reflex tests similar roots. Take care not to percuss the radial sensory nerve (location and palpation discussed in chapter 7) at the distal end of the radius. It is quite likely to be sensitive in conditions where cervical nerve roots are damaged.

For the **jaw reflex**, (cranial nerve V, mandibular branch of the trigeminal nerve) press down with your index finger on the patient's chin while her mouth is open a little and relaxed. You then percuss your finger. There is obviously no other side to compare with here. Sometimes a response is difficult to achieve, however, when it can be readily obtained without reinforcement it can be said to be abnormal (Mayo Clinic 1991).

Plantar reflexes have been described by a number of authors. These are elicited by tapping the heads of the fourth and fifth metatarsals (Grieve 1981) with the patient's foot in plantar flexion and inversion. It is very similar to the plantar strike technique described above.

The **thigh adductor reflex** can be evaluated by tapping on your finger or thumb on a slightly abducted thigh about 5cm above the medial condyle of the tibia (DeJong 1979). While the adductors share the same root supply as the more easily tested knee jerk, the motor supply is different - the femoral nerve supplies the patella tendon and the knee extensors, the obturator nerve supplies the adductors. Therefore with pathology such as an obturator hernia, the knee jerk may be present yet the adductor reflex may be absent (Hannington-Kiff 1980). You will need to compare with the other side.

ANALYSIS AND RECORDING OF REFLEX BEHAVIOURS

Neither areflexia nor hyperreflexia can be regarded as absolute evidence of abnormality, nor do normal reflexes exclude a neurological lesion. Findings must be correlated with other neurological observations, findings and reports, and compared with other ipsilateral and contralateral stretch reflexes (Mayo Clinic 1991). Minor changes can usually be neglected although asymmetry should always be noted. Note also that considerable variability in inter-observer and intra-observer reliability has been shown.

A hypoactive or diminished stretch reflex can result from changes in various components of the circuit, such as the muscle, the sensory or motor neurones. Hyperactive reflexes always result from central changes which allow increased excitatory input to motor neurones (Kandel et al. 1995).

Fading reflex responses identified by six successive percussions on the tendon have been suggested by Grieve (1981) and Magee (1997). There appears to be no neurophysiological rationale for this. Fading reflexes may occur due to changes in excitatory and inhibitory currents related to the examiner/patient relationship, and the diminishing novelty of the stimulus. Ageing will decrease the responsiveness of the patellar tendon jerk and also the responsiveness of the Jendrassik manoeuvre (Burke et al. 1996), but ageing alone will not eliminate muscle-stretch reflexes (Impallomini et al. 1984).

Zero to 5 scales have been proposed by Nolan (1996). The Mayo Clinic (1991) suggests a 9 scale rating from -4 to +4 and there is the National Institute of Neurological Disorders and Stroke (NINDS) myotatic reflex scale. Substantial intra and inter-observer reliability of the NINDS scale was shown by Litvan et al. (1996), however a study by Manschot et al. (1998) revealed that inter-observer agreement among doctors testing both scales was never better than "fair". These researchers suggested a verbal description was best with terms such as "absent, low, average, brisk, some clonus" and with a separate record for asymmetry.

I suggest that reflexes are descriptively recorded as absent, decreased, normal or increased with asymmetrical changes noted.

OTHER REFLEXES

SUPERFICIAL SKIN REFLEXES

Some reflexes can be evoked by receptors in the skin rather than in the muscles. Like the muscle-stretch reflexes, these are normally occurring phenomena that help preserve the functional status of the individual. They rarely require testing and they are very difficult to elicit in obese patients. For the abdominal reflexes, the patient lies on their back with the knees slightly bent. Use the blunt end of the reflex hammer or the tip of a wooden applicator tip to provide a firm noxious stimulus. Move from the side of the abdomen towards the midline at both upper and lower abdominal levels. Keep the stimulus within a dermatome as much as possible. The normal response is an ipsilateral contraction of the abdominal muscles and a deviation of the umbilicus towards the stroke. Applying the stimulus from medial to lateral will result in a mechanical deformation of the umbilicus and thus be far less specific. The reflexes are reasonably easy to elicit in normal individuals. A loss suggests corticospinal system disease (Nolan 1996).

The cremasteric reflex (L1-2) is the elevation of the testicle from stimulating the proximal and inner aspect of the thigh. The reflex is lost in lesions of the upper lumbar spine and corticospinal lesions. There is no female equivalent.

CENTRAL NERVOUS SYSTEM REFLEXES

When there are suspicions of central nervous system disease or injury, it is worthwhile performing reflexes that test the function of CNS neurones.

Clonus is repetitive muscle jerks at 5 to 10 per second in response to rapid stretch. It is usually tested in the calf muscles, (Fig. 9.16) although it may occur in any muscle. To test clonus, make sure the lower limb is relaxed as in either of the ankle reflex testing positions described, then abruptly dorsiflex the ankle and maintain the pressure. According to the Mayo Clinic (1991) this test has the same significance as hyperreflexia of the muscle-stretch reflexes, and is not necessarily indicative of a disease state in the central nervous system.

Clonus may also be elicited at the jaw and in the quadriceps. Clinicians may note that quadriceps clonus can sometimes be made worse when the body is in a slump position.

If the plantar surface of an adult's foot is firmly stroked with a solid object such as the end of a reflex hammer as in figure 9.17A, the toes normally flex and fan inwards. The **Babinski response** (dorsiflexion of the four lateral toes and adduction of the great toe - a fanning as shown in 9.17B) is a pathological reflex, part of the flexion withdrawal reflex, which only appears when the inhibitory currents associated with the corticospinal tracts are lifted. It is a response that may indicate central nervous system disease in adults. The Babinski sign can be observed in babies although the reflex is normally integrated by 12 months of age. The Babinski response is recorded as positive (upgoing) or negative.

THE CRANIAL NERVES

All clinicians should be aware of quick tests for the cranial nerves, particularly those clinicians acting as first contact practitioners. Where there is a suspicion that there is a problem with the cranial nerves, a full medical examination by an appropriate specialist is necessary. Quick tests are discussed below. For closer details consult any of the following references; Wilson-

Pauwels (1988), Sapira (1990), Brazis et al (1990), Mayo Clinic (1991), Goldberg (1992), and Nolan (1996). A relevant text for movement therapists is von Piekartz and Bryden (2000).

OLFACTORY (I)

Test the ability to identify familiar odours, one nasal passage at a time. The eyes must be closed. Try common non-irritating odorants such as orange, coffee, tobacco, and vanilla. The appreciation of smell is more important than the actual identification of the odorant. Deficits are usually related to local nasal disease, such as the common cold or the normal olfactory losses associated with aging. However a frontal lobe lesion or damage to the olfactory tracts, as could occur from a fall onto the back of the head, could cause a decrease in the sense of smell, in addition to a visual loss (Brazis et al. 1990).

OPTIC (II)

Visual complaints following trauma are always indications for appropriate referral. However, there are two quick tests which therapists can carry out. Visual acuity can be tested by asking the patient to read signs or describe pictures about 6 metres (20 feet) distant. Test both eyes, asking her to cover one eye at a time.

Peripheral vision may be tested by a confrontation test. Sit in front of the patient, ask her to cover her left eye with her palm and look at your nose. Cover your right eye, thus using your own visual field as a control. A static visual stimulus or either one, two or three fingers is presented to the patient in each of the four diagonals. She indicates the number of fingers

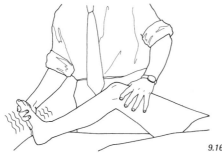

9.16 Clonus

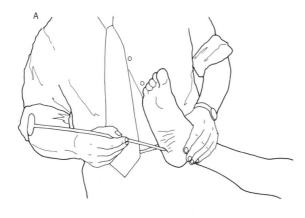

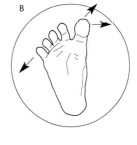

9.17 Babinski response
A Testing for a Babinski response
B A positive response

while looking at the your face. The test should be repeated a number of times (Nolan 1996). Any suspicion of change may require a more sophisticated examination.

OCULOMOTOR (III), TROCHLEAR (IV) AND ABDUCENS (VI)

These three nerves are controlled as a group by higher centres in the cortex and brainstem. Their integrated action is necessary for eye movement and ocular alignment. Strabismus refers to an abnormality of ocular alignment. The best and quickest test is to ask the patient to follow your finger while she keeps her head in the mid-position (Barker 1995). Test up, down, left, right and in the oblique direction. Watch for symmetry and speed of motion of eye movement and for the presence of nystagmus when her head is still. In addition to a somatic motor component, the oculomotor nerve also carries the parasympathetic supply to the pupillary and ciliary muscles of the eyes. It is thus important for pupillary responses of dilation and constriction.

TRIGEMINAL NERVE (V)

This is the major sensory nerve of the face with three major divisions as seen in figure 8.6. A sensory examination as described above can be used. Make sure that the zones of all three nerves are tested. A central nervous system lesion may involve all three divisions. Intranasal and corneal sensitivity are likely to relate to the trigeminal nerve. Quick tests of the muscles of mastication are difficult. The masseter and temporalis muscles can be palpated bilaterally as the patient bites down. Terminal branches of the trigeminal nerve can be palpated where the nerve exits the cranium, maxilla and mandible. This is described in the previous chapter.

FACIAL NERVE (VII)

The facial nerve is responsible for motor supply to the muscles of facial expression, for taste on the anterior two thirds of the tongue and sensory supply to part of the external ear. The patient's face should be observed for symmetry, especially the nasolabial folds and the corners of the eyes and mouth during movements and tests. Flattening of the nasolabial fold may be the first indications of a neuropathy. Voluntary facial movements are controlled by the motor facial nucleus. The whole face needs to be inspected as lower and upper facial muscles can be selectively affected. Upper motor neuron lesions may only affect the lower part of the face, hence the typical cerebral stroke results in mouth weakness yet the patient can still frown and wrinkle her brow. Lower motor neuron involvement such as Bell's palsy affects the whole of one side of the face. There are also involuntary movements associated with emotions. Involuntary and voluntary movement may be clinically dissociated, thus suggesting separate pathways with involuntary movements linked to the right cerebral hemisphere, hypothalamus and thalamus (Brazis et al. 1990). To test the upper face ask the patient to wrinkle her brow or close both her eyes tightly, and to test the lower part ask the patient to smile, puff out their cheeks, or show both upper and lower teeth.

VESTIBULOCOCHLEAR NERVE (VIII)

Vestibular sensation (balance) and audition (hearing) are carried by the eighth cranial nerve from special sensory receptors in the inner ear. Patients may complain of hearing problems or tinnitus (ringing in the ear). Dizziness, nausea and balance problems may be other complaints. The quick test for a hearing deficiency is for you to rub both index finger and thumb together next to the patient's ears and then to slowly move them away from her ears. Ask her when she can no longer hear. Side to side variations may be due to conductive deficits such as wax in the ear. A 256 Hz tuning fork can also be used. Place the vibrating fork on the patient's forehead and ascertain her ability to hear the buzzing noise equally with the left and right ear (Weber's test). She should hear the buzzing louder in the normal ear. Patients with any deficits need to seek appropriate referral. The vestibular system should be a consideration when testing gross function. The "finger to nose to examiner's finger test" also tests aspects of balance (see tests of proprioception earlier in this chapter). Some patients with vestibular disease report dizziness or vertigo when they march on the spot with their eyes closed (Nolan 1996).

GLOSSOPHARYNGEAL NERVE (IX)

Cranial nerve IX supplies the sensation of taste to the posterior third of the tongue, as well as sensation from the middle ear, eustacian tube and pharyngeal mucosa (Brazis et al. 1990) and thus the sensory component of the gag reflex. There are no quick tests. Patient may complain of numbness at the back of the throat (Nolan 1996).

VAGUS NERVE (X)

The vagus nerve is the major parasympathetic nerve in the body. A nasal quality of voice may emerge when the nerve is affected. The vagus nerve provides the motor control of the gag reflex. Observation of ease and control of swallowing is all that is necessary to observe here.

ACCESSORY NERVE (XI)

Cranial nerve XI provides motor supply to the upper trapezius and the sternocleidomastoid muscle. The upper trapezius muscle can be tested by resisting shrugging of the shoulders (see figure 9.12B). The sternocleidomastoid is tested by asking the patient to rotate her neck to one side and then you resist flexion of the neck. Simple observation of symmetry and palpation of muscle bulk may also add useful data. In some patients, the accessory nerve can also be palpated at the base of the neck, anterior to the upper trapezius muscle (see chapter 8 on nerve palpation).

HYPOGLOSSAL NERVE (XII)

The hypoglossal nerve is the motor nerve to the tongue. Fibrillations may be observed in the tongue, and the test for the nerve is to ask the patient to poke her tongue out. Observe for deviations. Strength can also be assessed by asking the patient to push her tongue to the left and right against the pressure of a tongue blade. A patient may complain of difficulties manipulating food in her mouth, and there may be some speech difficulties with the lingual sounds (N,T, D, L). This nerve is rarely affected, but testing is extremely simple and quick.

TESTS OF AUTONOMIC FUNCTION

The autonomic nervous system is difficult to measure without the appropriate equipment and laboratory. However therapists should be aware of obvious signs and symptoms that may indicate injury or disease in the system. This may necessitate referral for further medical attention.

THE EYE AND HORNER'S SYNDROME

The eye is the most well developed receptor in the body and pupil responses offers a unique view of autonomic nervous system activity in response to various inputs. Pupil size and shape is a product of complex combined sympathetic/parasympathetic activity, although the sympathetic nervous system is more involved in dilation. Manual therapists should note the long and complex oculosympathetic pathway in figure 9.18 and consider how it is related to the cervical and upper thoracic spines, the lung, tissues anterior to the cervical spine and a number of cranial nerves.

Horner's syndrome can occur due to interruption at any part along the sympathetic nervous system pathway. Cervical, thoracic and lung trauma may cause the syndrome. The clinical signs are unilateral miosis (constricted pupil), ptosis (drooping of the upper eyelid) and perhaps enopthalmos (eye retracted in the orbit). Sometimes there is a lack of sweating (anhidrosis) on the affected side (Farris 1991; Loewenfeld 1993). Ptosis or "lazy eye" is a 1-2mm drooping of the upper eyelid due to paralysis of Müller's muscle, a sympathetically innervated muscle in both eyelids. Sometimes a lower lid ptosis occurs but this is not as obvious.

There is also a "reverse Horner's syndrome" (Cole and Berghuis 1970; Cross 1993). This is an irritation of sympathetic pathways rather than paralysis. In this state there is intermittent or constant pupillary dilation (mydriasis) sometimes associated with increased sweating (hyperhidrosis) and facial flushing. The large pupils often noted during migraines could be due to sympathetic irritation. (Drummond 1990).

Pupillary alterations may be quite subtle, but the following examination is suggested.

1. Examine the pupils in dim light

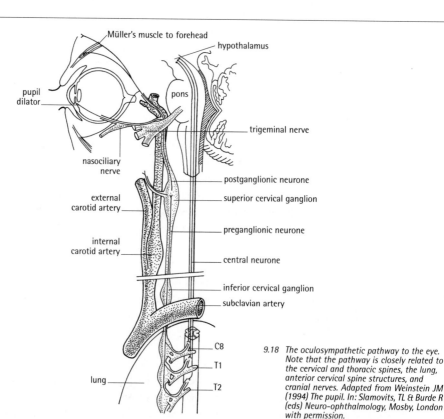

9.18 The oculosympathetic pathway to the eye. Note that the pathway is closely related to the cervical and thoracic spines, the lung, anterior cervical spine structures, and cranial nerves. Adapted from Weinstein JM (1994) The pupil. In: Slamovits, TL & Burde R (eds) Neuro-ophthalmology, Mosby, London with permission.

2. Compare left and right sides. Be aware that unequal pupils (anisocoria) are present in 20% of the population (Farris 1991)

3. The affected side will be slow to dilate

4. Clinicians may note that some movements will influence the pupils, usually causing dilation. I have noted pupillary dilation during a test such as the upper limb neurodynamic test, sometimes on evoking pain and other times when resistance is felt. I have also noted the pupil may become oval shaped during periods of spinal pain, usually on the ipsilateral side. Normally the pupillary control mechanisms are robust enough not to alter with cervical spine movements (Butler 1996), so any alterations may indicate some pathological changes.

Suggested indications are complaints of facial and neck sweating changes, cervical trauma especially to the anterior neck, hints of cranial nerve damage to the trigeminal and oculomotor nerve, C8 and T1,2 nerve root disorders, and lung disorders.

OBSERVATION AND PALPATION OF THE SKIN

Injured sympathetic fibres affect the innervation of blood vessels and sweat glands in the same area of skin supplied by the sensory fibre of the nerve (Stewart 1993). As clinicians, you may have noted the occasional vasomotor, sweating and trophic changes in neural zones when peripheral nerves and roots are injured.

Vasomotor changes include redness and sweating changes in the area. These are nearly always less prominent than sensory and motor changes. They may however be quite prominent in patients with a diagnosis of complex regional pain syndrome.

Alterations in sweating are commonly seen in patients and are often a cause of worry and discontent. You may notice sweating from one axilla but not the other during a physical evaluation. Ask your patient whether sweating is a problem or has altered since the injury/disease. Question her about dryness and wetness of socks and whether it is the same bilaterally. Hyperhidrosis is the term for sweating that is excessive for a given stimulus. In partial nerve injuries, excessive sweating may reflect regeneration or irritative phenomena. Gentle stroking with the examiner's fingers can pick up sweating changes. Stroking across neural zones will pick up sweating changes in peripheral neural zones.

Trophic changes occur with alterations in the sympathetic nervous system, especially in the extremities. Early changes you might see include pitting oedema and later, shiny and inelastic skin. The nails may show signs such as clubbing or become brittle and thick. Other complaints that clinicians may hear or extract from patients are changes in bladder, bowel and sexual function (usually erectile failure). Patients may need a medical opinion/treatment in these cases.

APPENDIX 9.1

REMEMBERING NERVE ROOTS AND THEIR FUNCTION

This appendix draws heavily on the work of Dr. Tony Pohl (1997). Many students use this simple system to remember the motor and sensory nerve root innervations. This is a classification for nerve roots. Tests for peripheral nerves and for the CNS will be different.

Trunk

This is the simplest place to start. There are no plexuses. The nerve roots on the trunk are sensory and follow the cutaneous field (see figures 9.2,3).

The nipple in men is around T4 and the belly button is around T9 presuming the belly is where it should be.

Lower limb nerve roots – motor

There are only five facts necessary to remember which muscles are innervated by which nerve roots in the lower limb.

1. In the leg everything starts at L2.

2. The muscles that move each joint are innervated by four nerve roots. Therefore the muscles around the hip are innervated by L2,L3,L4 and L5.

3. As you move down one joint, you move down one nerve root. Therefore the muscles controlling the knee are innervated by L3,L4,L5 and S1, the muscles controlling the ankle are innervated by L4,L5,S1 and S2.

4. "Front before back". This means that the muscles in the front of the joint are innervated "first". There will be two nerve roots innervating muscles in front and two behind. Therefore, at the hip, muscles innervated by L2 and L3 (iliacus and psoas) are in front and the gluteals innervated by L4 and L5 are behind (see table 9.4). At the ankle, the muscles in front such as

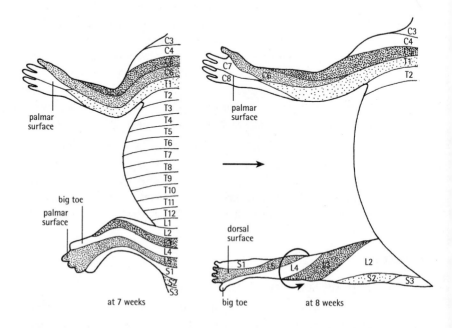

9.19   *By 8 weeks the lower limb rotates and gives the characteristic spiralling of the lower limb dermatomes. Adapted from Netter FH (1987) The CIBA Collection of Medical Illustrations, Volume 8, The Musculoskeletal System, CIBA-Geigy, Summit, New Jersey*

tibialis anterior will be innervated by L4 and L5 and those behind (gastrocnemius, soleus) are innervated by S1 and S2.

I hope you agree that it is all very simple. There is however point 5.

5. The nerve roots which control inversion and eversion also being at the ankle, begin at L4 of course, although they are asymmetrical. Inversion is L4 and eversion is L5,S1. I always remember that you have to go in before you go out.

I can't believe that it so easy, yet so many people forget !

Lower limb sensory innervation

The dermatomes have been described above in the familiar patterns, but how to remember them? As Pohl (1997) points out, they are easier to remember if we recall embryologically (Fig. 9.19) that our knees once pointed backwards early in utero. The knee rotated anteriorly as we developed and hence we have the spiralled dermatomes.

Upper limb nerve roots- motor

The upper limb nerve root innervation to muscles is a little more complex, but there are only four principles to follow, so stay with me.

1. The muscles that move the shoulder and the elbow are innervated by the same 4 nerve roots (C5-C8).

2. In the shoulder innervation is assymetrical: abduction is innervated by C5 and adduction by the rest. At the elbow, flexion is C5 and C6 and extension is C7 and C8.

3. As you progress down the arm you drop down a nerve root, but each joint movement is innervated by only 2 roots. At the wrist both flexors and extensors are innervated by C6 and C7 and at the metacarpophalangeal joints, both flexors and extensors are innervated by C7 and C8.

4. For an easy finish, all of the small muscles in the hand are innervated by T1.

Upper limb Sensory system

An easy way to remember the C7 dermatome is that the nerve arising from the longest spinous process (C7) innervates the longest finger !

Imagine a line down the front of the arm, forking to either side of the middle finger and crossed below the elbow. The arm is now quartered. The lateral upper is C5, the lateral lower is C6. The middle finger is C7. The medial lower is C8 and the medial upper is T1. The dermatomes thus go in a circle from shoulder to axilla (also refer back to figure 9.2 A,B).

Reflexes

Reflexes are simple - counting from the heels to the elbows

1,2 = ankle

3,4 = knee

5,6 = biceps

7,8 = triceps

Practice this a couple of times and you will never forget it.

REFERENCES CHAPTER 9

Andersson GBJ & Deyo RA (1997) Sensitivity, specificity, and predictive value: a general issue in screening for disease and in the interpretation of diagnostic studies in spinal disorders. In: Frymoyer JW (ed.) The Adult Spine: Principles and Practice, 2nd edn. Lippincott-Raven, Philadelphia.

Aronson HA & Lee BC (1963) Herniated upper lumbar discs. Journal of Bone and Joint Surgery 45A: 311-317.

Barkauskas VH (1994) Health and Physical Assessment, Mosby, St. Louis.

Barker S (1995) Screening for nervous system disease. In: Boissonault WG (ed.) Examination in Physical Therapy Practice, 2nd edn. Churchill Livingstone, New York.

Bell JA (1978) Sensibility evaluation. In: Hunter JM, Schneider LM, Macklin EJ et al. (eds.) Rehabilitation of the Hand, C.V. Mosby, Philadelphia.

Benassi G, D'Alessandro R, Gallassi R, et al. (1990) Neurological examination in subjects over 65 years: an epidemiological survey. Neuroepidemiology 9: 27-38.

Bovie J, Hansson P & Lindblom U (1994) Touch, Temperature, and Pain in Health and Disease: Mechanisms and Assessment, IASP Press, Seattle.

Brazis PW, Masdeu JC & Biller J (1990) Localisation in Clinical Neurology, 2nd edn. Little, Brown and Company, Boston.

Burke JR, Schutten MC, Koceja DM, et al. (1996) Age-dependent effects of muscle vibration and the Jendrassik maneuver on the patellar tendon reflex response. Archives of Physical Medicine and Rehabilitation 77: 600-604.

Butler DS (1996) Pupillary responses to posture. Thesis, School of Physiotherapy University of South Australia, Adelaide.

Byl NN & Melnick M (1997) The neural consequences of repetition: clinical implications of a learning hypothesis. Journal of Hand Therapy 10: 160-174.

Chaplan SR & Sorkin LS (1997) Agonizing over pain terminology. Pain Forum 6: 81-87.

Cohen LA (1958) Analysis of position sense in human shoulder. Journal of Neurophysiology 21(550-562).

Cole M & Berghuis J (1970) The reverse horner syndrome. Journal of Thoracic and Cardiovascular Surgery 59: 603-606.

Council. MR (1976) Aids to the examination of the peripheral nervous system. Memorandum No 45., HMSO, London.

Cross SA (1993) Autonomic disorders of the pupil, ciliary body and the lacrimal apparatus. In: Low PA (ed.) Clinical Autonomic Disorders, Little, Brown and Company, Boston.

Daniels L & Worthingham C (1972) Muscle Testing, 3rd edn. Saunders, Philadelphia.

DeJong RN (1979) The Neurologic Examination, 4th edn. Harper & Row, New York.

Delwaide PJ & Toulouse P (1981) Facilitation of monosynaptic reflexes by voluntary contraction of muscles in remote parts of the body. Brain 104: 701-719.

Deville WLJM, van der Windt DAWM & Dzaferagic A (2000) The test of Lasegue. Spine 25: 1140-1147.

Drummond PD (1990) Disturbances in ocular sympathetic function and facial blood flow in unilateral migraine headache. Journal of Neurology Neurosurgery and Psychiatry 53: 121-125.

Dubuisson D (1994) Nerve root damage and arachnoiditis. In: Wall PD & Melzack R (eds.) Textbook of Pain, 3rd edn. Churchill Livingstone, Edinburgh.

Farris BK (1991) The Basics of Neuro-ophthalmology, Mosby, St. Louis.

Felsenthal G & Reischer MA (1982) Asymmetric hamstring reflexes indicative of L5 radicular lesions. Archives of Physical Medicine and Rehabilitation 63: 337-338.

Foerster O (1933) The dermatomes in man. Brain 1: 1-39.

Goldberg S (1992) The 4-minute Neurological Examination, MedMaster, Miami.

Grieve GP (1981) Common Vertebral Joint Problems, Churchill Livingstone, Edinburgh.

Gross J, Fetto J & Rosen E (1996) Musculoskeletal Examination, Blackwell Science, Cambridge.

Haddox JD (1999) Neuropsychiatric physical examination. In: Aronoff GM (ed.) Evaluation and Treatment of Chronic Pain, Williams & Wilkins, Baltimore.

Hakelius A (1970) Prognosis in sciatica. Acta Orthopaedica Scandinavica (Suppl) 129: 1-70.

Hannington-Kiff JG (1980) Absent thigh adductor reflex in obturator hernia. Lancet 1:180.

Haymaker W & Woodhall B (1953) Peripheral Nerve Injuries: Principles of diagnosis, 2nd edn. WB Saunders, Philadelphia.

Hirabayashi S, Kumano K, Ohnishi I, et al. (1995) Relationship between the anatomic and dermatomal levels of spinal cord tumors in the thoracic region. Journal of Spinal Disorders 8: 93-102.

Hoppenfeld S (1976) Physical Examination of the Spine and Extremities, Apple-Century-Crofts, New York.

Impallomini M, Kenny RA, Flynn MD, et al. (1984) The elderly and their ankle jerks. Lancet 1: 670-672.

Jendrassik E (1883) Beitrage zur lehre von den sehnen-reflexen. Deutch Arch Klin Med 33: 177-199.

Jendrassik E (1885) Zur untersuchung des Kniephanomens. Neurol Zentralb 4: 412-415.

Jensen MC, Brant-Zawadzki MN, Obuchowski N, et al. (1994) Magnetic resonance imaging of the lumbar spine in people without back pain. The New England Journal of Medicine 331: 69-73.

Jensen OH (1987) The level-diagnosis of a lower lumbar disc herniation: the value of sensibility and motor testing. Clinical Rheumatology 6: 564-569.

Jensen OH (1987) The medial hamstring reflex in the level diagnosis of a lumbar herniation. Clinical Rheumatology 6: 570-574.

Kandel ER, Schwartz JH & Jessell TM (1995) Essentials of Neural Science and Behaviour, Appleton & Lange, Norwalk.

Keegan JJ & Garrett FD (1943) The segmental distribution of the cutaneous nerves in the limbs of man. Anatomical Record 102: 409-437.

Kendall HO, Kendall FP & Wadsworth GE (1971) Muscle Testing and Function, Williams and Wilkins, Baltimore.

Kerr RS, Cadoux-Hudson TS & Adams CB (1988) The value of accurate clinical assessment in the surgical management of the lumbar disc protrusion. Journal of Neurology, Neurosurgery and Psychiatry 51: 169-173.

Kirkpatrick CT (1982) Extensor digitorum brevis-a predictor of neuropathy in the leg. British Medical Journal 284: 238.

Knuttson B (1961) Comparative value of electromyographic, myelographic and clinical-neurologic examinations in diagnosis of lumbar root compression syndrome. Acta Orthopaedica Scandinavica (Suppl) 49.

Kortelainen P, Puranen J, Koivisto E, et al. (1985) Symptoms and signs of signs of sciatica and their relation to the localization of the lumbar disc herniation. Spine 10: 88-92.

Liguori R, Krarup C & Trojaborg W (1992) Determination of the segmental sensory and motor innervation of the lumbosacral spinal nerves. Brain 115: 915-934.

Little P, Smith L, Cantrell T, et al. (1996) General practitioner's management of acute back pain: a survey of reported practice compared with clinical guidelines. British Medical Journal 302: 485-488.

Litvan I, Mangone CA, Werden W, et al. (1996) Reliability of the NINDS myotatic reflex scale. Neurology 47: 969-972.

Loewenfeld IE (1993) The Pupil, Iowa State University Press, Ames.

Mackinnon SE & Dellon AL (1988) Surgery of the Peripheral Nerve, Thieme, New York.

Madden PJ & Lazaro RP (1997) Drooping of the big toe: another diagnostic marker for L-5 radiculopathy. Southern Medical Journal 90: 209-210.

Magee D (1997) Orthopedic Physical Assessment, 3rd edn. W.B. Saunders, Philadelphia.

Maigne JY, Lazareth JP, Guerin S, H., et al. (1989) The lateral cutaneous branches of the dorsal rami of the thoraco-lumbar junction. Surgical and Radiologic Anatomy 11: 289-293.

Manschot S, van Passel L, Buskens E, et al. (1998) Mayo and NINDS scales for assessment of tendon reflexes: between observer agreement and implications for communication. Journal of Neurology, Neurosurgrey and Psychiatry 64: 253-255.

Marin R, Dillingham TR, Chang A, et al. (1995) Extensor digitorum brevis reflex in normals and patients with radiculopathies. Muscle & Nerve 18: 52-59.

Mayo Clinic (1991) Clinical Examinations in Neurology, 6th edn. Mosby, St. Louis.

Merskey H & Bogduk N (1994) Classification of Chronic Pain, 2nd edn. IASP Press, Seattle.

Murphy RF (1987) The Body Silent, WW Norton, New York.

Nitta H, Tajima T, Sugiyama H, et al. (1993) Study on dermatomes by means of selective lumbar spinal nerve block. Spine 10: 1782-1786.

Nolan FM (1996) Introduction to the Neurological Examination, F.A. Davis, Philadelphia.

O'Keefe ST, Smith T, Valacio R, et al. (1994) A comparison of two techniques for ankle jerk assessment in elderly subjects. Lancet 344: 1619-1620.

Omer GE & Bell-Krotoski J (1997) Sensibility testing. In: Omer GE, Spinner M & Van Beek AL (eds.) Management of Peripheral Nerve Problems, 2nd edn. WB Saunders Company, Philadelphia.

Peeters GG, Aufdemkampe G & Oostendorp RA (1998) Sensibility testing in patients with a lumbosacral radiacular syndrome. Journal of Manipulative and Physiological Therapeutics 21: 81-88.

Pohl AP (1997) Assessment of nerve root function in the upper and lower limb. Modern Medicine of Australia 40: 148-151.

Postacchini F & Perugia D (1992) Changes in the ankle reflex related to posture. Journal of Bone and Joint Surgery 74B: 155.

Ross ED, Kirkpatrick JB & Lastimosa ACB (1979) Position and vibration sensations: Functions of the dorsal spinocerebellar tract. Annals of Neurology 5: 171-177.

Sapira JD (1990) The Art and Science of Bedside Diagnosis, Urban & Schwarzenberg, Baltimore.

Seidel HM, Ball JW, Dains JE, et al. (1995) Mosby's Guide to Physical Examination, 3rd edn. Mosby, St. Louis.

Sherrington CS (1906) The Integrative Action of the Nervous System, Yale University Press, New Haven.

Smorto MP & Basmajian JV (1980) Neuromotor Examination of the Limbs, Williams and Wilkins, Baltimore.

Spangfort EV (1972) Lumbar disc herniation: a computer aided analysis of 2504 operations. Acta Orthopaedica Scandinavica (Suppl) 142: 1-9.

Stam J, Speelman HD & van Crevel H (1989) Tendon reflex asymmetry by voluntary mental effort in healthy subjects. Archives of Neurology 46: 70-73.

Stam J & van Crevel H (1990) Reliability of the clinical and electromyographic examination of tendon reflexes. Journal of Neurology 237: 427-431.

Stewart JD (1993) Focal Peripheral Neuropathies, 2nd edn. Raven Press, New York.

Sunderland S (1978) Nerves and Nerve Injuries, 3rd edn. Churchill Livingstone, Melbourne.

Tarkka IM & Hayes KC (1983) Characteristics of the triceps brachii tendon reflex in man. American Journal of Physical Medicine 62: 1-11.

Thivolet C, el Farkh J, Petiot A, et al. (1990) Measuring vibration sensations with graduated tuning fork. Simple and reliable means to detect diabetic patients at risk of neuropathic foot ulceration. Diabetes Care 13: 1077-1080.

Toft E, Sinkjaer T & Rasmussen A (1991) Stretch reflex variation in the relaxed and the pre-activated quadriceps muscle of normal humans. Acta Neurologica Scandinavica 84: 311-315.

Tsuruike M & Koceja DM (1999) Conditioned patellar tendon-tap reflexes in patients with ACL reconstruction. International Journal of Sports Medicine 20: 263-266.

Uysal H, Mogyoros I & Burke D (1999) Reproducibility of tendon jerk reflexes during a voluntary contraction. Clinical Neurophysiology 110: 1481-1487.

van den Hoogen JMM, Koes B, van Eijk JTM, et al. (1995) On the accuracy of history, physical examination and erythrocyte sedimentation rate in diagnosing low-back pain in general practice. Spine 20: 318-327.

von Piekartz H, Bryden L (2000) Cranial Dysfunction and Pain. Butterworths Heinemann, London.

Vastamaki M & Goransson H (1993) Suprascapular nerve entrapment. Clinical Orthopaedics and Related Research 297: 135-143.

Williams RP & Sugars W (1998) Lumbar root innervation of the medial foot and ankle region. Australian and New Zealand Journal of Surgery 68: 565-567.

Wilson-Pauwels L (1988) Cranial Nerves, B.C. Decker, Toronto.

Wolf JK (1981) Segmental Neurology, University Park Press, Baltimore.

Zabelis TN, Karandreas NT, Constantinidis TS, et al. (1998) The effect of Jendrassik manoevre on the latency, amplitude and left-right asymmetry of tendon refexes. Electromyography and Clinical Neurophysiology 38: 19-23.

CHAPTER 10

NEURODYNAMIC TESTS
IN THE CLINIC

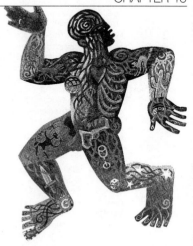

INTRODUCTION

THE BASE TEST SYSTEM

RELATIONSHIP BETWEEN BASE TESTS

CONCEPTUALLY, IT IS A DYNAMIC EXAMINATION

ACTIVE AND PASSIVE MOVEMENTS

A CLINICAL CATEGORISATION

CONCEPT OF STRUCTURAL DIFFERENTIATION

ANALYSIS OF STRUCTURAL DIFFERENTIATION - CARE NEEDED
TAKING THE BASE TESTS FURTHER - GO "JAZZY" IN THE CLINIC
WHEN AND HOW MUCH NEURODYNAMIC ASSESSMENT TO DO
RECORDING

ANALYSIS OF NEURODYNAMIC TEST FINDINGS

A SENSITIVE MOVEMENT DOESN'T PROVIDE MUCH INFORMATION
DETERMINING THE RELEVANCE OF THE TEST
IDENTIFICATION OF SOURCE
UNEXPECTED RESPONSES
THE ART OF GOOD HANDLING

REFERENCES CHAPTER 10

INTRODUCTION

The next two chapters explore neurodynamic tests and are the "how to" chapters. This chapter is the basis of performance and analysis of the tests. I hope you will refer back to it after chapters 11 and12

THE BASE TEST SYSTEM

You need to start somewhere with a neurodynamic evaluation. I have previously proposed a base test system (Butler 1991), utilising a series of tests which cover large tracts of neural tissues and inevitably other tissues. The base test system is a clinically intuitive system that evolved for ease of handling and to fulfill a perceived clinical demand. Where possible it is based on existing tests and the basic principles of neurodynamics (chapter 5). Whether the tests are refined or adapted or even used, depends on reasoned diagnoses and the clinical presentation. The base tests have been made as simple as possible with minimal components. This allows for ease of handling and accurate clinical test-retest. It also makes for easier research methodology.

The proposed base tests are passive neck flexion (PNF), straight leg raise (SLR), the prone knee bend (PKB), the slump test and 4 varieties of upper limb neurodynamic test (ULNT). All are described in chapters 11 and 12. The SLR, PKB and PNF are well established tests for an orthopaedic or neurological examination. The Slump and ULNT tests are still relatively new, but are logical extensions of the more traditional tests.

While the base tests may have a bias to a particular nerve trunk, root or section of meninges, they cannot be specific. Inevitably, loading in other neural structures will occur and neural/non-neural tissue relationships will alter. For example the relationship of nerve roots to disc pathology will alter. Hopefully from the early chapters you are already thinking past the pure physical input. Base tests such as a slump test will challenge the central nervous system's ability to accommodate inputs which may be painful, novel, feared or a reminder of a stressful incident. Movement will elicit motor responses depending on the meaning of the test to the person. Consider that the motor system responses may have been established prior to the test, it is not something which is test specific.

RELATIONSHIP BETWEEN BASE TESTS

It may seem that an all-inclusive test such as the slump test would preclude the necessity of testing SLR and PNF. While the slump test has been shown to be more sensitive than the SLR in patients with low back pain (Massey 1985), it is a repeated clinical observation that the responses will differ. It is possible to observe patients who have a sensitive SLR yet the slump is not sensitive, and vice versa. The anatomy and neurobiomechanics involved in the tests and the performance environment of the tests are very different.

A slump test and an SLR are not the same. Therapists and doctors persist in the fallacy that responses should be the same and sometimes when there are differing results in the two tests, suspicions of the organic nature of the patient's complaints often emerge. A pilot study (Dibden 1996) has shown that responses to the seated SLR and the supine SLR are not comparable in a large group of asymptomatic subjects.

SLR and slump responses could be different because:

• The components of the tests are performed in a different order.

• The slump test involves spinal flexion while the SLR is performed with the spine in a more neutral or even extended position.

• Patients may be more familiar with the SLR, which, depending on experience, could enhance or diminish responses. If it has been performed aggressively in the past, then apprehension and fear are likely to contribute to the test's sensitivity and range of movement.

• The patient is in more control during a slump test, SLR is out of the patient's control as it is more passive.

• The SLR involves the spreading of legs, the slump is a more "private" test and patients may feel more comfortable and relaxed.

CONCEPTUALLY, IT IS A DYNAMIC EXAMINATION

Neurodynamic evaluations have usually focused on elongating and gliding neural tissues. However, you should also consider the relationship of the nervous system to surrounding structures and the possibility of pinching forces being placed upon the system. In the clinic, think about whether the system can accommodate being shortened (as in spinal extension) and neighbouring structures pinching or "closing down" on it. For example, the structures of the cubital tunnel of the elbow close down on the ulnar nerve during flexion. The size of the intervertebral foramen in the lumbar spine is smaller in extension. "Dynamic roominess" is a useful term introduced by Penning (1992) and one which inspires clinical awareness. The concept is spreading to diagnostic studies as well. Examples are nerve conduction tests in various positions (eg. Kupfer 1998, Bronson 1997), flexion/extension myelography for spinal stenosis (Coulier 2000) and dynamic magnetic resonance imaging (Muhle 1998).

A design exists to accommodate pinching and compressive forces (chapter 5). However the "dynamic roominess" may be overextended by degenerative and or inflammatory changes in the structures of the spinal and intervertebral canals. It would also be dependent on the mechanosensitivity of the contained neural tissues. In the case of the cervical spine, the tests of lower cervical nerve root's abilities to cater to pinch forces is often referred to as Spurling's test. It involves cervical extension and lateral flexion and rotation towards the test side (chapter 15). Others may know the test and its correlate in the lumbar spine as quadrant tests (Maitland 1986). "Dynamic roominess" should serve as a reminder that when considering the physical health of nerves, you need to be aware of the neighbouring structures around the nervous system in both a static and a dynamic sense.

ACTIVE AND PASSIVE MOVEMENTS

All tests can be performed actively, although the SLR presents some difficulties. Where possible, I suggest that the tests can be performed actively before passively. It may be that a finding of good range and movement quality in a particular movement precludes passive performance of a test. There will usually be a greater range of passive motion than active. Where a passive evaluation follows an active evaluation, the patient should be better informed allowing better performance of the test. Protocols for active neurodynamic test evaluation are suggested for all of the tests (chapters 11,12). I like to encourage as much active use of the tests as possible including active structural differentiation.

A CLINICAL CATEGORISATION

When you are evaluating a patient, try to think about the mechanisms behind the sensitivity to your inputs. Is it more of a primary (tissue based) sensitivity or are there more secondary (central) influences.

An SLR in an asymptomatic person will usually cause some discomfort. This normal response is a product of peripheral and central mechanisms. The peripheral components could be muscle and fascia (non-neural) and/or peripheral nerve (neural). These are quite normal **physiological responses** of neural and non-neural tissue origin operating with the central nervous system in a control state (chapter 4).

If a person in pain has a limited and sensitive SLR, thus enhanced mechanical sensitivity (hyperalgesia), this will also be a product of peripheral and central nervous system processing. The peripheral component could be non-neural (eg. muscle or joint) or neural (eg. nerve root). These are **clinical responses** of neural and non-neural tissue origin. However they will also include varying degrees of central nervous system up or down regulation. Depending on the state of the CNS, responses can be enhanced or decreased (Fig. 10.1).

CONCEPT OF STRUCTURAL DIFFERENTIATION

An SLR evoked response, say in the buttocks, which is worsened by the addition of ankle dorsiflexion is said to confirm the role of the nervous system in the disorder (eg. Breig and Troup 1979; Butler 1991). During the slump test, a hamstring area symptom response eased by neck extension is said to be neurogenic. If a person with an ankle injury has pain on plantar flexion and inversion of her foot, this pain could be predominately due to peripheral mechanisms related to tissues at the foot. However, if the foot position could be held and a straight leg raise added, resulting in an increase of pain, then the inference would be that there was some physical involvement of the nervous system. Perhaps small branches are embedded in organising scar and are sensitive and starved of blood. This examination technique is illustrated in figure 11.6. Further clinical data would need to be collected to

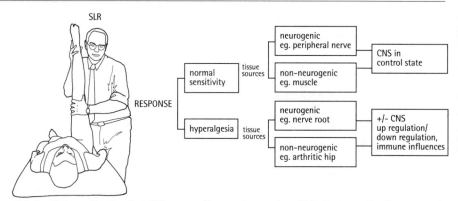

10.1 Sensitivity considerations in an SLR response. There may be normal sensitivity due to neural and/or non-neural sources and the CNS in control state. A hyperalgesic state could be due to neural and/or non-neural injury and be modified by the state of the CNS.

strengthen or reject such a hypothesis and to determine where and how the nervous system was involved.

Structural differentiation can be used actively. Some patients diagnosed with de Quervain's disease may have a local neuropathy of the musculocutaneous or superficial radial nerve rather than a tendon/tendon sheath disorder (Mackinnon and Dellon 1988). Finkelstein's test (Finkelstein 1930) of thumb flexion and wrist ulnar deviation should therefore be considered a test of all lateral wrist tissues. However, if the "Finkelstein position" is maintained and the elbow extended (Fig. 10.2), symptoms which alter are suggestive of a neurogenic origin. Even better, you could check the effect of shoulder girdle elevation and depression. Perhaps the most commonly performed active structural differentiation procedure is illustrated in figure 10.3. Here the patient with spinal pain stands with her hip flexed. This is quite common in acute nerve root disorders. For active structural differentiation, ask her to keep her back still and then ask her to carefully flex her neck. If this alters the evoked lumbar pain then you would expect some nervous system involvement. In some patients, cervical extension will "unload" pressures on neural structures and the hip and knee will flex further.

ANALYSIS OF STRUCTURAL DIFFERENTIATION – CARE NEEDED

The clinical examples mentioned above are attractive and often exciting findings for patients and clinicians. However if you find that a remote movement alters an evoked symptom this does not mean much in terms of biological mechanisms. It may well preferentially "unload" one tissue and assist in a clinical diagnosis. It should not lead to an instant diagnosis of "neural tension" or "altered neurodynamics". Be modest (though quietly excited!) with your finding. It comprises one more piece of data to add to others to support or reject the hypothesis that the nervous system is sensitive and/or physically compromised in that person's particular pain state.

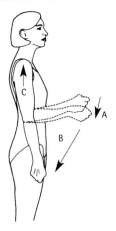

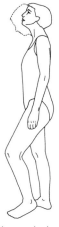

10.2 The Finkelstein test (A) could be a test of soft tissues (including nerve) at the wrist. If the elbow were extended, with the wrist position maintained as in B, then an alteration in symptoms may suggest a neurogenic origin. Further clarification will be provided if shoulder girdle elevation as in C alters symptoms.

10.3 Patients with severe back pain, apparently of nerve root origin, often stand with a flexed knee. Cervical flexion may worsen symptoms and extension will lessen symptoms.

The mechanisms behind structural differentiation probably depend on the processing state of the nervous system (chapters 3 and 4). If your patient's symptoms are related to a central sensitisation state, then the addition or removal of normal input may still make a difference. The nervous system may not even be physically compromised. Recall from chapter 3 that when the central nervous system is in a sensitised state, that A beta input can gain access to the pain processing system. Hence an SLR may evoke spinal pain and the addition of ankle dorsiflexion may increase it by adding further normal input to an already sensitised system. This is not physically compromised nerve per se, it is sensitised nervous system. However the same SLR plus dorsiflexion responses could occur if the pain state was due to low lumbar nerve root irritation/compression. They are both positive tests, but positive due to different mechanisms. Management is likely to differ.

There will also be structural differentiation difficulties and perhaps confusion when there is multiple tissue injury and sensitivity. So for example, an SLR may hurt in the spine and the addition of dorsiflexion increases symptoms in the upper thigh or elsewhere. It's still a sign of nervous system involvement, but not the nice clear response sometimes seen. The finding may mean that you have a bit more evaluation to do. There may be other tissues involved surrounding the nervous system.

A clinical scenario also exists, say spinal stenosis or post lumbar surgery, where extensive peridural scarring occurs, tethering the meninges but without a great deal of sensitivity. In this case, SLR may evoke symptoms but neck flexion does not alter them. Perhaps there is no force transmission past the scarred area.

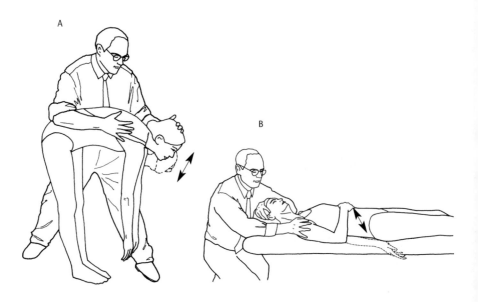

10.4 A and B. Frequently used structural differentiation tests. In A, the patient has complained of low back pain on flexion. With skilled handling, the thoracic and lumbar spines can be held stationary and the effects of cervical extension assessed. In B, the length of the upper trapezius muscles are being tested. To see if there is any sensitivity related to the physical abilities of the nervous system, the test is performed first with the elbow in flexion and then in extension. A further confirming step would be to add wrist extension.

I believe that if we can apply a broader scientific perspective, the concept of structural differentiation can be extremely useful. Further useful examples of structural differentiation are shown in figure 10.4.

TAKING THE BASE TESTS FURTHER - GO "JAZZY" IN THE CLINIC

The base tests are merely the starting point. As a clinician you may perform a number of tests including refined base test derivatives, in others for various reasons, none. In many clinical situations, the base tests will need to be varied and adapted to accommodate clinical variations.

THERE MAY BE NO NEED TO EXAMINE THE FULL TEST

In more sensitive and acute disorders, you will not need to perform the entire test. For example, if shoulder depression elicits wrist pain, then that may provide enough information. If your patient sits in a chair and when she extends her knee out it increases their back pain then that is probably enough neurodynamic examination. Some patients with severe low back pain of nerve root origin cannot lie supine with their knees extended. There is no need to attempt a straight leg raise here - just extending one knee will be enough information.

Take a look at figure 10.5. I have obviously evoked some discomfort with the test. If this were shoulder discomfort, I could release the hand position. If it were hand or forearm pain, I could carefully release the shoulder position.

EXAMINE THE OPPOSITE SIDE

For best handling, it is always advisable to test the opposite or least troublesome side first. It's good for communication especially on the initial visits. Your patient's central nervous system will know a little more what to expect of you. In sensitive disorders, movements, of the "good" side will often evoke symptoms, even in the opposite limb. This would probably be related to sensitive nerve roots on the opposite side and/or central sensitisation. You may like to place a patient's painful limb just short of a sensitive position and test the effect of a neurodynamic test on the other side. There has been one study where asymptomatic students were placed in an upper limb neurodynamic test position to the point of symptoms. When a similar test was performed on the other side, the original symptoms frequently disappeared (Rubenach 1985).

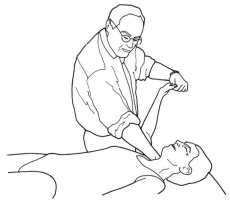

10.5 "It hurts". Refer to text for more details.

ADD MORE SENSITISING MANOEUVRES

To place further load on the nervous system, more sensitising manoeuvres can be used. For example, a typical hamstrings stretch performed by countless sportsmen and women is to stand straight and place their leg on a rail and then bend forward. The symptomatic response will be very different if this is performed with hip adduction and medial rotation. Ankle dorsiflexion or plantar flexion and cervical flexion could also be added. People often perform this stretch with their chin poked forwards. Tucking the chin in and flexing the neck will often increase the stretch sensation in the hamstring area.

In chapter 15, in the section on foot disorders there are further examples of using sensitising manoeuvres to access foot disorders such as plantar fasciitis and Morton's metatarsalgia.

PERFORM THE TESTS IN DIFFERENT COMPONENT ORDERS

The base tests as proposed may not be the best way to perform the tests. These tests can be performed in different orders of component addition. For example, an upper limb neurodynamic test could be performed beginning at the wrist first (chapter 12). Responses will usually be different depending on the order of movement. This is a clinical and logical finding and one borne out of clinical endeavour to access minor neuropathies. It also provides a framework for gentle evaluation (ie. movements can be tested some distance away from the presumed sources of problems). Additionally, it allows a conceptual basis to present movement to the central nervous system in different and perhaps more acceptable forms.

Movement will accumulate, meaning that available movement in one part of the body will depend on the position elsewhere. For example, the range of knee extension in sitting will depend on the spinal position. The range of shoulder girdle depression is dependent on the hand and wrist position (Johnson and Chiarello 1997; Coppieters et al. 1999).

MAKE UP YOUR OWN TESTS

Listen carefully to your patients and you can quickly adapt and make up your own tests. The simplest way to do this is when a patient exhibits a painful position. Try to move a remote part (within reason). Adding cervical flexion to a pain evoked lumbar position is probably the most common clinical procedure. If your patient has shoulder area pain while placing her hand behind her back, you could compare the effects of hand movements while keeping her shoulder and elbow still.

If your patient has a painful arc on shoulder movement, compare the movement with the neck in neutral and then in lateral flexion, either away from or towards the test side.

ADD PALPATION OR MUSCLE CONTRACTION

In any of the tests, you could add nerve palpation. There are some examples of this in the carpal tunnel examination in chapter 15. You could also get patients to contract muscle around nerves when a relevant pain has been evoked.

WHEN AND HOW MUCH NEURODYNAMIC ASSESSMENT TO DO

The answer to this lies in the data collected principally from the precautions, dysfunction, and pathobiology reasoning categories.

I believe that at least some evaluation should be performed for all patients, where a physical evaluation is carried out. Common clinical indicators for performing a more detailed neurodynamic examination would be peripheral neurogenic pain mechanisms and sources. Worthwhile clues to the amount of detail required in a physical evaluation may emerge from a subjective evaluation. For example, if a patient reported that her low back hurt while getting into a car, then I would be inclined to perform a slump test, an SLR, even a passive neck flexion. In another patient where the history sounded like local lumbar spinal joint pathology, an SLR alone may suffice. Some clinical examples follow.

PATIENT 1 - SPRAINED ANKLE

Your patient sprained her ankle 6 weeks ago and it still causes some problems on the lateral aspect of the ankle. The neurodynamic component of the evaluation may include:

- SLR
- Ankle plantar flexion/inversion plus SLR
- Ankle dorsiflexion/inversion plus SLR.
- All responses compared to the other side.

This would be enough to test the peroneal and sural nerves (chapter 11). I would perform a slump test if I thought there was some coexistent nerve root involvement. In this patient my thoughts are related to likely peripheral neurogenic mechanisms with structural sources in the ankle. I would also palpate the sural and peroneal nerves and perform a sensory evaluation. Please don't be totally nerve focused. Depending on the presentation, I would be likely to evaluate muscle and joints, consider stability tests and explore occupational and sporting contributing factors to the pain state.

PATIENT 2 - POST LUMBAR LAMINECTOMY

This patient had a lumbar laminectomy 8 weeks ago. Original symptoms in the leg are now reappearing as well as headache and a "tennis elbow". If you ask her to flex her spine, she can reach about 20 cm above her patellae and then she has to extend her neck to ease the pain. A forward head posture has developed in the last month.

In this patient the suggested neurodynamic part of the physical evaluation would include:

- Test of effect of cervical movement when she flexes her spine
- SLR
- Passive neck flexion
- Slump test
- Slump long sitting test
- Upper limb neurodynamic tests for the median and radial nerves
- Compare both sides

In this patient, attention to muscle and joint contributions and psychosocial aspects such as fear of movement and blame may be relevant, but she still needs a comprehensive physical investigation. Her sensitivity to movement may be related in part to unhealthy neural tissues and in part to the central nervous system. It is quite common for people to extend their necks to allow less painful back movement. I may look at the ULNTs in the slump long sitting position. The slump long sitting position as described in chapter 11 can be an excellent base for self mobilisation in these patients.

PATIENT 3 - THE ALL OVER PAINS

This patient has had chronic "all over" pains for 15 years and has been recently diagnosed with fibromyalgia. On a standard physical evaluation, he moves reasonably well. However, there are great restrictions in work and leisure activity levels and he reports difficulties sleeping.

This patient needs a more general examination which may include functional tests such as balance, in and out of chair movements, and gait analysis. However, some neurodynamic tests could be performed.

- SLR

- Slump

- PNF

- If there were problems getting out of a chair, the slump test could be modified and performed in this position.

With this patient, I am not expecting to find relevant signs peripherally, thus the tests are more general and more an examination of general sensitivity rather than a specific peripheral sensitivity. More specific evaluation, if required, can be left for later.

Some examples of common pain evoking postures and possible neurodynamic evaluations are exhibited in table 10.1.

PROVOCATIVE MOVEMENT/POSTURE	POSSIBLE NEURODYNAMIC EVALUATION
Back pain getting into a car	Slump test
Left hip pain rotating spine to the left	SLR including left hip medial rotation
Shoulder pain drying back	ULNT 3
Left groin pain hurdling cervical	Slump plus right SLR plus left PKB and extension
Wrist pain with pushup	ULNT (median) with wrist position first
Thoracic pain on correction of forward head posture	Neck retraction in long sit slump
Straining hurts lumbar spine	Strain in slump position
Lateral upper arm pain in hemiplegic arm	ULNT2 (radial)
Serving in tennis catches shoulder	Modified ULNT 1 (mimic serve position)
Squatting hurts medial knee	Palpate infrapatellar branches saphenous nerve
Spinal pain when rowing	Slump long sit

Table 10.1 Examples of pain evoking situations suggestive of a particular neurodynamic evaluation

RECORDING

Recording of physical dysfunction must include what you did and the responses to your inputs. Some relevant quotes from your patient and a note on the relevance of the responses can also be helpful. To record neurodynamic tests, I recommend a simple method using abbreviations and indicating the order of movement. For example, if I placed a patient's foot in plantarflexion/inversion, did a straight leg raise, and then I adducted the hip, I would document it as PFI/SLR/HAd. Symptoms evoked and range of movement from each component of the manoeuvre could be placed under the component. See table 10.2. Recording styles vary. Some clinicians can quickly draw slump tests and ULNT tests and illustrate clearly what they have done.

If a neural movement is challenged either via passive or active means, the IN:DID system works well. That is, you can record the position and symptoms that your patient was in before you performed the test and you could include the technique. For example, if you were performing some vigorous right knee extension manoeuvres in hip flexion and right spinal lateral flexion away from the treatment side, you could record it as IN: lat flex (R)/Hip flex 90 DID: KE 10 x 111+. The 111+ is part of the grading system used by Maitland (1986). Use what ever grading system is familiar to you, as long as you have some idea of, and can record the forces used and relationship to symptoms.

Record keeping in manual therapy can be highly personal. Although records may show that two therapists performed similar management strategies, other non-specific factors in the management process will have an effect. I think it is important to have a note regarding all the reasoning categories in the history.

ANALYSIS OF NEURODYNAMIC TEST FINDINGS

With a bit of practice, especially on the upper limb neurodynamic tests, everyone can perform similar tests to the ones described in this book and elsewhere. Analysis is the next step.

A SENSITIVE MOVEMENT DOESN'T PROVIDE MUCH INFORMATION

Without a subjective and physical assessment, all a test can inform you of is that your patient has a sensitive movement. Alone, it says nothing about sources of symptoms, nor does it

PFI	/SLR	/HAd
Slight pain lateral ankle lateral foot	/increased pain at 40 degrees	/increased pain

Table 10.2   Recording suggestions. This recording would read as follows. Ankle plantarflexion inversion caused a lateral ankle pain which increased with straight leg raise of 40 degrees and which increased again when some hip adduction was added.

impart any information about mechanisms behind the symptoms, or where along the nervous system pathologies may lurk. Perhaps a few pins and needles may point to a neural contribution, but further clinical data will be necessary to make judgements about the clinical relevance. It is important to realise that discomfort reproduced during the test is not necessarily indicative of any pathological processes occurring. It could be quite normal and you will have to compare responses to the opposite side, to expected normals and place it in the big reasoning picture.

Some clinical data should already be at hand from a subjective evaluation and the use of external evidence such as scans. Indeed, if this is so, you will have an expectation of certain findings on physical evaluation. Examples of support data may include area of symptoms, kind of symptoms, physical findings, aggravating and easing movements, and tests such as nerve conduction tests.

DETERMINING THE RELEVANCE OF THE TEST

The neurodynamic tests are not pathognomic, nor can they ever be called tests for syndromes such as the carpal tunnel test. The tests will only provide information about one aspect of the wider truth. Even the best researched of the tests, the SLR, can only provide supporting evidence for a nerve root or discogenic problem (eg. Supik and Broom 1994).

We will all have varying sensitivity to the straight leg raise or the upper limb neurodynamic test and so will patients. The following guidelines may help determine the relevance of a test. Read these and try to imagine particular patients.

THE POSITIVE TEST

A test such as a SLR can be considered positive in a clinical sense if:

It reproduces symptoms or associated symptoms, *plus* structural differentiation supports a neurogenic source, *plus* there are differences left to right and to known normal responses, *plus* there is support from other data such as history, area of symptoms, imaging tests (Fig. 10.6).

You may also get some proof in retrospect. For example, with a nerve block the movement may change, or surgical release may prove your assessment findings (eg. Shacklock 1996).

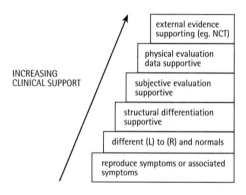

10.6 *The accumulation of data to help infer a neurodynamic test is positive for the nervous system. NCT = nerve conduction test.*

However this process of additive hypothesis support or rejection is just the first step to a clinical diagnosis. The more of the above then the stronger the support that a sensitive/mechanically unhealthy nervous system is involved. Each needs to be analysed individually. For example, asymmetry by itself is not necessarily a problem unless it is marked and appears clinically relevant (see below). The "associated symptoms" may or may not be relevant either. Relevance of findings is the critical issue.

POSITIVE AND RELEVANT TESTS

A test may appear positive but is it relevant? The key question to ask yourself is this - is it a movement which would be worthwhile addressing to reduce sensitivity, improve quality of movement and function? Also, if used as a reassessment tool – would a change in this movement be a worthwhile indicator of progression?

There are no protocols here. These guidelines are suggested.

• Base relevance to your patient's general dysfunction. If your neurodynamic test is improved will it help the patient function better? To make this judgement, detailed knowledge about general dysfunction including goals and current activity levels is required. So is a skilled physical examination. For example, minor limitations and hyperalgesia in a test which loads the radial nerve and which is different from the other side may well make the test relevant in a professional tennis player. Similar minor findings in a sedentary patient with post traumatic shoulder pain may not be as relevant. A 65 year old woman may have buttock pain on right straight leg raise at 110 degrees. However the left is 160 degrees and she wishes to keep up her dancing classes which include the can-can. I would say that the physical dysfunction was definitely relevant in this case.

• A clinical decision on pain processes in operation may help. For example, a judgement that more central mechanisms are in play and the tissues are unhealthy but have had plenty of time to heal may support a clinical diagnosis of a central sensitivity state. In management it would be better to investigate ways of altering threshold control of the CNS, in addition to getting tissues healthier. Your finding may not be as relevant. More peripheral pathobiological processes would suggest that more time be spent on analysis of tissue function and health.

• Finally, when considering which tissues are involved, consider all tissues. For too many years clinicians have had favourite hypotheses which usually focus on one tissue. Any innervated tissue, particularly well innervated ones, are a potential source of symptoms. Modern clinicians need a clinical appreciation of all tissues and all processes related to pain. A certain modesty about clinical findings can be helpful.

IDENTIFICATION OF SOURCE

When a pain state is dominated by peripheral neurogenic mechanisms, it may be possible to identify the source of the pain. In clear cut nerve root disorders, this can be obvious from the area of symptoms and a neurological examination. Where there is multiple spinal level and tissue involvement, and where the CNS is maladaptively sensitive, it is more difficult.

For peripheral neurogenic pain, accepting the above provisos, these features may help identify a source of symptoms.

• Area. Symptoms in a dermatome or cutaneous neural zone may assist identification.

Symptoms in a cutaneous zone are more nerve trunk in origin, those in a dermatome, more nerve root (chapter 9).

• Motor loss. A loss of reflex may point to a nerve root. Specific muscle loss may point to a nerve root or nerve trunk (see chapter 9 and figure 9.11, the muscle innervation map).

• History. It may be quite simple - the site of injury may be the source of the peripheral neurogenic mechanisms.

• Palpation. You may be able to put your finger right on the site of an abnormal impulse generating site.

• Skilled examination of surrounding tissues. You may find physical dysfunction in joints, muscles, fascia or skin which acts as container tissue to the nervous system. Remember to think "along the nerve" and to appreciate that mechanical and sensitivity changes elsewhere along the nerve may be a contributing factor. Can you appreciate that irritation of the median nerve from a tight pectoralis major muscle may contribute to a carpal tunnel syndrome?

Levels of meningeal irritation may also be identified by root involvement, history of trauma, scanning, health of surrounding tissues and response on testing.

UNEXPECTED RESPONSES

WHEN RELEASE OF A COMPONENT MAKES THE PAIN STATE WORSE, OR ADDITION OF COMPONENT MAKES IT BETTER

These two clinical scenarios are quite common. Imagine in your clinic that you have just evoked a low back pain on SLR and your patient flexes her neck and the pain goes. Or, in the slump test, neck extension which usually makes evoked pain better, makes it worse. On first consideration, this is not supposed to happen. One would think that with more mechanical loading, symptoms might increase. However, the symptoms may be due to the nervous system's particular movement relationship with surrounding container tissues. For example, an SLR could pull neural tissue containing an abnormal impulse generating site onto scar or osteophyte and then the neck flexion pulls it away (Fig. 10.7). In the case of the slump test, the neck extension may allow more migration of neural tissues out of the lumbar foramina. These

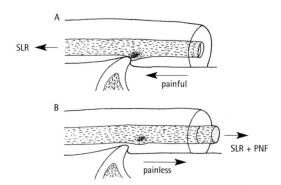

10.7 Possible explanations for odd responses during a neurodynamic test. In A, the SLR has pulled a segment of nerve root onto an osteophyte causing symptoms. In B, the addition of passive neck flexion has pulled the sensitive piece of nervous system away from the osteophyte. From: Butler DS (1991) Mobilisation of the Nervous System, Churchill Livingstone, Melbourne, with permission.

are hypotheses only. My clinical suggestion would be to try to make surrounding tissue as healthy as possible, in addition to trying to quieten down the abnormal impulse generating site.

WHEN THERE ARE ULNAR SYMPTOMS ON A MEDIAN BIASED ULNT

If you are performing a ULNT1 for the median nerve, some patients may complain of ulnar based symptoms such as paraesthesia in the little finger. There is no need to be puzzled. This is an example of the crudity of the tests and there are a number of possible reasons for this. The ulnar nerve could be joined to the median nerve in the forearm (Martin-Gruber connection - see chapter 8). Your patient's particular brachial plexus arrangement may create an abnormal focus on ulnar based cords. With the ulnar response to the test, you could check out the effect of elbow flexion in addition to assessing elbow extension as in the routine test.

With spread of pathology, this kind of response often happens. For example, prone knee bend is often sensitive when SLR on the same side is sensitive and restricted. Sometimes to get people moving, treating the less sensitive physical dysfunction can be beneficial.

WHEN PAIN RESPONSES SEEM BIZARRE

Through most of my clinical life, when symptoms evoked on movement were really weird I used to neglect them or sometimes wonder what was going on in my patient's mind. For example, shoulder girdle depression will often aggravate low back pain and after whiplash injury, toe movements can worsen neck and head pains. More than once, I have had patients flex and extend their wrists in front of their face, commenting that it hurts, then with their neck in another position, the same movement doesn't hurt. Prone knee bend can cause headaches. A patient once reported to me that the knee extension phase of the slump test evoked pain on the tip of his penis. This was eased by neck extension. On retest another day when his entire nervous system seemed less sensitive, the symptom had gone.

Listen to the story, encourage patients to tell you about the odd things that they think others will consider too weird. More and more there are now explanations for the more weird pains and many of these explanations are to be found in chapters 2 to 5.

THE ART OF GOOD HANDLING

I believe that if you are going to perform a physical evaluation, then do it well and under a framework of best available science.

• Establish what hypotheses you have generated before testing. That is, based on the best evidence - external and internal, is it worthwhile performing the test and what state is the nervous system in?

• Tell the patient exactly what you are going to do and what to expect. Make him/her feel comfortable about reporting pain anywhere in the body.

• If possible and appropriate, get your patient to perform the test actively first.

• Perform the test on the less painful side or non-painful side first if appropriate, or if little difference, perform the test on the left side first. It just makes it easier to remember when recording.

• Starting position should be consistent each time (ie. if SLR is performed with a pillow under the neck, make sure that the pillow is used for subsequent testing).

• Note symptom responses including areas and nature of response.

• Watch for antalgic postures during the test. Common examples are hip hiking or cervical extension during a SLR. There is no need to control them but they give great visual feedback about the effects of the input.

• Test for symmetry between sides.

• Explain your findings to the patient, appropriate to the pathobiology and management hypothesis.

• Appreciate that the body is not a passive recipient of input. There will be outputs depending on the way you perform the test. Most notable will be muscle protective responses. There will also be passive resistance from various tissues, there may be visible autonomic effects and there will be cognitive and emotional responses.

• Appreciate resistance and don't simply "symptom hunt". Respect the tightness and resistance offered back by the body.

• Perform the tests well with good handling, communication and understanding of the patient's sensitivity or don't perform them.

REFERENCES CHAPTER 10

Breig A & Troup J (1979) Biomechanical considerations in the straight leg raising test. Spine 4: 242-250.

Bronson J, Beck J, Gillet J. (1997) Provocative motor nerve condition testing in presumptive carpal tunnel syndrome unconfirmed by traditional electrodiagnostic testing. Journal of Hand Surgery 22A: 1041-1046.

Butler DS (1991) Mobilisation of the Nervous System, Churchill Livingstone, Melbourne.

Coppieters MW, Stappaerts KH & Staes FF (1999) A qualitative assessment of shoulder girdle elevation during the upper limb tension test 1. Manual Therapy 4: 33-38.

Coulier B (2000) Evaluation of lumbar canal stenosis: decubitus imaging methods versus flexion-extension myelography and surface measurements versus the diameter of the dural sac. Journal Belge de Radiologie 83: 61-67.

Dibden K (1996) A comparison of straight leg raising manoeuvres in supine and sitting in an asymptomatic population. Thesis, School of Physiotherapy University of South Australia, Adelaide .

Finkelstein H (1930) Stenosing tenovaginitis at the radial styloid process. Journal of Bone and Joint Surgery 12A: 509-539.

Johnson EK & Chiarello CM (1997) The slump test: the effects of head and lower extremity position on knee extension. Journal of Orthopedic and Sports Physical Therapy 26: 310-317.

Kupfer DM, Bronson J, Lee GW (1998) Differential latency testing. Journal of Hand Surgery 23A: 859-864.

Mackinnon SE & Dellon AL (1988) Surgery of the Peripheral Nerve, Thieme, New York.

Maitland GD (1986) Vertebral Manipulation, 6th edn. Butterworths, London.

Massey A (1985) Movement of pain sensitive structures in the neural canal. In: Greive GP (ed.) Modern Manual Therapy of the Vertebral Column, Churchill Livingstone, Edinburgh.

Penning L (1992) Functional pathology of lumbar spinal stenosis. Clinical Biomechanics 7: 3-17.

Rubenach H (1985) The upper limb tension test: the effect of the position and movement of the contralateral arm. In: In: Proceedings, Manipulative Physiotherapists Association of Australia, 4th biennial conference., Brisbane.

Shacklock MO (1996) Positive upper limb tension test in a case of surgically proven neuropathy. Manual Therapy 1: 154-161.

Supik LF & Broom MJ (1994) Sciatic tension signs and lumbar disc herniation. Spine 19: 1066-1069.

CHAPTER 11

NEURODYNAMIC TESTING
FOR THE SPINE AND LOWER LIMB

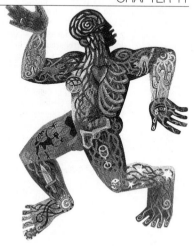

INTRODUCTION

MANUAL HANDLING

HANDLING GUIDELINES FOR ALL NEURODYNAMIC TESTS

STRAIGHT LEG RAISE

INTRODUCTION
SLR PERFORMANCE
THOUGHTS ON SLR PERFORMANCE
NORMAL RESPONSES
SENSITISING TESTS
OTHER STRAIGHT LEG RAISES
INDICATIONS AND SOME CLINICAL THOUGHTS
A QUICK REMINDER OF THE BIGGER PICTURE

PASSIVE NECK FLEXION

PNF PERFORMANCE
VARIATIONS AND LINKS TO THE SLR
NORMAL RESPONSES/RESEARCH
CLINICAL USE
LHERMITTE'S SIGN

THE SLUMP TEST

INTRODUCTION
PERFORMANCE OF THE SLUMP TEST
FREQUENTLY USED VARIATIONS
NORMAL RESPONSES
INDICATIONS
PRECAUTIONS RELATED TO THE SLUMP TEST

SLUMP TEST IN LONG SITTING

PERFORMANCE OF THE TEST
REFINED TESTING
SLUMP LS NORMAL RESPONSES
DO IT YOURSELF

PRONE KNEE BEND

PERFORMANCE OF THE TEST – PKB
NORMAL RESPONSES AND ANALYSIS
VARIATIONS

REFERENCES CHAPTER 11

INTRODUCTION

This chapter and the following one are the suggested "how to do it" chapters for an examination of the nervous system's physical abilities, that is, its ability to slide and strain and cope with chemical and physical events in neighbouring structures. While the chapter focuses on the physical aspects of examination, any analysis will require consideration of temporal and spatial aspects of the overall sensitivity setting.

Where possible I have discussed something of the history of the test, the performance of the test and possible variations, normal responses and related research, indications for testing and handling thoughts. As in previous chapters and in the illustrations, I am the examiner and the patient is referred to as female. I have described her as if she were a subject, thus inferring no pathology and therefore the neurodynamic tests are described to their final positions.

Clinicians who have leapt to this chapter on opening the book are asked to curb their enthusiasm and review some of the earlier chapters, in particular the assessment strategies chapter, chapter 7.

MANUAL HANDLING

This chapter is all about manual handling and how it is a combination of clinical reasoning skills, patient communication skills and actual physical handling skills.

These tests have been described in many textbooks, but there are very few with an adequate graphic or written description of the test. Even a seemingly simple test such as the straight leg raise is poorly described in texts and the actual methodology is rarely described in research studies. Others share this belief (Haddox 1999). Remember that what you find via physical handling is likely to be an expression of the same pathobiology which is represented on a scan, an imaging test or in your patient's pain self report. This is a plea for skilled manual handling and analysis.

HANDLING GUIDELINES FOR ALL NEURODYNAMIC TESTS

This is a summary of the detailed discussion in chapter 7. Let's recap.

• Establish hypotheses in all reasoning categories prior to testing, especially pathobiology, likely specific dysfunctions on examination, precautions and sources.

• Tell your patient exactly what you are going to do and what she may expect. Make her feel comfortable about reporting any responses to your testing, anywhere in her body.

• Perform the test on the less painful side or non-painful side first. Where there is little difference, perform the test on the left side first to aid later recall of movements and responses.

• Starting position should be consistent each time. Any variations from normal practice should be noted.

• Note symptom responses including areas and nature.

• Watch for antalgic postures and other motor responses during the test (eg. hip hiking or cervical extension during a SLR, or trapezius activity during a ULNT).

- Test for symmetry between sides.

- Explain your findings to your patient.

- Repeat the test a number of times before taking an actual measurement.

The extent and finesse of handling will depend on the likely pathobiological processes in operation. Fine detail may be necessary for some patients (eg. obscure hamstring pain), yet in others (eg. widespread pain as in fibromyalgia) more functional tests (eg. walking, bending sitting) may be more appropriate.

STRAIGHT LEG RAISE

INTRODUCTION

In 1951, Charnley stated in regard to back pain, that "the straight leg raise was more important than all of the other clinical and radiological signs put together" (Charnley 1951). He may have been close to the truth, even with the advances of imaging. The SLR is the most frequently performed neurodynamic test and has been shown to have reasonable validity, especially in its ability to diagnose disc herniation (Hakelius 1970; Spangfort 1972; McCombe et al. 1989; Deyo et al. 1992). Kosteljanetz et al. (1988) makes a fair summary of the SLR research, based on their findings of specificity 0.87 and sensitivity 0.33 in diagnosing a prolapsed disc. They state that although it is "......a reasonably good clinical test, the significance of the presence or absence of the sign should not be overstated".

In disc herniation, the SLR has a strong correlation with parameters such as night pain, pain at rest and analgesic consumption. If it is positive postoperatively, then an inferior surgical outcome is likely (Jonsson and Stromqvist 1995).

Nearly all research on the SLR focuses on its role to diagnose disc pathology. However the SLR has a variable chemical and mechanical relationship to disc pathology. A research direction for the SLR test should be its ability to detect a site of abnormal impulse generation in the nervous system that may or may not be associated with an injured disc.

The SLR is quick and safe and can provide useful clinical information. A good clinician will be aware of the likely responses to the test after collecting information on the patient's pain provoking and easing movements and after watching her flex her spine.

SLR PERFORMANCE

This is the only test, along with passive neck flexion, where the responses are best assessed passively, although walking and swinging a leg is to some extent an active representation of the test. Lifting a patient's leg in the air should be easy but it is often performed badly. Look at figure 11.1.

1. Lie your patient close to your side of the bed with both legs extended. This closeness will allow supportive handling and stop the frequent error of allowing the leg to fall into lateral rotation.

2. Stand facing your patient and place one hand under the ankle avoiding pressure on the peripheral nerves where they are superficial and place the other hand above the patella.

3. Keeping the knee extended, flex the hip in a perpendicular plane.

4. The leg is taken short of, to, or into sensory or motor responses depending on prior reasoned hypotheses of pathobiological processes involved.

5. Be aware of symptom responses before, during and after the test.

This simple and easily reproducible protocol was suggested by Breig and Troup (1979). There is no need to abduct or medially rotate the hip at this stage, as may have been traditionally taught some years ago.

THOUGHTS ON SLR PERFORMANCE

You should have a fairly good idea what the responses will be prior to the test. Clues will come from an examination of active movements, especially lumbar flexion and there might be good information gleaned in the subjective evaluation. Have your patients look up at the ceiling while you are performing the test. If they look at you there may be some upper cervical flexion and in some chronic pain patients, the visual input may enhance responses.

While some patients may only have a few degrees of SLR, some hypermobile individuals may have excellent ranges of SLR, yet the movement may still hide some pathology. Dancers and gymnasts come to mind. With a smaller person you may be able to control the leg and "walk up with it" as in figure 11.2. With a larger person, you could place her leg on your shoulder and "walk up with it".

A pillow or not? Cadaver studies have demonstrated that cervical flexion will mechanically influence the neural tissues of the lumbar spine (Breig and Marions 1963; Tencer et al. 1985), as have in-vivo studies (Lew and Puentedura 1985) and animal cadaver studies (Lew et al. 1994). Thus for accurate test-retest scores, the same position (ie. a pillow or no pillow) should be maintained.

Clinicians often forget that the SLR begins in a significant amount of neural loading. In supine, the knee is already extended. People with an injured nervous system may lie with the knee in some degree of flexion and thus have a minus degree of SLR. The degree to which they can extend their knee can be measured. This can be a range measurement or the distance from the knee crease to the bed.

It may be worth performing the test with the knee and hip of the opposite leg flexed. This

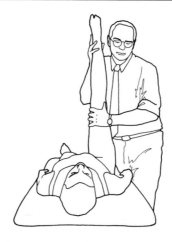

11.1   The basic straight leg raise test.

may be more comfortable for patients with a "touchy" problem and it probably allows a little more lateral migration of neural tissue in the spinal and intervertebral canals. In a study on healthy subjects, Cameron et al. (1994) found that opposite side hip flexion would increase the SLR range. They also noted in the same study group that passive range of SLR will be greater than active range.

NORMAL RESPONSES

Clinicians quickly realise that the range and responses to a SLR are extremely variable in healthy individuals. My SLRs are about 45 degrees on both sides, but I have no back pain and this range is adequate to get me through life. There is no evidence that such a range sets me up for a problem later in life, although it is clear that rowing, gymnastics and hurdling are events that I should steer clear of. Some dancers appear to have quite normal straight leg raises of around 150 degrees. My clinical impression is that the hypermobile patients who lose their range of movement through injury, lack of use or fear, appear to have more musculoskeletal problems later.

The straight leg raises of 500 English postal workers aged 22 to 63 years were examined by Sweetham et al. (1974), who found a minimum of 56^0, a maximum of 115^0 and a mean of 83.4 degrees. Given that occupation may alter SLR (Ramamurthi 1980) these figures should be taken with caution and the wide range be accepted.

There are variations throughout the day in the range of the SLR (Porter and Trailescu 1990; Gifford 1994). The diurnal range of SLR does not alter as much as range of spinal movement, although mean variations may be as much as 10 degrees with a rise during the day and a fall at night (Gifford 1987). In the presence of lumbar disc protrusion/radiculopathy, the variations are greater, with mean increases in SLR range up to 17^0 with most of the increase in the first hour out of bed (Porter and Trailescu 1990). There are obvious ramifications for the use of range of motion scores to measure improvement.

It is very rare to find a study where the symptomatic response has been documented. The three main symptom areas are posterior thigh, posterior knee and posterior calf extending into the foot. A "deep stretch sensation" is usually reported in the posterior thigh which may extend to the posterior calf and foot (Slater et al. 1994).

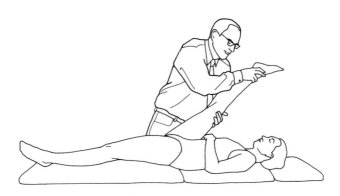

11.2   Straight leg raise in a more mobile patient.
"Walk up with the leg".

SENSITISING TESTS

The term "sensitising test" refers to an additional body movement that is likely to place more mechanical forces upon the nervous system. For example, ankle dorsiflexion is a sensitising manoeuvre for an SLR. Sensitising tests are derived anatomically by observing the relationship of nerves to the axis of movement. In figure 11.3, possible sensitising tests for the SLR are listed.

Sensitising tests can be added at different times during the examination. For example, dorsiflexion can be added first and then the SLR can be performed or vice versa. This order is suggested to obtain the optimal physical challenge on the nervous system, and to vary the input into the CNS. See chapter 5 on neurodynamics and chapter 10 on assessment strategies for a full discussion of order of movement.

ADD ANKLE DORSIFLEXION + EVERSION (DF/EV)

Clinicians have added ankle dorsiflexion to the SLR for many years. It is regarded as an essential part of the SLR, and is usually referred to as a "qualifying sign" for root tension (Troup 1981). The addition of dorsiflexion to the SLR is sometimes called Bragard's manoeuvre.

To add dorsiflexion first requires some handling skills. This is clearly shown in figure 11.4. I have grasped the patient's right foot with my right hand so I can hold the foot in ankle dorsiflexion and guide it towards eversion. My left hand comes around the medial side of her ankle with my fingers towards or around the heel. This can assist the dorsiflexion a little, but in particular it keeps the foot in ankle eversion by keeping the hindfoot in abduction. My right

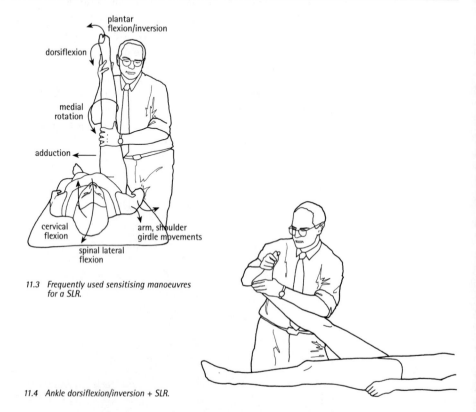

11.3 Frequently used sensitising manoeuvres for a SLR.

11.4 Ankle dorsiflexion/inversion + SLR.

hand can also add supination and pronation as needed. Pronation will place a bit more load on neural structures including the plantar nerves. Once in this position, I have placed my left arm on the shaft of the tibia, controlling knee extension. The leg is now well controlled right through the straight leg raise.

A major error occurs during dorsiflexion because the foot naturally falls into inversion, thus lessening some of the load on the system. It is especially important to include eversion for neuropathic contributions to plantar fasciitis and posterior tarsal tunnel syndrome. You can review your anatomy of the tibial nerve at the medial ankle in chapter 8 if required.

A problem with the technique above is that control for smaller therapists with patients with large heavy legs can be sacrificed and another problem occurs if more than 50 to 60 degrees of DF/Ev/SLR is required. However, remember that most patients will have less range of SLR with DF/Ev added than in the base test. To solve this problem, I usually kneel on the bed, place the patient's leg on my shoulder and then lift the straight leg up (Fig. 11.5). It can be difficult to control the eversion and your left arm will be needed to control the knee and stop it flexing. This is also a good position to add an ankle dorsiflexion/eversion to a SLR (SLR/DF/Ev) thus altering the order of movement.

Palpation of the tibial nerve can also be performed in this position if required. The position shown in figure 11.4 and 11.6 makes it quite easy to perform. With good handling you may be able to palpate a sensitive spot on any nerve at the foot and then add the SLR to see if the sensitivity alters.

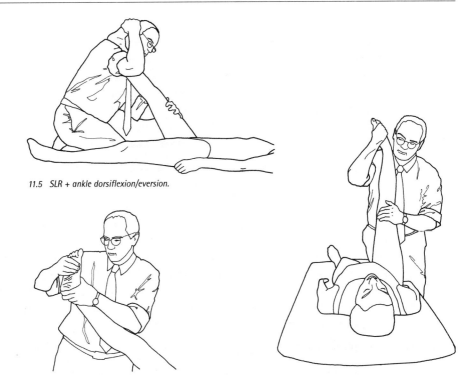

11.5   SLR + ankle dorsiflexion/eversion.

11.6   Ankle plantar flexion/inversion + SLR.

11.7   SLR + ankle plantar flexion/inversion.
       Leg on shoulder technique.

ADD PLANTARFLEXION AND INVERSION (PF/IN)

The position is similar to adding dorsiflexion to an SLR. Note in figure 11.6 that my right hand holds her foot in plantarflexion and inversion, aided a little by my left hand. This gives good control of the foot and fine variations can be added if needed. My left arm lies along the shaft of the tibia and allows good control of the knee.

Alternately, the foot position can be added after the SLR. This is demonstrated in figure 11.7. The process is again similar to adding dorsiflexion to the SLR. It is best to place the leg on the shoulder and then add the plantarflexion/inversion. In figure 11.7, I have my right knee on the bed and I am thus providing good support. This will help the shorter therapist/larger patient dilemma. Palpation of the superficial peroneal branches of the nerve on the dorsum of the foot may be possible. Note that the nerve loses its lateral mobility when the leg is in the PF/In/SLR position.

In the absence of published data, theses are the next best thing. The normal responses have been tested by students at the University of South Australia. Shacklock (1989) reported that the typical area of responses in 50 asymptomatic young volunteers was a stretching pain in the anterolateral leg and foot with plantarflexion/inversion which always increased with the addition of more hip flexion. There was a spread of pain to the posterior thigh in 24% and a few reported posterior knee and calf pain when further SLR was added. In a control group (N=30, 18-30 year volunteers) for a sprained ankle study, Molesworth (1992) found that ankle plantarflexion/inversion plus SLR will result in symptomatic responses on the anterolateral shin and ankle, and the dorsal aspect of the forefoot with some spread to the posterior thigh.

ADD DORSIFLEXION/INVERSION (DF/IN)

In the search for better clinical access to patients with ankle "impingement" syndromes and persistent Achilles tendon problems, the sural nerve and its branches were considered as possible sources (Butler 1991). Although regarded as an uncommon neuropathy (see "sprained ankles" chapter 15), injury to this nerve appears quite common in ankle sprains and it only takes half a minute to perform a test. The sural nerve runs laterally to the achilles tendon and then inferior to the lateral malleolus (chapter 6). Thus, if the ankle was dorsiflexed and the foot inverted this would place a load on the nerve as well as other lateral structures.

Use the same position and handling as for the dorsiflexion/eversion/SLR manoeuvre described above, except invert rather than evert the foot (Fig. 11.8). A straight leg raise can then be added to this position.

A normal response to ankle dorsiflexion/inversion + SLR to a painful limit was tested by Molesworth (1992) in 30 volunteers aged 18 to 30 years. Symptoms were evoked in the posterior calf and posterolateral ankle area with some reporting symptoms in the lateral border of the foot and some reporting a spread to the posterior knee and thigh. The foot, ankle and calf symptoms are in the field of the sural nerve and this nerve is a likely source of the symptoms. In this sample there were some differences in the area of strongest responses, perhaps due to common variations in sural nerve anatomy.

ADD HIP MOVEMENTS IN VARIOUS ORDERS

Hip movements can be added before or after the SLR. These will be useful to place more load on neural structures and to help differentiate sources of ankle problems.

Hip adduction (Fig. 11.9) is a powerful sensitising position to add to the SLR (Breig and Troup 1979). A quick review of the anatomy of the sciatic nerve and its relationship to the hip joint will reveal why. The sciatic tract is well lateral to the axis of hip abduction and adduction and thus the adduction will load the nervous system. If you are examining patients with a lot of hip adduction it may be better to stand on the other side of the bed.

Another option is to medially rotate the hip as in figure 11.10 (Breig and Troup 1979). The handling can be a bit difficult and I sometimes find myself just keeping the leg fixed to my shoulder and then rotating my body to take the leg into medial rotation. It would appear anatomically and clinically that the peroneal division of the sciatic nerve and the peroneal nerve may be more loaded during this position. It does not appear as sensitive as the hip adduction movement.

These sensitising manoeuvres can also be considered during general physical examination. In the example in figure 11.11, with lumbar rotation and feet firmly planted, the patient complains of a right hip pain. This may be due to the effect of medial rotation on hip area structures or on neural structures. You could also check here whether cervical flexion and extension altered the evoked pain response.

Remember that the order of adding components can change. For example, if during the subjective evaluation, you became aware that your patient had buttock pain on rotating her body to the right (thus medially rotating the right hip), you may consider performing the right SLR with hip in medial rotation first and then straight leg raise.

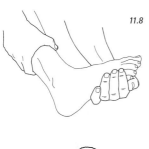

11.8   Ankle dorsiflexion/inversion + SLR (focus on the sural nerve).

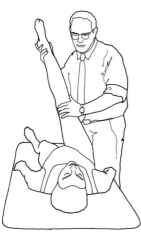

11.9   SLR + hip adduction.

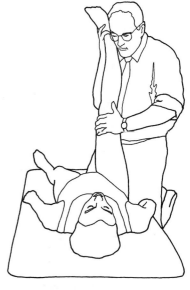

11.10 SLR + Hip medial rotation.

A commonly performed test is to flex the hip and then add knee extension. This is a reversal of the order of movement for the base test. It can be a gentle way to explore SLR and is often a nice way to get a patient to begin to move neural structures. It can also be used for differentiation. In figure 11.12A, I have flexed my patient's hip. Note the handling and the control it gives. I have her foot supported so that I can add foot movements and the hip and knee are controlled so that I can extend the knee or add flexion/extension, abduction/adduction or rotations to the hip. If this position was symptomatic, and could be held still, the addition of knee extension (Fig. 11.12B) will add further loading to the nervous system and may implicate the nervous system in a pain state.

ADD CERVICAL FLEXION

In the SLR position you could check out the effects of adding cervical flexion. This has to be done actively of course. Try asking your patient to just nod at first thus seeing if upper cervical flexion and extension alters evoked symptoms. Then ask her to flex her neck. Don't be surprised if flexion eases SLR evoked symptoms (see chapter 10 for a discussion). Sometimes cervical rotation can also influence the SLR response. Don't forget to explain what you have found to your patients.

PRELOAD THE NERVOUS SYSTEM PRIOR TO THE SLR

Instead of adding a sensitising manoeuvre to the SLR, the patient's body could be placed in a neurally loaded position first. After all, when the patient lies with her knees extended, she is already in a neurally loaded position and it is just a matter of adding further loading.

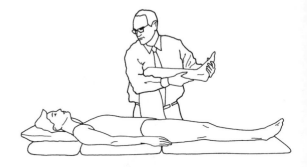

11.12A In hip flexion with good control, further sensitising manoeuvres can be added.

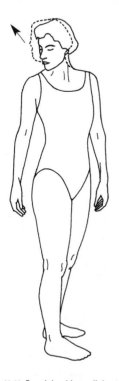

11.11 Examining hip medial rotation during lumbar rotation.

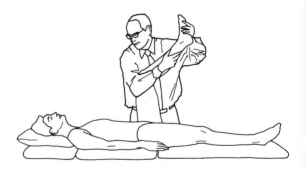

11.12B With position A held, knee extension is added.

There are a number of options here. The cervical spine could be flexed, but a clinically useful test is to perform the SLR with or without sensitising manoeuvres with your patient in some spinal lateral flexion (Fig. 11.13). You will need to be careful with your handling here. Make sure that the SLR is still performed perpendicular to the pelvis. It is very easy to perform the test with the hip in some abduction, thus lessening the tension on the system.

OTHER STRAIGHT LEG RAISES

Various straight leg raises have been described and readers will be familiar with a number of tests and names.

BILATERAL STRAIGHT LEG RAISE (BSLR)

Bilateral SLR can be a useful form of SLR. It is best to either kneel on the bed and elevate your patient's legs or, as in figure 11.14, I have my patient slightly diagonal on the bed and then I can "walk up" with the legs. Once in the BSLR position, either leg can be taken further if needed and you can check out the effects of ankle movements. Of course, the slump long sitting position (discussed later in this chapter) offers a less energetic form of BSLR, although the neurobiomechanics involved in the test are surely different.

CROSSED SLR

The crossed straight leg raising test is a SLR test of the "good leg". There is nothing special about the technique once you have mastered the base SLR; it's all in the analysis. The test has been shown to be a useful indicator of a disc prolapse (Hudgins 1979; Khuffash and Porter

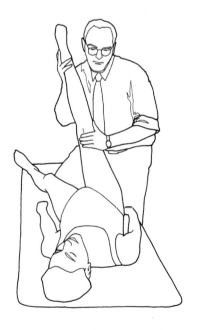

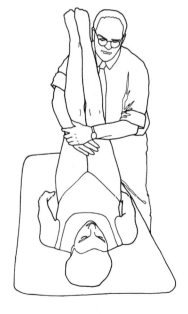

11.13 With the spinal lateral flexion position held, SLR can be performed.

11.14 Bilateral SLR.

1988; Vucetic and Svensson 1996). This is probably because the irritated dural theca is pulled across the damaged disc as well as tensioned. In Spangfort's large study (1972) on disc herniation and radiculopathy, the crossed SLR had a very high specificity (.95) but low sensitivity (.11). Similar findings were reported by Hsieh et al. (1983). This means it won't pick up all the disc herniatios, but if the test shows positive by reproducing symptoms then your patient is highly likely to have a disc lesion which is affecting nerves. Note that these sensitivities and specificities were the opposite for the base test SLR in these studies.

BOWSTRING TEST

In this test, the straight leg is raised to a point of symptom response and then the knee is flexed back to a point where the symptoms ease. In this position the tibial nerve at the knee crease is palpated. If pressure evokes pain or paraesthesia radiating up or down the leg, then the test can be regarded as positive (Macnab 1977; Waddell 1998). I believe that any information that this test gives can be obtained in the other tests. It is called the bowstring test because the tibial nerve is "bowstrung" in the popliteal fossa in the test position. The handling for a bowstring test is somewhat difficult and I find that careful use of the base SLR and the sensitising manoeuvres provides enough clinical information already.

LASEGUE'S TEST

The base SLR is sometimes called Lasegue's test after Professor Charles Lasegue at the University of Paris. The history of the test is detailed in Dyck (1984) and Wiltse (1997). In this test, which was described in 1865, hip area pain provoked by an SLR could be inferred to be from a hip source if the hip flexion position was held and flexion of the knee did not alter symptoms. It is simple and crude structural differentiation. Straight leg raise is a far more descriptive name than Lasegue's test and thus should be used in preference.

INDICATIONS AND SOME CLINICAL THOUGHTS

The SLR is probably the key neurodynamic test for the spine and legs and is universally used as a marker for the effectiveness of many interventions. Other than its use in diagnosing lumbar disc lesions, it appears useful for thoracic, lumbar, pelvic and lower limb neurogenic disorders, although what research there is on the test has focused on the lumbar disc. You will note that the SLR will occasionally evoke head and neck pain and occasionally shoulder pain. This may cause some clinicians to believe they have discovered a new Waddell's non-organic sign. Such a finding could perhaps be due to some mechanical transmission in the nervous system, but it would appear more likely if the entire nervous system is sensitised.

For readers where the concepts of the mobile nervous system and neurodynamics is new, it would be worthwhile beginning at the feet. Here the positive neurodynamic tests are very obvious, especially with the various foot positions as described above. The sprained ankle slow to heal, plantar fasciitis, medial foot pain in runners, calcaneal pain are all worth an examination based on SLR. With careful handling it only takes a few minutes.

A QUICK REMINDER OF THE BIGGER PICTURE

An opinion was sought by a young man for a longstanding ankle area pain problem after a crush injury at work. The unfortunate fellow was pinned under a forklift for a period of time. His foot was always painful and if I just performed the base SLR without any sensitising additions, the foot pain worsened at about 30 degrees of SLR. Hip adduction made the evoked pain worse. The addition of any foot movements, especially dorsiflexion first would increase his resting pain and then just a few degrees of SLR would increase it. Nerve palpation, especially over the tibial nerve was extremely sensitive, however I soon realised that he was tender to palpation everywhere, it was not specific. My reasoning in the category of pathobiology was that although there was sure to be multiple unhealthy and sensitive tissues here, he probably had an upregulated CNS as well. It didn't matter what I did or what structure I tried to test, it was all input, perhaps normal input, which could be turned into pain due to maladaptive CNS processing. My management therefore had to consider and deal with CNS processes which may have lowered the CNS threshold to input, in addition to improving the health of tissues in the leg.

PASSIVE NECK FLEXION

This test is considered a base test on its own merits, even though it is often added to the Slump and SLR tests. Most clinicians regularly perform a SLR, but this test "from the other end" is often forgotten.

Cervical flexion creates inputs from many tissues and structures including joints, muscles, balance organs and the eyes. It also creates a physical loading force on the connective and conducting tissues of the nervous system as described in detail in the neurodynamics chapter (chapter 5). As it is a passive test, there are additional inputs related to the person performing the test and the atmosphere of the test. Many of the neurodynamic tests have been derived by observation of patients with meningitis in the days before antibiotic management. Painful passive neck flexion (PNF) was listed by O'Connell (1946) as one of the clinical signs of meningitis.

PNF PERFORMANCE

Lie your patient supine and remove the pillow from under her neck unless she has problems in extension. Keep her arms by the side and legs extended if possible, although her knees could be flexed if she is particularly sensitive. Remember the continuum of the nervous system and that arm and leg movement will have influences on her neck.

The test can be broken down into upper cervical flexion, lower cervical flexion and a combined upper and lower passive neck flexion. Upper cervical flexion causes significant neural loading

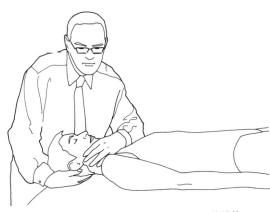

11.15 Upper cervical passive neck flexion.

and displacement of the lower brainstem, upper cervical cord and meninges. It is also a frequently used test for the length and sensitivity of the upper cervical extensor muscles and for the upper cervical joints. There is an anatomical link between the rectus capitus posterior muscle and the dura mater, reviewed in chapter 5. It is obviously impossible to perform the test for one structure at the expense of others. Patterns of symptoms may suggest that one structure is dominating the sensitivity picture. Although a comparison of the responses to cervical flexion with knees flexed or extended, or shoulders depressed or elevated may allow some structural differentiation, the meningeal-muscle connection and the likelihood of multi-tissue sensitivity calls for care in analysis.

Upper cervical flexion can be done actively. Simply ask your patient to keep her head on the pillow and nod or tuck her chin in. The test performed passively may reveal stiffness and perhaps different symptoms without the muscular effort. In figure 11.15, I have held her chin with my left arm while my right hand is cupped around the base of her occiput. In this position her head can be gently nodded.

The neck can also be flexed without the chin tuck and this is a gentle way to test a PNF. Make sure that you don't cover your patient's ears with your hands – this will certainly hinder effective communication.

The full test as shown in figure 11.16 involves upper and lower cervical flexion. Keep the chin tucked in during the flexion movement and be aware and responsive to any need for her to extend her neck and poke her chin out during the manoeuvre. The addition of cervical lateral flexion to load the convex side is also possible. If symptoms were evoked in the thorax, low back, or arm, some consideration would have to be given to the possibility that the nervous system may somehow be involved. As with all tests, the examiner should be aware of the responses including symptoms evoked and the resistance to the test.

VARIATIONS AND LINKS TO THE SLR

Any neck movement will have physical repercussions for the nervous system (Breig 1978). You may want to perform the PNF in some lateral rotation or flexion if the patient's history suggests that it would be worthwhile. Perform it with the knees flexed if the patient is sensitive. I occasionally cradle the cervicothoracic junction and do a passive neck/upper

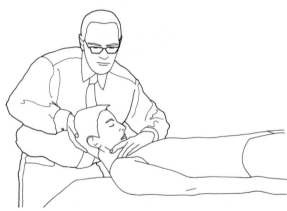

11.16 Upper and lower cervical passive neck flexion.

thoracic flexion if I suspect that there may be some physical disorder in the nervous system and the initial PNF has not picked it up.

It is often tempting in the clinic to see what effect a SLR will have on a PNF evoked lumbar symptom. Lew and Peuntedura (1985) tested this some years ago finding that the addition of cervical flexion to a SLR would change the symptom response and range of the SLR. Note the technique in figure 11.17. Ask your patient to cross her legs and then ask her to extend her knee to see the effect on the PNF evoked symptoms. The other option is to get an assistant to perform the SLR.

NORMAL RESPONSES/RESEARCH

The PNF test has had little research, even on clinical signs of bacterial meningitis (Attia et al. 1999). It is in widespread use and is recommended by most major orthopaedic, neurological and manual therapy texts. I feel that the test should not evoke any symptoms in asymptomatic individuals although a stretching of soft tissues, especially at the cervico-thoracic junction may be quite normal. Troup (1981) noted that it was positive for low back pain in 22% of all cases of back and sciatic pain seen in an industrial survey and 35% of those who were referred to hospital. These figures came from testing in the sitting position and it would seem likely that those who tested positive may have had a discogenic or spinal stenosis problem. I suspect that the results would be similar if the test was performed in supine. There is cadaveric work demonstrating that flexing the neck moves neural tissue in the lumbar spine and in the upper sciatic tract (Breig and Marions 1963; Breig 1978; Tencer et al. 1985), detailed in chapter 5. Experienced clinicians who take time to listen to patients will be aware that neck movements quite often affect the low back. Sometimes patients may feel uncomfortable about reporting what to them may seem like a strange symptom. I have also noted, particularly in widespread spinal pain, that PNF quite commonly elicits paraesthesia in the feet. This may be a "red flag", particularly in the presence of other symptoms (chapter 7).

CLINICAL USE

Passive neck flexion as a base test promotes an awareness of cervical neuromeningeal displacement and strain. The movement can be incorporated into active and passive movement and postural awareness.

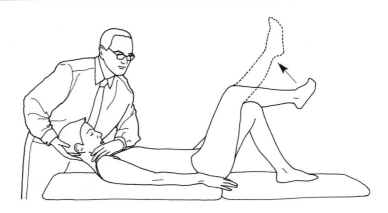

11.17 Checking the effect of straight leg raise on symptoms evoked by passive neck flexion.

The PNF test helps to explain some aspects of pain to patients. For example, the frequent finding of passive neck flexion pulling in the lumbar spine can help to explain dural irritation/adherence from lumbar injury. It could help form part of the rationale for why a patient may get headaches and it might help encourage a patient to get her whole spine as physically healthy as possible. Take care with explanations about nerve damage (see chapter 14) and make sure your patient knows that findings such as lumbar pain from passive neck flexion are very common and there is no need to panic.

LHERMITTE'S SIGN

Lhermitte's sign is the brief electrical like shock sensation that goes down the legs or spine of a person when the neck is flexed. Sometimes it could travel down the arms. Lhermitte's sign could also occur during cervical rotation and coughing. It is usually considered to be due to spinal cord damage, in particular in the dorsal columns of the cervical spinal cord (Gutrecht et al. 1993; Newton and Rea 1996).

Lhermittes's sign could be thought of as a very mechanosensitive positive PNF. Positive signs have often been noted in multiple sclerosis sufferers (Gutrecht et al. 1993). Lhermitte's sign has also been seen in cancer patients, either due to a space invading lesion (Newton and Rea 1996) or following radiation therapy and cisplatin chemotherapy (Newton and Rea 1996; van den Bent et al. 1998), although it is self limiting in most reports or it stops when chemotherapy ceases. It has also been noted in herpes zoster (Vollmer et al. 1991) and delayed onsets have been reported after head and neck injuries (Chan and Steinbok 1984).

A study of 42 consecutive cancer patients who reported electric shock like symptoms revealed that 43% had Lhermitte's sign and 24% also had a Lhermitte's sign on abducting the arm. (Lossos and Siegel 1996). This is a reminder of the possibilities of peripheral nerve injury from radiation therapy and the continuous nature of the nervous system. The self-limiting nature of the sign following irradiation and chemotherapy will be useful information for patients. Gentle activity should be promoted.

THE SLUMP TEST

INTRODUCTION

The slump test is about performing the SLR in a seated position. In this way head, neck and trunk movements can be added to the test, which will add more loading to the tissues and more input into the CNS. For lumbar pain it is often more sensitive than the other neurodynamic tests (Massey 1985), although not always. The slump test is a more functionally relevant test than an SLR and it is easy to convert a test into active and meaningful activity. Geoffrey Maitland (1985; 1986) was the predominant individual responsible for introducing the test into manual therapy and medicine.

Woodhall and Hayes (1950) suggested that the slump test was used as early as 1909. No doubt though, through history, many sufferers and clinicians would have noted or heard that in the sitting position, extending the knee and flexing the neck can sometimes evoke or aggravate spinal pain. Maitland noted that patients would complain of low back pain while getting into a car, particularly when they flexed their necks (Maitland 1985). This position is quite similar to the slump test and in the clinic, would be an indication to perform the test.

Inman and Saunders (1942) also discussed and experimented with slump manoeuvres. In their cadaver studies, they demonstrated that flexion of the spine will move upper lumbar nerves and SLR will move lower lumbar nerves and they suggested that this may be a way to localise a site of injury to either above or below the L4 level. Cyriax (1942) was another ahead of his time, examining spinal flexion as well as the SLR.

Still, among clinicians who take time to listen to their patients' complaints, there can be few who have not heard of spinal pain in sitting influenced by both neck and leg positions.

PERFORMANCE OF THE SLUMP TEST

The test is performed actively first and then if required, the knee extension part may be performed passively.

A. STARTING POSITION

Ask your patient to sit up straight and well back on the bed with her ankles uncrossed. The knee creases should be at the edge of the bed. Ask her to place her knees together and then to relax her legs. Her hips will abduct a little. Ask her to link her hands behind her back. Hands behind back is not absolutely necessary, but it has become a traditional part of the slump test and it does keep the patient's arms out of the way of testing. Sit next to her as in figure 11.18A with your hands ready to guide the movement.

B. SPINAL SLUMP

Ask her to slump or "sag in the middle" while still looking forward (Fig. 11.18B). Sometimes a gentle push in the stomach will facilitate this. Try to guide the movement so that the pelvis doesn't rotate backwards. If you ask your patient to "keep tall and sag your spine" it will help. There is usually no need to add extra pressure down the spine, although this can be done later if needed. Check to see if this movement brings on any symptoms or alters symptoms that were present at the beginning of the test.

C. NECK FLEXION

With the spinal slump position maintained, ask her to bend her head down, "chin to chest". You can gently guide this with one hand on her occiput. Note this in figure 11.18C. This gentle pressure means that if the neck flexion is painful, she has enough control to extend her neck if required. Note how she flexes her neck. Some patients will bend their head down, but their upper cervical spine will extend. Just watch how she performs the test and if you think that more load could be placed on the nervous system, then ask her to tuck her chin in and then flex the neck. For patients where slump testing is a novel experience, this gentle limited hands-on method should not be threatening.

D. KNEE EXTENSION

Now ask her to extend her knee (Fig. 11.18D). I usually have patients extend the less or non-painful side first or if there is no side dominance, I ask them to extend the left side first. Be aware of and compare responses between the left and right sides. Some patients will automatically dorsiflex their ankle, but just ask them to keep the ankle relaxed. Feel if there is any transmission of forces up to her neck and head and make sure she is comfortable about reporting any symptoms, even those remote from her knee. There will be great variation in knee extension in this position. Some mobile patients will be able to fully extend their knees without any symptoms and will need further sensitising manoeuvres to be added (see

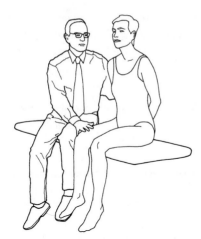

11.18A Slump test starting position.

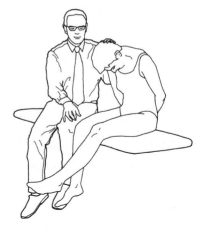

11.18D Slump test, knee extension stage.

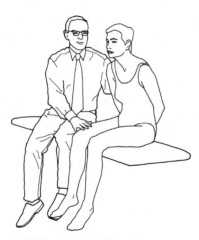

11.18B Slump test, spinal flexion stage.

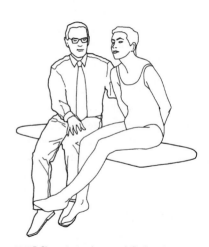

11.18E Slump test, release neck flexion stage.

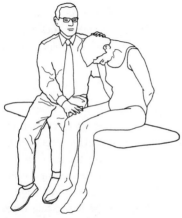

11.18C Slump test, neck flexion stage.

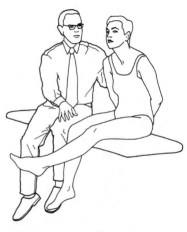

11.18F Slump test, extend knee further stage.

variations for hypermobile patient, page 288). The range as shown in figure 11.18D is quite common in mild to moderate radiculopathy, but could still be quite normal. You may also provoke symptoms on the opposite side, which could be considered a crossed slump test, similar to the crossed SLR test.

E. RELEASE NECK FLEXION

Have her maintain the above position and just ask her to extend her neck or to "look up a little". It is best to explore the effect of upper cervical extension first and then to ask her to extend her neck back completely as in figure 11.18E. Use your left hand to help guide her neck back and be aware of any change in symptoms. If a small amount of upper cervical extension alters say, lumbar pain, then the nervous system is quite clearly very sensitive. So, to refine the test, ask her to slowly extend the neck back and at the same time check when symptoms change.

F. EXTEND KNEE

With the above position held, ask her if she can straighten her knee any further than she can in figure 11.18F. This will often be the case. Check to see if it brings symptoms on again. Explain your findings to her and make her aware, if appropriate, that she can alter symptoms from movements at "both ends."

FREQUENTLY USED VARIATIONS

TAKE OVER AND DO IT PASSIVELY

There will be times when you will want to feel the range of movement passively and treat passively. You will also need to consider a passive movement evaluation when your patient can fully extend her knee and can be taken into some hip flexion. Notice in figure 11.19, that I have kept my hand on her head and taken over the knee extension passively. Note also that I am on the opposite side of the leg tested. This is useful in cases where there is a significant amount of hip flexion available and it also allows the easy addition of hip adduction to the movement. There will be some occasions when better spinal control is necessary. In this case, position yourself closer to your patient and place a downward pressure on the spine (Fig.11.20). Note how I am applying an equal pressure down both shoulder girdles. I have knelt on the bed and have my left axilla on her right shoulder and my left forearm on her left shoulder.

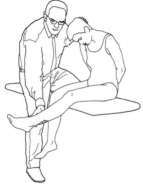

11.19 The slump test with a passive knee extension. Note how I am standing on the opposite side of the test side.

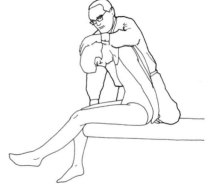

11.20 To apply further pressure down the spine, get close to the patient and place a spinal flexion force down through both shoulders.

ADDITION OF ANKLE MOVEMENTS

Ankle and foot movements can be easily incorporated into the slump test. Once she has extended her knee as in figure 11.18D, you could ask her to either dorsiflex or plantarflex her ankle. Try the commands "toes up to your face" or "toes to the floor." The addition of ankle movements may be useful if she can fully extend her knee (Fig. 11.21A,B), and it may also be useful for detecting peripheral neuropathy in the leg. The key handling point is to keep her body still while only the ankle movements are added.

BILATERAL KNEE EXTENSION

After the routine slump test, it may be worth asking your patient to extend both knees (Fig. 11.22). This will allow a comparison between left and right sides. There may be clinical clues that the slump/bilateral knee extension is worth examining, for example in central spinal pain on lumbar flexion or activities that require bilateral leg extension such as rowing or gymnastics.

VARIATIONS FOR THE HYPERMOBILE PATIENT

When your patient is very flexible such as the woman flexing forwards in figure 11.23A, it will be clear that the slump as described above will be inadequate to fully examine her nervous system. Adaptation based on knowledge of neurodynamics is needed. I suggest that you will need to stand on the opposite side to the side tested and use sensitising manoeuvres such as the hip flexion/adduction and ankle plantar flexion/inversion demonstrated in figure 11.23B.

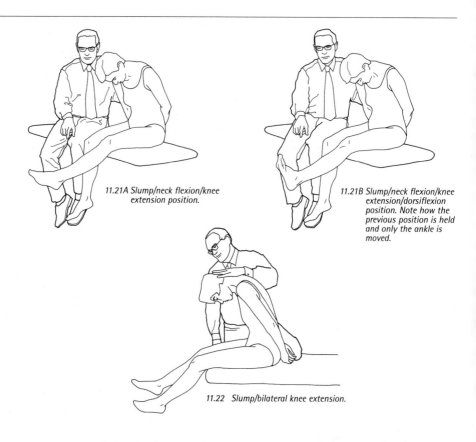

11.21A Slump/neck flexion/knee extension position.

11.21B Slump/neck flexion/knee extension/dorsiflexion position. Note how the previous position is held and only the ankle is moved.

11.22 Slump/bilateral knee extension.

Other possible additions could be more hip flexion, spinal lateral flexion to the left side, upper cervical flexion and shoulder girdle depression. In the position shown in figure 11.23B, an evoked response, say in the buttocks, could be structurally differentiated by extending the head or moving the foot and the responses could be compared to the other side. You'll need careful handling and good communication to control all the components.

VARIATIONS IN ORDER OF MOVEMENT

The test can be performed in any desired order of movement. For example, your patient could take up the foot component first and then consecutively add loading. Or the test could be performed as in the "do it yourself example" below where the patient has taken up the components from the head end first.

GET YOUR PATIENT TO DO IT

Most neurodynamic tests such as the slump test can be performed as active movements. For example my patient could easily perform a slump test herself and this may be a useful self mobilisation and pain exploration for her. In figure 11.24A, she has flexed her upper cervical spine and neck, in figure 11.24B, she has slumped, thus flexing her spine and in figure 11.24C she has extended her knees bilaterally. Of course, she could extend one knee at a time if desired.

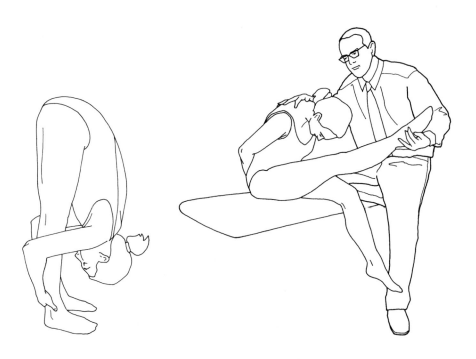

11.23A Lumbar flexion in a hypermobile patient.   *11.23B Slump test for the patient in 23A.*

NORMAL RESPONSES

Normal responses to the slump test as described above, in large groups of South Australian University students are available, offering some information on what could be expected in other population groups.

These studies have been summarised in Butler (1991). The three most important normal responses to note are:

• Half the subjects (mean age approximately 20 years) experience a central T8-9 area pain when neck flexion is added to the slump position. This is less common in older patients.

• Most subjects will be unable to fully extend their leg in the knee extension position due to symptoms usually experienced in the posterior thigh and knee area.

• The knee symptoms usually ease when the cervical spine is extended and the knee can be extended a little more.

Experimental support for cervical flexion effecting knee extension being a normal response was also provided by Johnson and Chiarello (1997). These authors also showed that hip medial rotation and ankle dorsiflexion in the slump position would decrease the range of knee extension in the slump position. There is thus a cumulative effect on the slump test by adding additional components known to physically challenge neural structures.

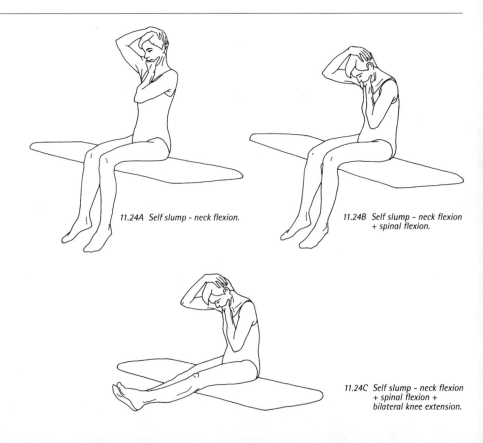

11.24A Self slump - neck flexion.

11.24B Self slump - neck flexion + spinal flexion.

11.24C Self slump - neck flexion + spinal flexion + bilateral knee extension.

The mechanisms behind the normal slump responses are unknown. I suggest that the symptomatic responses may be due to mechanically induced ischaemia, or stretch activated ion channel activation in a segment of peripheral nerve in addition to likely inputs from surrounding muscle and fascia. Pain or fear of pain will cause a muscle response which will be variable in individuals and across time and space. Neck extension easing lumbar symptoms could be due to an easing of physical forces upon the nervous system and/or the reduction of neck related inputs. These responses will all be dependent on the threshold control offered by the central nervous system.

There is a normal sensitivity to the slump test. Try it yourself and feel the characteristic dragging spreading sensation in the posterior thigh, knee and calf and feel how most of it eases when the neck is extended. Clinically what is sought is a difference in sensitivity between sides or what is considered normal (refer back to chapter 10 for analysis of findings, in particular the relevance of findings).

Because of the total body nature of the test, great care must be taken in analysis. Don't let your thoughts that you are performing a "slump test for neural tissues" bias you. The test physically stresses many tissues. The posterior spinal fascia in particular is a continuous structure, innervated, and quite capable of transmitting tension (Barker and Briggs 1999). It is also capable of interfering with the mechanical abilities of the nervous system. Other clinical data may need to be collected to infer neurogenic or non-neurogenic contributions.

INDICATIONS

The slump test is not necessary on all people and of course many people have recovered without a slump test ever being performed. The suggested indications are:

- spinal symptoms

- symptoms of lumbar and thoracic radiculopathy

- symptoms which could be related to the sciatic tract

- provocation patterns that indicate that a slump test will be positive, for example, pain on kicking or back pain when getting into a car.

- in the routine examination, lumbar flexion responses worsened with the addition of neck movements.

PRECAUTIONS RELATED TO THE SLUMP TEST

There is a general list of precautions in the discussion on "red flags" in chapter 7. Techniques of manual examination have become more refined and specific during the last 10 years. In particular, advances in identifying pain mechanisms, the potential of a latent reaction following nerve injury, an awareness of the effect of noradrenaline on injured nerves and a growing awareness of the importance of bio-psycho-social factors as contributing factors to pain maintenance have surely combined to allow better physical assessment and treatment. By performing the test actively first and with less pressure on the spine than was suggested previously (Maitland 1985; Butler 1991), a gentle and safe test is possible.

On a clinical note, you may notice what appears to be clonus in the quadriceps muscles at the knee extension stage of the slump test. It will often ease with neck extension. Proceed with care, raising your index of suspicion of a "red flag".

Remember too, that the entire test doesn't have to be performed. A patient may slump a little and experience lumbar symptoms that are made worse by neck flexion and this may be enough movement to provide sufficient information.

SLUMP TEST IN LONG SITTING

Although not listed as a base test, the slump in long sitting is included here as it is such a comfortable way to examine neural tissues in the head, neck and thorax as well as the lumbar spine. In addition, it is a useful position to initiate an active movement programme for a variety of disorders such as post spinal surgery troubles (see chapter 15). Some authors suggest that is a better test than PNF for meningitis (Vincent et al. 1993) and the suggestion certainly has a good anatomical base to it. There is no history to the test and in the past most authors have referred to the "toe touch" test as a measure of hamstring length. Hamstrings clearly are just one of many tissues involved in this test. Below is a suggested protocol for the test although, in the clinic I am sure you will want to alter and experiment with the order of movement.

PERFORMANCE OF THE TEST

A. STARTING POSITION

Sit your patient on the bed with both her knees and hips flexed. I often place my knee behind my patient's lumbar spine to stabilise the sacrum. Ask her to sit up straight and look ahead (Fig. 11. 25A). Be aware of any symptoms.

B. SPINAL SLUMP

With your patient looking forward, ask her to slump her body. Sometimes a gentle push in the stomach will facilitate this. Watch that she doesn't roll her pelvis back and either physically or verbally encourage her to keep it vertical. Check for any change in symptoms or new symptoms (Fig. 11.25B).

C. NECK FLEXION

Ask her to carefully flex her neck as in figure 11.25C. Note how difficult or easy the action is. You may need to ask her to hold her chin in as she flexes her neck. Check for a change in symptoms or any new symptoms anywhere in the body.

D. KNEE EXTENSION

Now ask her to slowly extend out her knees, one at a time and compare the symptoms evoked (Fig. 11.25D). Many patients cannot sit like this of course and adaptations will be needed, for example, you may need to place a pillow under her knees. In this position, ankle dorsiflexion or plantarflexion can be added.

REFINED TESTING

The slump LS test offers much better and more precise handling of the cervical and thoracic spine compared to the slump test in sitting. Further refinement to the testing can be made.

OPPORTUNITIES FOR STRUCTURAL DIFFERENTIATION

The test offers plenty of opportunities for structural differentiation. For example, if leg, lumbar or pelvic symptoms were evoked in the slump/knee extension position, you could

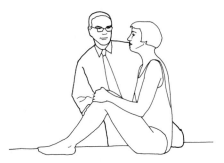

11.25A Slump long sitting test – starting position.

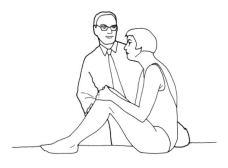

11.25B Slump LS spinal slump.

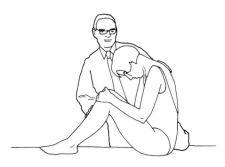

11.25C Slump LS neck flexion stage.

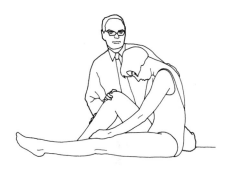

11.25D Slump LS knee extension stage.

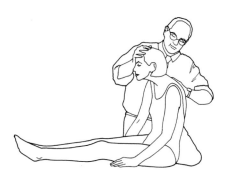

*11.26A Structural differentiation in slump
LS – upper cervical extension.*

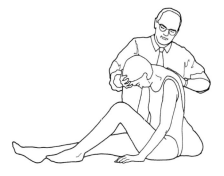

*11.26B Structural differentiation in slump
LS – knee extension.*

carefully extend her head (Fig. 11.26A). Or, if symptoms were evoked in her neck, head or thorax, you could carefully flex her knees, one at a time as in figure 11.26B. Try small amounts of movements. If a small amount of movement alters a remote symptom, your clinical inferences of mechanical and/or sensitivity changes in the nervous system will be well supported.

The slump long sit position also offers excellent opportunities for assessing what appears to be middle and upper thoracic neurogenic disorders. Note in figure 11.27A, an assessment technique that I find useful for what clinically appears to be upper thoracic neural disorders. Get your patient into the slump long sitting position, adapted as necessary with knee flexion. Pinch the C7 spinous process and stabilise it. Then check cervical lateral flexion to the left and right, making sure it is the neck on thorax that you are moving, not just head on neck. Tight muscles and stiff joints might limit the movement of course, but so can responses to mechanosensitive neural structures. Structural differentiation such as knee flexion can be used here to see if a response can be inferred to be neurogenic. You may notice catches and tightness in the interscapular area. For management, attention to joints, muscles and fascia may help and change the slump LS finding, or the slump test could be used as an active and/or passive mobilising technique.

Thoracic lateral flexion or rotation in the slump long sit position can be examined here also. Sit your patient close to you. I like to place my sternum on the patient's shoulder and then laterally flex the entire spine (Fig. 11.27B). Make sure you aren't pushing the patient away and

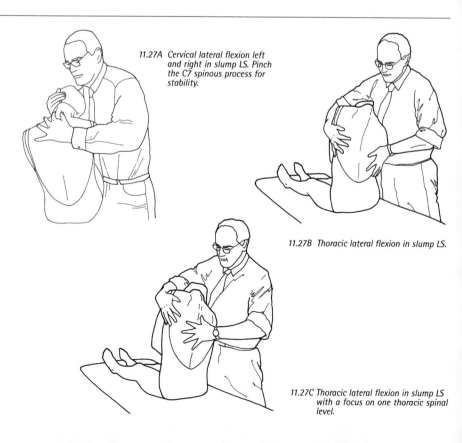

11.27A Cervical lateral flexion left and right in slump LS. Pinch the C7 spinous process for stability.

11.27B Thoracic lateral flexion in slump LS.

11.27C Thoracic lateral flexion in slump LS with a focus on one thoracic spinal level.

that the movement is one of thoracic/lumbar lateral flexion. Explain why you are doing such a technique to your patient so that she may feel at ease. With your thumb against the spinous process (Fig. 11.27C) you may be able to localise the lateral flexion. This test may evoke some local pain of joint and meningeal origin and what could be thoracic root pains. Use the knee flexion to structurally differentiate if needed.

Please don't make this some relentless chase for symptoms and signs to push and challenge. Many of us probably have a few catches in the thorax. Ask yourself "so what?" and consider the relevance of the response. Once again, refer back to chapter 7 and the section on specific physical dysfunction.

ORDER OF MOVEMENT

The basic and very broad principle is to load first the area that you want to give the most challenge to. The slump LS protocol as suggested above allows more load on the spine as this is the first component added. This will allow more spinal flexion. You may want to start with upper cervical flexion first. Just ask the patient to tuck her chin in, hold it in and then flex the spine and extend the knees. This would be a good way to examine upper cervical structures including the physical health of the occipital nerve.

You could start off with the neck placed in a lateral flexion and rotation position and then consecutively add the spinal flexion, if lateral flexion and rotation appear to be symptomatic movements.

THE HYPERMOBILE PATIENT

The slump test in long sitting is a useful position to examine your more hypermobile patients as I have shown in figure 11.28. Stand on the opposite side to the side being tested so you can flex and adduct the hip towards you. You may need to employ all the possible neural sensitising manoevres here. Order of movement means you can load the area suspected of housing the mechanosensitive tissues first. Sensitising additions could include upper cervical flexion and lateral flexion away, thoracic lateral flexion away, hip flexion, adduction and medial rotation and either ankle dorsiflexion or plantarflexion.

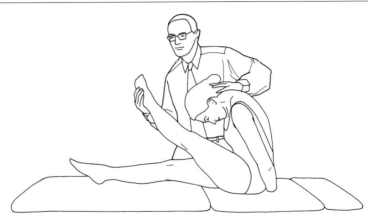

11.28 Slump LS for a hypermobile individual.

THE OBTURATOR NERVE

There is one major nerve that has not been addressed to this point and that is the obturator nerve. This nerve is medial to the axis of abduction and adduction and thus hip abduction will place a pressure on the nerve and its surrounding tissues. I suggest that in the slump LS position, the leg is taken out to symptom reproduction and then the spine is slumped and the neck flexed. Similarly, abduction in the slump knee bend test described and illustrated later in the chapter logically loads the obturator nerve. This nerve may be worth considering as part of chronic groin sprain. I have also noted this test and thus presumably the nerve, to be reactive in some patients long after kidney surgery.

SLUMP LS NORMAL RESPONSES

The normative symptomatic reponses to a slump LS test have not been documented. However there has been quite a lot of attention to the toe-reach test as a measure of flexibility, particularly of the hamstrings. However, in this test there is usually no control of the head and few researchers consider the possibility that the head position will affect the response to the test.

DO IT YOURSELF

This test is not difficult to perform by yourself. The only piece of equipment needed is a wall. Try it yourself. With knees and hips in flexion and back against the wall, position your bottom as close as possible to the base of the wall. Then you can slump, add neck flexion and extend the knees.

PRONE KNEE BEND

The Prone Knee Bend (PKB) test must be included as one of the base tests. It is clear from clinical observation and by reviewing the anatomy, that a load can be placed upon the upper lumbar nerve roots by flexing the knee. Although discogenic and radicular disorders are more common in the lower lumbar spine neurogenic disorders, this test may evoke symptoms in middle and upper lumbar radiculopathy and also sensitive lower lumbar radiculopathy.

Kreitz (1996) described a case study where PKB and a crossed PKB were positive in a patient with a surgically proven far lateral disc herniation at L3-4. In a large imaging study of 100

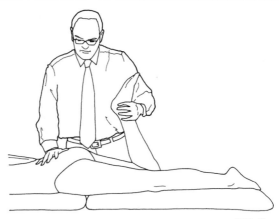

11.29 Prone Knee Bend base test.

patients with femoral neuralgia, Asquier et al. (1996) found that a herniated disc was responsible for the symptoms in 79 patients (83 herniated discs) and spinal stenosis for the other 21. Disc lesions were most common at L4-5 (40) followed by L3-4 (35) and then L2-3 (8). Foraminal herniations were very likely to present with a positive PKB. This supports Christodoulides' (1989) observations of positive PKBs in 40 patients with suspected L4-5 lateral disc protrusions.

PERFORMANCE OF THE TEST - PKB

Position your patient close to the side of the bed, ask her to do the movement actively first and then take over and perform it passively as is shown in figure 11.29. If you have a hand on her back you will feel the tension generated in multiple tissues and the spine will often extend a little. Compare the responses on left and right sides. Perform it bilaterally if you consider it warranted.

NORMAL RESPONSES AND ANALYSIS

The normal responses have never been documented. However it appears that in asymptomatic people, their heels should be able to touch or come close to the buttocks and be equal on both sides. A pulling or drag in the quadriceps is a common response.

It should be clear that many tissues are being stressed in this position, in particular anterior thigh fascia and muscles. It cannot be considered a complete femoral nerve loading test either, because the saphenous nerve runs posterior to the axis of flexion and extension. Thus the load placed on the nerve occurs due to the connection in fascia and muscle and perhaps the infrapatellar branch of the saphenous nerve.

VARIATIONS

CHANGE HIP AND FOOT POSITION

Extending the hip with the knee flexed as a further sensitising manoeuvre has often been suggested (O'Connell 1946; Macnab 1977; Grieve 1981; Corrigan and Maitland 1983). In normal asymptomatic university students, the PKB neutral was more sensitive for symptom reproduction than the test in extension (Davidson 1987). However, by reviewing the anatomy and listening to patient's complaints, if the femoral nerve or lateral femoral cutaneous nerve is injured or altered, then the addition of hip extension is likely to aggravate symptoms.

Clinicians who experiment in the clinic have sometimes noted that when a patient is in the PKB position, foot movements can alter test evoked pains. This is quite a common finding even in asymptomatic individuals. No clinical assumptions can be drawn from this. Perhaps a little more pressure is placed on the fascial tract or it may just be just another input into the nervous system, on top of what is already a novel inputs for the person tested.

SLUMP KNEE BEND POSITION

The slump knee bend position utilises the additional loading that can be placed on the PKB by spinal flexion (Fig. 11.30A). Call it the slump knee bend test rather than slump prone knee bend test for obvious reasons. The sensitivity which is apparent in the sitting slump test will not be present in this test and many of the responses will be due to soft tissue.

For the starting position for the test on the left side, ask your patient to hold her right knee and "cuddle up to it". This should prompt neck flexion, but make sure she doesn't completely flex her hip because she won't be able to flex her spine if her femur is held onto her chest. Note my position in the figure. I have her foot resting on my right hip, and my left arm supports the weight of her leg and my right hand stabilises her pelvis (Fig. 11.30A).

Now flex her knee a little, then extend her hip to the point of evoked symptoms. With this position held, you will be able to assess the effect of head and neck movements on the symptoms. When you have evoked symptoms, ask her to extend her neck as in figure 11.30B and note if there are any changes in resistance or symptoms. Sometimes you can feel a lessening of tension in the leg due to neck movements. Note also that there are no tight fascial links that could do this; the mechanism is likely to be neural. Neck extension will frequently change the responses in the anterior thigh in healthy individuals (Davidson 1987). In some patients, for example with an L3 nerve root lesion, the responses can be quite sharp and dramatic.

Note the way her foot is placed on my hip. You could try either hip. The model pictured is quite flexible, however in some patients it may be easier to dorsiflex the foot and place it on your hip as I have done in figure 11.31.

Mumenthaler (1991) has described a similar test and described it as a reversed Lasegue sign although the test as described above seems to be much better controlled.

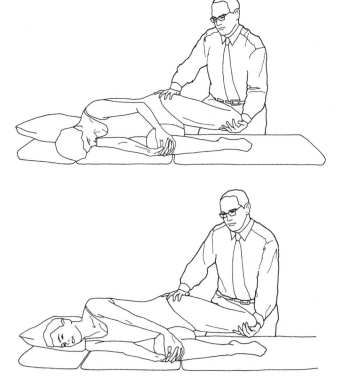

11.30A Slump knee bend test with cervical flexion.

11.30B Slump knee bend test with cervical extension.

THE LATERAL FEMORAL CUTANEOUS NERVE TEST

Kopell and Thompson (1963) practically described this test when they noted that adduction of the hip and a lateral flexion or shift away from the test side would tense the nerve. To place a physical challenge on the lateral femoral cutaneous nerve, use the above position, but add adduction to the manoeuvre. I have shown a slight variation of this is figure 11.31. I have performed the slump knee bend test with the test side down and then adducted her hip. This position is a little more comfortable and it makes it easier to add hip rotation to the test. The syndrome where this nerve becomes entrapped is known as "meralgia paraesthetica".

THE OBTURATOR NERVE

Some thought could be given to the obturator nerve and its representations during the slump knee bend test. My suggestion is that the hip is abducted in this position (Fig. 11.32). Any responses could be structurally differentiated by flexing or extending the neck.

THE SAPHENOUS NERVE TEST

Because the saphenous nerve is located posterior to the axis of flexion and extension of the knee (see figure 8.34) in the palpation and orientation chapter), it seems obvious that knee flexion as in the PKB test will slacken the nerve at the knee and that knee extension will tighten the nerve. Thus the peripheral neural component of the PKB test and a slump knee bend test is really a test of the femoral nerve above the knee, presumably tensioned by its connections to fascia and muscle. To test the saphenous nerve, the following is suggested for the right side (Fig. 11.33). Position your patient prone. Extend her hip and place it on your knee or on a hard pillow. Extend the knee, dorsiflex and invert her foot and then externally rotate the hip. You can palpate the saphenous nerve in this position and compare its sensitivity with alterations in hip or foot position. External rotation should be added. It is often reported as painful in those with clinical signs of saphenous entrapment (Nir-Paz et al. 1999). A similar combination of movements could be performed with the patient in supine.

The saphenous nerve is infrequently damaged, but if it is culpable, then this test may evoke symptoms. Kopell and Thompson (1963) report patients with surgically evident entrapments who complained of symptoms during knee extension. The infrapatellar branch of the saphenous nerve, by its location will be loaded during knee flexion, thus kneeling and squatting will tighten the nerve and test its physical abilities.

The next chapter focuses on the neurodynamic testing of the upper limb.

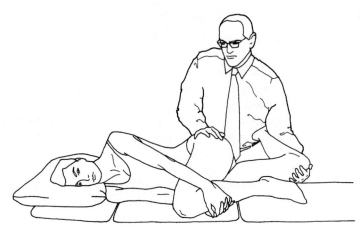

11.31 Test for the right lateral femoral cutaneous nerve.

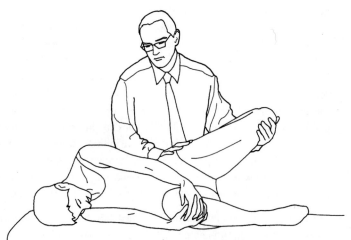

11.32 Test for the left obturator nerve.

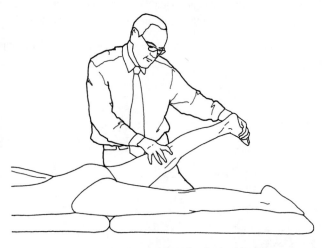

11.33 Test for the right saphenous nerve.

REFERENCES CHAPTER 11

Asquier C, Troussier B, Chirossel JP, et al. (1996) Femoral neuralgia due to degenerative spinal disease. A retrospective clinical and radio-anatomical study of one hundred cases. Revue du Rheumatisme (English Edition) 63: 278-284.

Attia J, Hatala R, Cook DJ, et al. (1999) Does this adult have acute meningitis? Journal of the American Medical Association 282: 175-181.

Barker PJ & Briggs CA (1999) Attachments of the posterior layer of fascia. Spine 24: 1757-1764.

Breig A (1978) Adverse Mechanical Tension in the Central Nervous System, Almqvist and Wiksell, Stockholm.

Breig A & Marions O (1963) Biomechanics of the lumbosacral nerve roots. Acta Radiologica 1: 1141-1159.

Breig A & Troup J (1979) Biomechanical considerations in the straight leg raising test. Spine 4: 242-250.

Butler DS (1991) Mobilisation of the Nervous System, Churchill Livingstone, Melbourne.

Cameron DM, Bohannon RW & Owen SV (1994) Influence of hip position on measurements of the straight leg raise test. Journal of Orthopedic and Sports Physical Therapy 19: 168-172.

Chan RC & Steinbok P (1984) Delayed onset of Lhermitte's sign following head and/or neck injuries. Report of four cases. Journal of Neurosurgery 60: 609-612.

Charnley J (1951) Orthopaedic signs in the diagnosis of disc protrusion with special reference to the straight leg raising test. Lancet 1: 186-192.

Christodoulides AN (1989) Ipsilateral sciatica on femoral nerve stretch test is pathognomonic of an L4/5 disc protrusion. Journal of Bone and Joint Surgery 71B: 88-89.

Corrigan B & Maitland GD (1983) Practical Orthopaedic Medicine, Butterworths, London.

Cyriax J (1942) Perineuritis. British Medical Journal: 578-580.

Davidson S (1987) Prone knee bend: an investigation into the effect of cervical flexion and extension. Manipulative Therapists Association of Australia, 5th biennial conference. Melbourne.

Deyo RA, Rainville J & Kent DL (1992) What can the history and physical examination tell us about low back pain? Journal of the American Medical Association 268: 760-765.

Dyck P (1984) Lumbar nerve root: the enigmatic eponyms. Spine 9: 3-6.

Gifford LS (1987) Circadian variation in human flexibility and grip strength. Australian Journal of Physiotherapy 33: 3-9.

Gifford LS (1994) Influence of circadian variation on spinal examination. In: Boyling J & Palastanga N (eds.) Modern Manual Therapy, 3rd edn. Churchill Livingstone, Edinburgh.

Grieve GP (1981) Common Vertebral Joint Problems, Churchill Livingstone, Edinburgh.

Gutrecht JA, Zamani AA & Slagado ED (1993) Anatomic-radiologic basis of Lhermitte's sign in multiple sclerosis. Archives of Neurology 50: 849-851.

Haddox JD (1999) Neuropsychiatric physical examination. In: Aronoff GM (ed.) Evaluation and Treatment of Chronic Pain, Williams & Wilkins, Baltimore.

Hakelius A (1970) Prognosis in sciatica. Acta Orthopaedica Scandinavica (Suppl) 129: 1-70.

Hsieh C-Y, Walker JM & Gillis K (1983) Straight-leg-raising test. Comparison of three instruments. Physical Therapy 63: 1429-1433.

Hudgins WR (1979) The crossed straight leg raising test. Journal of Occupational Medicine 21: 407-408.

Inman VT & Saunders JBC (1942) The clinico-anatomical aspects of the lumbosacral region. Journal of Radiology 38: 669-678.

Johnson EK & Chiarello CM (1997) The slump test: the effects of head and lower extremity position on knee extension. Journal of Orthopedic and Sports Physical Therapy 26: 310-317.

Jonsson B & Stromqvist B (1995) The straight leg raising test and the severity of symptoms in lumbar disc herniation. Spine 20: 27-30.

Khuffash B & Porter RW (1988) Cross leg pain and trunk list. Spine 14: 602-603.

Kopell HP & Thompson WAL (1963) Peripheral Entrapment Neuropathies, Williams and Wilkins, Baltimore.

Kosteljanetz M, Bang F & Shmidt-Olsen S (1988) The clinical significance of straight leg raising (Lasegue's sign) in the diagnosis of prolapsed lumbar disc. Spine 13: 393-395.

Kreitz BG, CÙtÈ P & Yong-Hing K (1996) Crossed femoral stretching test. Spine 21: 1584-1586.

Lew PC, Morrow CJ & Lew AM (1994) The effect of neck and leg flexion and their sequence on the lumbar spinal cord. Spine 19: 2421-2425.

Lew PC & Puentedura EJ (1985) The straight-leg-raise test and spinal posture. Fourth biennial conference, Manipulative Therapists Association of Australia. Brisbane.

Lossos A & Siegel T (1996) Electric shock-like sensations in 42 cancer patients: clinical characteristics and distinct etiologies. Journal of Neurooncology 29: 175-181.

Macnab I (1977) Backache, Williams and Wilkins, Baltimore.

Maitland G (1985) The Slump Test: Examination and Treatment. Australian Journal of Physiotherapy 31: 215-219.

Maitland GD (1986) Vertebral Manipulation, 6th edn. Butterworths, London.

Massey A (1985) Movement of pain sensitive structures in the neural canal. In: Greive GP (ed.) Modern Manual Therapy of the Vertebral Column, Churchill Livingstone, Edinburgh.

McCombe PF, Fairbank JCT, Cockersole BC, et al. (1989) Reproducibility of physical signs in low-back pain. Spine 14: 908-918.

Molesworth J (1992) The effect of chronic inversion ankle sprains on the dorsiflexion-inversion straight leg raise test and the plantarflexion-inversion straight leg raise test. Thesis. University of South Australia, Adelaide .

Mumenthaler M & Schliack H (1991) Peripheral Nerve Lesions, Thieme, New York.

Newton HB & Rea GL (1996) Lhermitte's sign as a presenting symptom of primary spinal cord tumor. Journal of Neurooncology 29: 183-188.

Nir-Paz R, Luder AS, Cozacov JC, et al. (1999) Saphenous nerve entrapment in adolescence. Pediatrics 103: 161-163.

O'Connell JEA (1946) The clinical signs of meningeal irritation. Brain 69: 9-21.

O'Connell JEA (1946) Sciatica and the mechanism of the production of the clincial syndrome in protrusions of the lumbar intervertebral discs. British Journal of Surgery 30: 315-327.

Porter RW & Trailescu IF (1990) Diurnal changes in straight leg raising. Spine 15: 103-106.

Ramamurthi B (1980) Absence of limitation of straight leg raising in proved lumbar disc lesion. Journal of Neurosurgery 52: 852-853.

Shacklock M (1989) The plantarflexion/inversion straight leg raise test. An investigation into the effect of cervical flexion and order of component movements on the symptom response. Thesis. University of South Australia, Adelaide .

Slater H, Butler DS & Shacklock MO (1994) The dynamic nervous system: examination and assessment using tension tests. In: Boyling JD & Palastanga N (eds.) Grieve's Modern Manual Therapy, 2nd edn. Churchill Livingstone, Edinburgh.

Spangfort EV (1972) Lumbar disc herniation: a computer aided analysis of 2504 operations. Acta Orthopaedica Scandinavica (Suppl) 142: 1-95).

Sweetham BJ, Anderson JA & Dalton ER (1974) The relationships between little finger mobility, lumbar mobility, straight leg raising and low back pain. Rheumatology and Rehabilitation 13: 161-166.

Tencer AF, Allen BL & Ferguson RL (1985) A biomechanical study of thoracolumbar spine fractures with bone in the spinal canal: part 111. Mechanical properties of the dura and its tethering ligaments. Spine 10: 741-747.

Troup JDG (1981) Straight-leg-raising (SLR) and the qualifying tests for increased root tension: their predictive value after back and sciatic pain. Spine 6: 526-527.

van den Bent MJ, Hilkens PH, Sillevis Smith PA, et al. (1998) Lhermitte's sign following chemotherapy with docetaxel. Neurology 50: 563-564.

Vincent J, Thomas K & Matthew O (1993) An improved clinical method for detecting meningeal irritation. Archives of Disease in Childhood 68: 215-218.

Vollmer TL, Brass LM & Waxman SG (1991) Lhermitte's sign in a patient with herpes zoster. Journal of Neurological Science 106: 153-157.

Vucetic N & Svensson O (1996) Physical signs in lumbar disc hernia. Clinical Orthopaedics and Related Research 333: 192-201.

Waddell G (1998) The Back Pain Revolution, Churchill Livingstone, Edinburgh.

Wiltse LL (1997) The history of spinal disorders. In: Frymoyer JW (ed.) The Adult Spine, 2nd edn. Philadelphia.

Woodhall B & Hayes BJ (1950) The well leg raising test of Fajersztajn in the diagnosis of ruptured intervertebral disc. The Journal of Bone and Joint Surgery 32A: 786-792.

CHAPTER 12

THE UPPER LIMB
NEURODYNAMIC TESTS

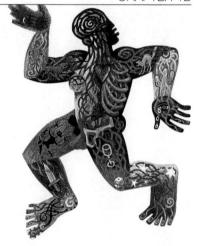

INTRODUCTION

WHAT'S IN A NAME
CONCEPT OF ULNT

ULNT1 (MEDIAN) BASE TEST - PERFORMANCE

ULNT1 (MEDIAN) - ACTIVE TEST
ULNT1 (MEDIAN) - PASSIVE TEST
ULNT1 - ALTERNATIVE HANDLING
GENERAL ULNT1 HANDLING COMPONENTS
ULNT1 (MEDIAN) - NORMAL RESPONSES
INDICATIONS AND SPECIAL CARE
ADAPTIONS, SENSITISING ADDITIONS
ANALYSIS OF INPUTS
THE REVERSE ULNT1 (MEDIAN) - TEST VARIATION

ULNT2 (MEDIAN) PERFORMANCE

ULNT2 (MEDIAN) - ACTIVE TEST
ULNT2 (MEDIAN) - PASSIVE TEST

PERFORMANCE OF THE ULNT2 (RADIAL)

ULNT2 (RADIAL) - ACTIVE TEST
ULNT2 (RADIAL) - PASSIVE TEST
HANDLING COMMENTS AND VARIATIONS FOR THE ULNT2 TESTS
NORMAL RESPONSES

ULNT3 (ULNAR) - PERFORMANCE

INTRODUCTION
ULNT3 (ULNAR) - ACTIVE TEST
ULNT3 (ULNAR) - PASSIVE TEST BEGINNING DISTALLY
ULNT3 - PASSIVE TEST BEGINNING PROXIMALLY
HANDLING COMMENTS/NORMAL RESPONSES/FURTHER SENSITISATION

MUSCULOCUTANEOUS NERVE TEST

MUSCULOCUTANEOUS NERVE - ACTIVE TEST
MUSCULOCUTANEOUS NERVE - PASSIVE TEST
HANDLING COMMENTS/NORMAL RESPONSES/FURTHER SENSITISATION

OTHER UPPER LIMB TESTS

AXILLARY
SUPRASCAPULAR NERVE

REFERENCES CHAPTER 12

INTRODUCTION

Neurodynamic tests for the upper limb are recent additions to orthopaedic and neurological assessment. They have been integrated into many undergraduate and post-graduate manual therapy programmes. Kenneally et al. (1988) drew attention to them, calling the upper limb tension test "The Straight Leg Raise of the Arm." This is an apt title, because the test appears as useful for examination and management of upper quadrant disorders as the SLR is for assessment and management of patients with disorders in the lower limbs. While clear diagnostic validity for the tests is still lacking (chapter 13), there are excellent neuroanatomical and neuropathological bases for the test. When the movements are sensitive, they can be integrated into management under the broad spectrum clinical reasoning base suggested in chapters 6,7,10 and 14.

Despite recent interest in the tests, promoted in particular by Elvey (1986) and Butler (1991), there are much older references to tests that physically challenge upper limb neural tissues. In Germany, Bragard (1929) clearly described a series of upper limb tension tests, similar to the ones described in this chapter. A version of upper limb tension test, including an abducted, elevated and extended arm was suggested by Chavany (1934). Smith (1956) performed a superb series of human and monkey dissections better known for their straight leg raising and spinal flexion examination, but he also included upper limb tension test like manoeuvres. Pechan (1973) described a test known as the ulnar nerve tension test, very similar to the test described later in this chapter. And of course, Cyriax, who was often ahead of his time, suggested that when a patient had a symptomatic wrist, the wrist should also be examined with the elbow extended (Cyriax 1978). Other manoeuvres used over the years seeking neurovascular compromise in the upper limb include Adson's test (Adson 1951) and Wright's manoeuvre (Wright 1945). In Wright's manoeuvre, the arm is placed in an abducted and externally rotated position and the patient turns her head away from the test side while taking a deep breath. Changes in the pulse are sought.

Concepts of dynamic examinations of carpal and cubital tunnel syndromes are widely recommended, for example, Novak (1994) and Rayan (1992). Tinel recommended performing the test that bears his name before and after Phalen's test or before and after full flexion of the elbow (Omer and Bell-Krotoski 1997). Clinicians who have taken the time to listen openly to their patient's stories over the years must have been aware of movement dependent mechanosensitivity of neural tissues. I sometimes marvel at how long it took for an upper limb equivalent of the SLR to emerge. There have been strong clues from the world of anaesthesia as well. Although their patients could only complain after the event, surgeons have been aware for many years that if the arms of anaesthetised patients were placed in certain positions, rather drastic neurological sequelae could follow. Abduction and depression of the shoulder girdle have been identified as the positions posing the most danger.

WHAT'S IN A NAME?

Well known Australian manual therapist, Robert Elvey first introduced the test known as the brachial plexus tension test (BPTT) to an international manual therapy conference in Melbourne (Elvey 1979). The term upper limb tension test (ULTT) was introduced by Kenneally et al. (1988) and numerous research projects were carried out under that name at the University of South Australia in the 1980s. ULTT was used in the "Mobilisation of the Nervous

System" text (Butler 1991). BPTT is still frequently used, for example, Selvaratnam (1994) and Balster (1997)

The term "neural provocation test" has also emerged (Elvey 1997). The term is also widely used by hand surgeons. It may be alright for assessment, but I prefer that it is not used in management. The test should rarely be a provocative test. Certainly don't tell a patient that you are about to perform a "neural provocation test", find a more acceptable name for it. Sir Sydney Sunderland (pers. comm. 1991) thought that the best term was ULTT as it relates to the entire upper limb neural tissues and doesn't necessarily infer that neural tissue is the only tissue physically challenged. In this book, I am using the term "upper limb neurodynamic test" (ULNT). As Shacklock (1995) rightly pointed out, the term neurodynamic is more encompassing than "tension". It encourages thoughts of the neurophysiological aspects of mechanosensitivity. The term neurodynamics can also encompass the recent awareness of the ULNT as a test of the stability of various upper limb representations in the central nervous system homonculi.

As long as clinicians and researchers are performing similar tests and clearly describing what they are doing, it probably doesn't matter much. Ultimately it is more important to see the test responses as an expression of the pathobiological processes occurring in your patients and to analyse the responses in relation to the patient's overall problem.

CONCEPT OF ULNT

Despite the discussion in the literature over the years, integration into manual therapy did not occur until the 1980's, much of it due to Elvey's pioneering work in Australia (Elvey 1979; Elvey et al. 1986). Tests for various nerves were suggested by Kenneally et al. (1988) and tests for the radial and ulnar nerves were described in Butler (1991) on anatomical and clinical grounds.

Four upper limb neurodynamic tests were suggested in Butler (1991). These tests evolved from Elvey's initial test and are derived from clinical experimentation, intuition and necessity. I believe four base tests are necessary to provide a basic overview assessment of the physical health of the nervous system in the upper limb. They include attention to the major neural pathways and the major sensitising movements.

I refer to the tests as:

- ULNT1 (median nerve bias)

- ULNT2 (median nerve bias)

- ULNT2 (radial nerve bias)

- ULNT3 (ulnar nerve bias)

The numbers simply refer to powerful sensitising movements. One is shoulder abduction, 2 is shoulder girdle depression and 3 is elbow flexion. The reason there are two tests for the median nerve is simply because this nerve is more commonly injured than the other nerves in the upper limb and it was felt that a test was required to evaluate shoulder girdle depression and glenohumeral elevation independently.

I recommend that all ULNTs be performed actively before passively. This may decrease patient's anxieties, but it may be that after active examination a reasoned decision is made not to perform the tests passively. And, if found sensitive, it is very likely that they will be used actively in therapy. ULNTs can also be performed in combination with other manoeuvres such as nerve palpation.

ULNT1 (MEDIAN) BASE TEST – PERFORMANCE

The examination technique, adapted from Butler (1991), is described, for a patient who has no problems with her upper quadrant, hence the test can be taken towards the end of range. As in previous technique descriptions, the patient is described as "she" and I am the examiner. I describe the test as if you were standing next to me with the patient. The key handling clues described in detail in the last chapter are summarised below for quick reference.

• Establish hypotheses in all reasoning categories prior to testing, especially pathobiology, likely specific dysfunctions to be found on examination, precautions and sources.

• Tell your patient exactly what you are going to do and what you want her to do. Make her feel comfortable about reporting any responses to your testing, anywhere in her body. Upper limb neurodynamic tests, especially those involving shoulder girdle depression occasionally evoke low back pains.

• Perform the test on the less painful side or non-painful side first. If little difference, perform the test on the left side first.

• Starting position should be consistent each time. Any variations from normal practice should be noted.

• Note symptom responses including areas and nature.

• Watch for antalgic postures and other motor responses during the test (eg. cervical movements or trapezius activity).

• Test for symmetry between sides.

• Explain your findings to your patient.

• Repeat the test a number of times before recording an actual measurement.

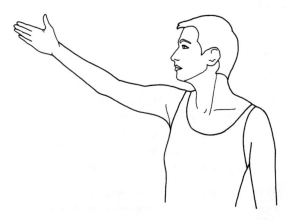

12.1 ULNT1 performed actively.
See text for full description

ULNT1 (MEDIAN) - ACTIVE TEST

If your patient has described a provocative position, get her to show you that position. Observe the mechanics involved and be aware of how she feels about bringing on symptoms. You may be able to perform a quick structural differentiation. For example, your patient may demonstrate a symptomatic position for her elbow pain. Get her to maintain that position and then ask her to move her neck to see if that alters the evoked symptoms.

I suggest a simple protocol for the active evaluation of neurodynamic tests. Have your patient look at her hand, then get her to perform the test and then add wrist and neck movements if required. So for the ULNT1 (median), ask your patient to look at the palm of her hand, extend her elbow, then get her to extend her arm out sideways with the hand held forward until it comes to just above her head (Fig. 12.1). Then ask her to extend her wrist and tip her head away from the test side. Compare with the opposite side.

Note the symptom responses and also note what happens to the shoulder girdle. Where the nervous system is sensitive the shoulder girdle will often elevate.

ULNT1 (MEDIAN) - PASSIVE TEST

I have described this test for my patient's right arm.

A. STARTING POSITION

Lie your patient in a comfortable supine position close to your side of the bed. Make sure she has her legs straight and left arm by her side. A pillow is not necessary unless neck extension is uncomfortable. Note my positioning in figure 12.2A. Get in a stride standing position and face your patient. See how I am holding her right hand in my left hand. Her fingers are straight including her distal interphalangeal joints and my thumb is on her thumb. (You could adapt here and use your index finger also). Keep her wrist in neutral. Her upper arm rests on my right thigh and is abducted a few degrees in the coronal plane for handling convenience. I have the bed at a height so that my hip is flexed a little and her arm can rest comfortably on my upper thigh. I am taking approximately half the weight of the arm on my thigh and half through her hand. With my right hand I form a fist and push into the bed to control the natural shoulder elevation during the shoulder abduction component of the test (but see alternative position later). Try and maintain both shoulder girdle positions equal. If you can achieve this controlled and comfortable starting position, then the handling will be easier and it should be more accurate for test-retest.

B. SHOULDER ABDUCTION

Now "walk the arm up" in the coronal plane. It is important that only the glenohumeral component is moved and also to keep the shoulder from elevating while abducting. The fist "punched " into the bed should prevent this. Abduct her arm to approximately 110 degrees or to any resistance or appreciable tightening of the tissues, or symptoms. The elbow is kept at 90 degrees flexion and the hand position is kept constant. Look at her, ask about and be aware of responses (Fig. 12.2B).

C. WRIST AND FINGER EXTENSION

With the shoulder abduction position maintained, extend her wrist and fingers (Fig. 12.2C). Be sensitive to any symptom changes and just take the movement into some tissue tightness.

D. FOREARM SUPINATION

Now, as in figure 12.2D, just carefully rotate her forearm into supination. You may prefer to add the wrist and finger extension after the supination. It doesn't really matter. As always, check responses. Make sure the shoulder position is held firmly and hasn't moved.

E. SHOULDER LATERAL ROTATION

With the above position held, laterally rotate her shoulder. Pay some attention to your handling here because the wrist and finger extension must be held firmly. The shoulder is carefully rotated to the onset of resistance or onset of any symptoms (Fig. 12.2E). Talk to the patient through the movement and tell her how the test is going. Shoulder lateral rotation can be a threatening movement for some, especially if there are memories of this movement as an injuring movement. You may need to coax her through the movement.

F. ELBOW EXTENSION

Extend her elbow now, keeping the wrist and shoulder position constant (Fig. 12.2F). Be ready, because the neural and soft tissues in this position will be challenged and there will probably be symptoms or a change in symptoms at this stage. Very few patients (and subjects) will be able to extend their elbows in this position. Ask about symptoms, particularly if you feel tightness. If she has some difficulty describing symptoms, ease the movement off so she can explain her responses. My patient is quite mobile and can nearly extend her elbow.

G. CERVICAL LATERAL FLEXION AWAY

With the test so far, if an appropriate symptom is reproduced at any stage, cervical spine movements can be added. In particular, test cervical lateral flexion. It is well worth demonstrating what you want your patient to do before asking her to perform it when she is in a full ULNT position. I find it useful to say, "look at the ceiling and move your ear to your shoulder". Also, if you demonstrate the lateral flexion component for the patient prior to the test there should be a better movement recall. In figure 12.2G, cervical lateral flexion away from the test side is demonstrated. Make sure it is neck on thorax lateral flexion, not head on neck, so that the test will challenge middle and lower cervical nerve roots.

H. CERVICAL LATERAL FLEXION TOWARDS

You could also check the responses to lateral flexion towards the test side (Fig. 12.2H). This cervical spine movement would be an appropriate thing to do if the patient had a particularly sensitive problem. Other cervical combinations can be tested if required such as extension, lateral glides, retraction and rotation. If your patient had a forward head posture, then it may be useful to see the response to symptoms if she retracted her neck. These situations and treatments are discussed in chapter 15.

ULNT1 - ALTERNATIVE HANDLING

Some clinicians prefer to use an examination technique using their elbow, bringing them much closer to their patient. See figure 12.3. Rather than maintaining the shoulder girdle position by my outstretched arm, I have moved much closer to her and leant on the bed with my elbow. She can now lie in the middle of the bed. Note how my left hand can cradle her arm just below the elbow. This can be a very supportive and secure position to help get a patient to move, particularly one who is frightened to move after injury. Precise hand control is still possible.

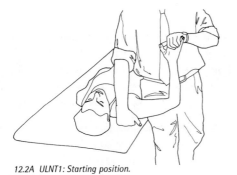

12.2A ULNT1: Starting position.

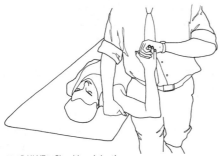

12.2B ULNT1: Shoulder abduction.

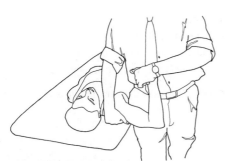

12.2C ULNT1: Wrist extension.

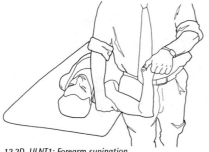

12.2D ULNT1: Forearm supination.

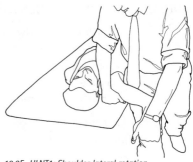

12.2E ULNT1: Shoulder lateral rotation.

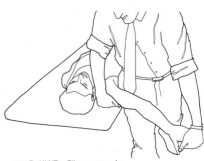

12.2F ULNT1: Elbow extension.

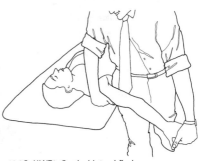

12.2G ULNT1: Cervical lateral flexion away.

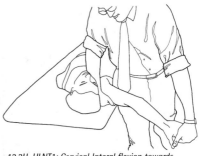

12.2H ULNT1: Cervical lateral flexion towards.

GENERAL ULNT1 HANDLING COMMENTS

The upper limb neurodynamic tests are gentle tests. With good communication and handling based on an accurate assessment, your patient's symptoms should never be aggravated. Accurate assessment means knowing what to look for and what to expect during the examination. This information should be gleaned from a subjective interview in particular and also the physical examination prior to testing. Review chapters 6 and 7 if necessary.

Elbow extension was performed last in this sequence. In earlier descriptions of the test (Kenneally et al. 1988), the wrist and finger extension were the last components performed. I recommend the sequence performed above. Range of movement is easier to gauge from elbow extension compared to wrist extension and in the case of rough handling or unexpected responses, the patient can protect the movement with biceps and brachialis activity.

Some clinicians "preload" tissues first by performing the test with the cervical spine in lateral flexion away from the test side and include shoulder girdle depression as part of the initial test. However, consider that in healthy young individuals, a symptomatic response and a restriction in elbow extension is nearly always achieved during the test as described above (see normal responses below). Preloading is rarely required for an initial ULNT1 assessment. In addition, test-retest reliability should be better if it is performed with the head in a neutral position.

And please, be aware of all responses to your input - both verbal and nonverbal. By nonverbal responses, I mean more than just a range of motion measurement. There could be motor adaptive responses elsewhere, a facial reddening, perhaps some sweating.

ULNT1 (MEDIAN) - NORMAL RESPONSES

A pattern of frequently reported and observed responses has been noted in young, asymptomatic, healthy South Australian university students. Presumably these responses are similar in other members of the community. "Stretching", "pulling", "pain", "tingling" are quite commonly reported sensations even in individuals who are asymptomatic prior to the test.

Kenneally et al. (1988) summarised the responses to the ULNT of 400 asymptomatic individuals as follows:

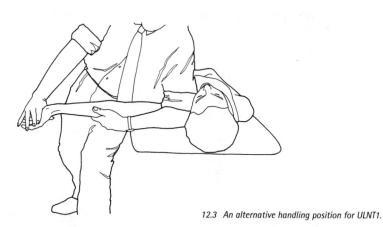

12.3 An alternative handling position for ULNT1.

• A deep stretch or ache in the cubital fossa (99% of volunteers) extending down the anterior and radial aspect of the forearm and into the radial side of the hand.

• A definite tingling sensation in the thumb and first three fingers.

• A small percentage felt stretch in the anterior shoulder.

• Cervical lateral flexion away from the side tested increased evoked responses in 90% of subjects.

• Cervical lateral flexion towards the side tested decreased the test response in 70% of subjects.

These sensory responses have been mapped out for easy reference in figure 12.4.

Pullos (1986) applied the test to 100 asymptomatic subjects, reporting that the range of elbow extension deficit during the test was 16.5 to 53.2 degrees. In testing thousands of students, it is only a rare, extremely hypermobile individual who has elbow extension which is full range and asymptomatic in this position.

The ULNT, like any neurodynamic test, is a threat to the patient. The more familiar the test, the better the patient understands what you are doing. The quality of your interaction will vary the threat. It is normal that there is some progressive muscular activity during the test, as has been shown in the trapezius muscle during the test by Balster & Jull (1997). Earlier, Edgar et al. (1994) had demonstrated that neural extensibility as defined by the ULNT was related to the extensibility of the trapezius muscle. There will inevitably be more hidden autonomic and endocrine activity depending on the "value" that your patient's CNS gives to your ULNT input.

Care is needed using these normal responses in the clinic and they must be considered a guideline only. There is a discussion on the use of normal responses in chapter 10. In chapter 13, Jim Matheson discusses research in relation to the ULNT.

INDICATIONS AND SPECIAL CARE

You would consider using a ULNT1 in the clinic where there is:

• a hypothesis of neurogenic pain in the upper limb.

• a hypothesis that the source of the disorder lies in the median nerve pathways and receptive fields.

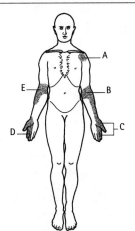

12.4 Normal responses to the ULNT1 in a large group of healthy university students. Subjects could feel symptoms in areas B and C, or area E, or area D. Symptoms were only occasionally experienced in area A (adapted from Kenneally et al. 1988).

• a pain provocative pattern which is similar to the test (eg. hanging washing on the line) or a part of the test, for example, forearm pronation and supination activities).

• objective tests such as a nerve conduction test, supporting nerve injury, especially the median nerve.

Some care is also required. Please read the general precautions, contraindications and "red flags" list in chapter 7. Clinically there are two benign neurogenic phenomena that require care. The first is acute nerve root injuries – they need to be handled gently or even not handled at all; the second is apparent central sensitivity. Excessive testing and repeated movements may lead to a long lasting aggravation.

Always take care with acute apparent neurogenic pain. Many patients with painful upper limbs may not have had their arm elevated to such position for months. Clinically it appears easier to aggravate upper limb disorders than lower limb.

ADAPTATIONS, SENSITISING ADDITIONS

The ULNT1 has just been described for a healthy subject. Adaptations will be required when the tests are performed on patients, the most frequent one being that the complete test may not be required. The most likely scenario is that you will perform part of the test, duplicate your patient's symptoms or something very similar and move a remote part to structurally differentiate.

You will need to think on your feet while performing the test. There is no set adaptations protocol because of the normal variability between subjects and the greater variability in patients with pathological changes. For example, you may be performing the test and during the shoulder abduction phase, your patient may complain of wrist pain. You could then ease off the shoulder movement and check a few times to see whether it was the shoulder movement which altered the wrist symptoms. Or, if you were performing a ULNT1 and your patient complained of ulnar based symptoms during the shoulder abduction stage, hopefully you would consider assessing the effect of elbow flexion to load the ulnar nerve, as well as assessing the effects of elbow extension.

More shoulder extension, more shoulder abduction, shoulder girdle in protraction, perhaps add a SLR; these are all possible additions to the test. You may gather clues to the value of adding these movements via the aggravating movements or postures that your patient complains of, and by thoughts about neuroanatomy in relation to joint axes of movement. In chapter 10 there is a section on taking base tests further.

ANALYSIS OF INPUTS

The upper limb neurodynamic tests are tests of aspects of the physical abilities of many tissues including neural structures, plus tests of the threshold controls of the CNS in relation to that specific input. Threshold control computations will include the meaning of the movement, the therapeutic relationship and various spatiotemporal characteristics involving both you and your patient. It must be a test of not only neural structures in the periphery but also the stability of the representations of the arm in the various brain homonculi.

If you find that the ULNT is sensitive, more so on one side than the other, then in the absence of any other data all you can infer is that the patient has a sensitive movement. Perhaps the area of pain and some paraesthesia may point to a neurogenic contribution. However there is no doubt that the test also places a significant physical challenge upon local neural tissues.

The basic principle is that the nerve will be loaded, depending on the relationship of the nerve with the joint axis. For wrist and elbow extension it is clear that the median nerve will have to adapt by straining and gliding (see chapter 5 for further details). The shoulder movements are more complex. During shoulder abduction the C5 and C6 roots in particular are strained (Elvey 1986; Selvaratnam et al. 1988; Kleinrensink et al. 2000). Buckle transducer studies in cadavers have shown that lateral and medial cords of the plexus are subjected to tension during the test (Reid 1987; Ginn 1989; Kleinrensink et al. 2000), although in a ULNT1 position Kleinrensink (2000) demonstrated that more tension was transmitted via the medial cord more than the lateral cord. In addition, a "pulley effect" occurs on the brachial plexus as it wraps around the coracoid process (Lord and Roseti 1971). You can easily visualise this as the arm is elevated.

During the test, the shoulder girdle position has to be held to maintain the elevation force from the abduction manouevre. It is a common clinical observation that patients with 5th and 6th cervical nerve root pain often obtain relief by elevating their shoulder girdle, or even by placing one hand on top of their head.

Lateral rotation of the arm will often alter evoked symptoms from the glenohumeral abduction position either by increasing or decreasing the position. Buckle transducer studies on two cadavers (Reid 1987) have shown that lateral rotation decreases tension on the cords of the plexus. However there may be gliding of the neural tissues and this position could be interpreted as threatening by the patient, hence the lateral rotation may be symptomatic.

Many other tissues are strained during upper limb neurodynamic tests and not just the obvious joints, muscle and skin. Wilson et al. (1994) have provided quantitative data from embalmed cadavers showing that strain is produced in segments of the subclavian artery during the ULNT and increased by contralateral lateral flexion. Moses and Carman (1996) performed an anatomical investigation of the lower cervical neural structures while considering the implications of the ULNT on the anatomy. The posterior longitudinal ligament anchors the nerve roots to the vertebral bodies and intervertebral discs and there are connections to the periosteum of the vertebral bodies and to the capsule of neighbouring zygapophyseal joints.

Research findings such as that of Moses & Carman (1996) are a reminder of the grossness of a test such as the ULNT, yet it is also a reminder of its complexity and completeness. It will always be extremely difficult to diagnose the tissue at fault and in many cases, particularly when maladaptive central sensitivity appears to be part of the patient's clinical picture, accurate tissue diagnosis may not be critical in assessment and in management.

THE REVERSE ULNT1 (MEDIAN) – TEST VARIATION

The base upper limb neurodynamic test will always need to be varied to adapt to patients. If you can perform the base test smoothly and safely, then variations will be easy to accomplish. A reversed ULNT1, that is, beginning the test from the wrist first, seems particularly useful. It is based on the clinical finding that patients with carpal tunnel syndrome have their symptoms reproduced more easily with this distal to proximal test.

A. STARTING POSITION

This is similar to the ULNT1, although there is no need to maintain the shoulder girdle position initially. In this particular case, I have given my patient a pillow (Fig. 12.5A). I often use one for this test because the neck is not as likely to be used as in the base test. Lie her in the middle of the bed, thus allowing her to rest her forearm on the bed. Observe my hand position. You can be very specific here with hand positioning as this test appears more sensitive than the base ULNT1 test for neurogenic disorders distal to the elbow. I have control to her fingertips and my left thumb is on her left thumb. For clinicians with smaller hands, try using your index finger to control her thumb.

B. WRIST AND FINGER EXTENSION

This should be easy from the starting position (Fig. 12.5B). If necessary more of a focus can be placed on an individual digit. Be aware of your patient's symptoms. This is similar to Phalen's test and it may evoke symptoms in many carpal tunnel syndrome sufferers. There will be many variations possible here. For example, you may wish to begin the test with one particular finger. I have discussed many variations and their handling in chapter 15 in the section on carpal tunnel syndrome.

C. FOREARM SUPINATION

Add forearm supination (Fig. 12.5C). Remember to be aware of your patient's symptoms and to maintain the wrist and finger extension.

D. ELBOW EXTENSION

Check this out in figure 12.5D. For the previous stages of the test, I have hardly utilised my right arm. With the wrist and forearm position maintained, add elbow extension. You can guide this movement via your right hand. I am between her arm and the bed and her arm is in approximately 30 degrees of abduction.

E. WHOLE ARM LATERAL ROTATION

This needs to be guided with both of my hands as in figure 12.5E. It is now easier if her arm is resting on my right thigh. Observe what happens during the movement, particularly at the shoulder girdle and always check for changes in symptoms.

F. SHOULDER ABDUCTION

Now is the time to stabilise her shoulder girdle with your right hand. Try the "punch grip" as used in the base test. Her arm can be carefully elevated now using your right thigh (Fig. 12.5F). Be careful here with the abduction as symptoms could come on quite quickly. If need be, although it is unlikely, lateral flexion movements of the cervical spine could also be added. Most of the structural differentiation can be performed via the shoulder.

ULNT2 (MEDIAN) PERFORMANCE

There is a complexity of neurodynamics in the upper limb that the ULNT1 as described above does not fully examine. The major neural sensitising movement that is missing is shoulder girdle depression, even though the shoulder girdle elevation is controlled. Also, consider that the ULNT1 is performed with surrounding tissues on some stretch and it may be difficult to fully examine the neural tissues. In some cases (eg. post shoulder surgery, acute trauma) it may

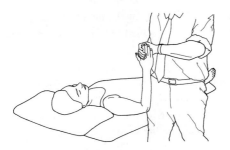

12.5A ULNT1 distal to proximal: Starting position.

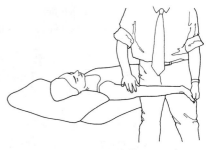

12.5D ULNT1 distal to proximal: Elbow extension.

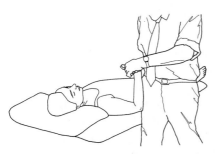

12.5B ULNT1 distal to proximal: Wrist extension.

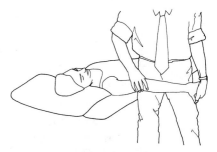

12.5E ULNT1 distal to proximal: Whole arm lateral rotation.

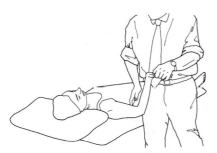

12.5C ULNT1 distal to proximal: Forearm supination.

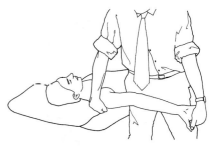

12.5F ULNT1 distal to proximal: Shoulder abduction.

not be appropriate to elevate the shoulder. The base test ULNT2 was developed utilising shoulder girdle depression. The clinical stimulus to develop the test came from a large number of keyboard operators experiencing ongoing pain and other symptoms from working at computers. There was something of an epidemic of this in Australia in the 1980s and early 90s triggering much debate about the organic validity of the presentations. At the time, I was trying to make some sense of their pain state and the ULNT2 tests appeared clinically useful.

ULNT2 (MEDIAN) - ACTIVE TEST

My suggestion for an active performance of the test is to ask your patient to hang her arm naturally by her side and to look at her thumb. Then ask her to point her thumb away, extend her wrist and then to push her hand towards the floor (Fig. 12.6), thus depressing the shoulder girdle. If need be, she can then laterally flex her cervical spine away from the test side. Compare with the other side.

ULNT2 (MEDIAN) - PASSIVE TEST

The test is described for my patient's right arm. Follow the sequence of figures in 12.7.

A. STARTING POSITION

I suggest that shoulder girdle depression can be easily performed using your thigh, although easy variations exist and are described below. Position your patient so that she lies slightly diagonal across the bed with her shoulder just over the edge of bed to allow contact with your thigh. Give her a pillow if she wants one. My left thigh now rests against the superior aspect of her right shoulder. My right hand holds her wrist, my left arm cradles and supports her forearm and I hold her elbow (Fig. 12.7A). It is something of a crossed arms position. This position means that at the end position of the test (Fig. 12.7F) minimal manoeuvering will be required. You can see an alternative view of this crossed arms starting position in figure 12.19A. Always ensure that you get your starting position correct and a well controlled test will follow. Remember the guidelines for checking symptoms at the start and then be aware of symptom and resistance changes throughout the test.

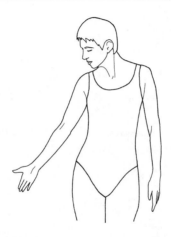

12.6 ULNT2 (median) performed actively. See text for full description.

B. SHOULDER GIRDLE DEPRESSION

Now, using your thigh, and with the patient's shoulder in about 10 degrees of abduction, carefully depress her shoulder girdle (Fig. 12.7B). Take it to symptoms or the point where you can feel some resistance, which ever comes first. There is no need to use much force at all. Your thigh can be remarkably sensitive. In this position it is quite easy to watch the patient's face for any nonverbal input. When the "thigh technique" is used it leaves two hands free for manipulation of the rest of the limb. If the patient is lying diagonally across the bed, then the test will be performed in approximately 10 degrees of abduction and the arm will be over the side of the bed, making for easy addition of further movements.

C. ELBOW EXTENSION

With the shoulder girdle depression maintained, the elbow can easily be extended as shown in figure 12.7C. Notice my hand positions haven't moved. Make sure you check symptoms and be aware of responses. This position will not usually be as provocative as the elbow extension in the ULNT1.

D. WHOLE ARM LATERAL ROTATION

The next step may need some practice. With your right hand, try to come under her wrist to hold the radial side of the wrist if possible. Then laterally rotate her whole arm (Fig. 12.7D). Do this using both hands, guiding and supporting with your left hand while ensuring that the depression force upon the shoulder girdle stays constant.

E. WRIST AND FINGER EXTENSION

Now you will need to extend her wrist and fingers. Your right hand could slip over her palm and do this. Or you could try slipping your thumb in her web space from the palm side (Fig. 12.7E). This is a useful grip because it gives control of her thumb. Check it out in the insert of figure 12.7E. You can then easily extend her wrist and fingers. Take care, it will be highly likely that there will be symptoms evoked during this stage of the test.

F. SHOULDER ABDUCTION

In this position, if necessary, some shoulder abduction can be added. This can be performed up to around 40 degrees until the shoulder girdle depression begins to lift (Fig. 12.7G). For this base test, keep the movement in the coronal plane.

Variations, sensitising manoeuvres, normal responses and handling thoughts for the shoulder depression based tests are discussed after the ULNT2 test for the radial nerve.

PERFORMANCE OF THE ULNT2 (RADIAL)

Consider this scenario. A patient has lateral elbow pain diagnosed as "tennis elbow". There are a number of aggravating movements such as gripping, but he also comments that he gets the pain while walking, but not running. An analysis of movement reveals that he runs with very flexed elbows but walks with extended elbows and during the extension he would internally rotate his arm a little. This would be a prompt to examine the radial nerve and its related pathways as part of the presenting disorder.

An examination of the relationship of the radial nerve with joint axes of movement reveals that internal rotation of the shoulder and pronation of the forearm will load the radial nerve. The clinical ramifications of this have been noticed by many clinicians such as Cyriax (1978)

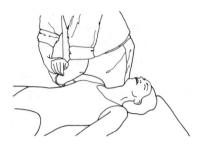

12.7A ULNT2 (median): Starting position.

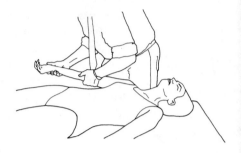

12.7D ULNT2 (median): Whole arm lateral rotation.

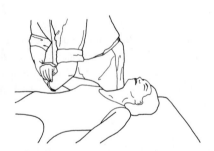

12.7B ULNT2 (median): Shoulder girdle depression.

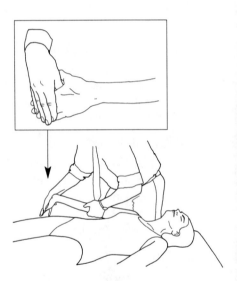

12.7E ULNT2 (median): Wrist and finger extension. Inset of hand position.

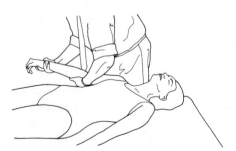

12.7C ULNT2 (median): Elbow extension.

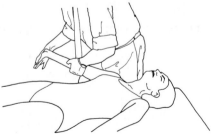

12.7F ULNT2 (median): Shoulder abduction.

and Mackinnon (1988) and I have used it routinely to examine "tennis elbow" (Butler 1989). The Mill's manipulation espoused by Cyriax but now out of vogue, probably gave a quick mobilisation to the radial nerve and surrounding tissues.

ULNT2 (RADIAL) – ACTIVE TEST

There are many ways to do this. Here is my suggestion. I ask my patient to hold her arm to the side, flex her wrist, look at her palm and then to internally rotate her arm so that she can look at her palm over her shoulder. Try it yourself. Then ask her to depress her shoulder girdle ("push wrist to floor") (Fig. 12.8) and "look away" to laterally flex her neck if needed. If warranted, ask her to hold the position for up to a minute. Some discrete pains related to the radial nerve may take some time to be reproduced. This is similar to an active test described by Mackinnon & Dellon (1988). You could, of course, perform these movements in any order. A similar active test for radial sensory nerve involvement in de Quervain's disease is described in chapter 10.

ULNT2 (RADIAL) – PASSIVE TEST

I prefer to test the radial nerve using the shoulder depression method described above. A variation is suggested at the end of this chapter and elsewhere (Elvey and Hall 1997). The following description is the way in which many colleagues have used the test and the way in which a number of normative studies have been carried out. The description is for my patient's right arm.

A. STARTING POSITION

The starting position is the same as for the ULNT2 previously described for the median nerve and related pathways. Position her slightly diagonally across the bed so that her right shoulder comes in contact with your left thigh (Fig. 12.9A). Note the "crossover arms" starting position. I have her right elbow in my left hand and my right hand holds her left wrist. Attention to this starting position will make for a smoother test with minimal manoeuvering. Remember the guidelines of checking symptoms at the start and then carefully rechecking responses throughout the test.

B. SHOULDER GIRDLE DEPRESSION

Using your thigh, carefully depress her shoulder girdle. See how I have positioned myself so I can still see her face (Fig. 12.9B). When the thigh is used it leaves two hands free for

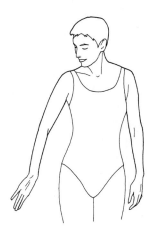

12.8 ULNT2 (radial) performed actively.

manipulation of the rest of the limb and this is particularly important for this test. If she lies diagonally across the bed, then the test will be performed in approximately 10 degrees of abduction and the arm will be over the side of the bed, making further manipulation easy. Check responses to the depression.

C. ELBOW EXTENSION

Now extend her elbow. Don't force it and make sure you keep the shoulder position stable (Fig. 12.9C).

D. WHOLE ARM INTERNAL ROTATION

This might be the hard bit. The above positions must be held and not moved while you add the rotation. Reach around to grasp the dorsal aspect of her wrist and then using your left hand to guide, let the arm come into internal rotation as is shown in figure 12.9D. You will know you are in the right position because when the internal rotation is taken up, it should be possible to lock her arm into elbow extension with your right arm. You may even be able to take your left hand away and still maintain good control over her arm with your right arm. That free left hand may be useful for refining the test or for techniques such as mobilising the radial head or deep frictioning of tissues around the elbow.

E. WRIST FLEXION

You can flex her wrist by asking her to perform it actively or by using your left hand. If you have a large hand you may be able to use your right hand. There is usually no need to flex the fingers as in this position there is insufficient tendon length to allow it. The radial sensory branch will be further loaded by flexion of the joints of the thumb and ulnar deviation of the wrist (Fig. 12.9E).

As in the ULNT2 for the median nerve, the arm can be abducted up to 40 degrees. Of course the neck position can be altered. Usually, the easiest structural differentiation manoeuvre is to carefully release the shoulder girdle depression position. Do this a little at a time to check responses.

HANDLING COMMENTS AND VARIATIONS FOR THE ULNT2 TESTS

THE THIGH ON SHOULDER GIRDLE STARTING POSITION

The thigh position is suggested because of the superior handling that it offers. It is also very good for structural differentiation as you only have to release just a few grams of pressure to see if there is any alteration in the evoked symptoms in the arm. The starting position is important and in figure 12.19 you can view it again from the opposite side of the bed.

Sometimes, for various reasons, you may not like the thigh on shoulder position. One reason may be that it is a bit uncomfortable for your spine, especially if you are short and your patient has long arms. You can easily adapt. Have her move towards the middle of the bed so that her arm is resting comfortably by her side and on the bed. Stand next to your patient and just coax and pull the arm down into shoulder girdle depression (Fig. 12.10). Then internally rotate the whole arm and flex the wrist. You can even do it sitting down. Elvey (1997) suggests adding the internal rotation after you have abducted the shoulder. This is another option worth trying. Some manual therapy beds have an insert at the shoulder level that could be used to maintain the depression.

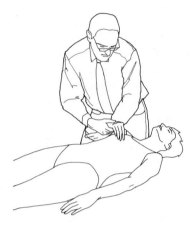

12.9A ULNT2 (radial): Starting position.

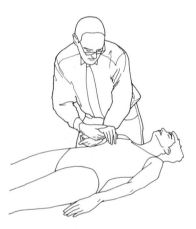

12.9B ULNT2 (radial): Shoulder depression.

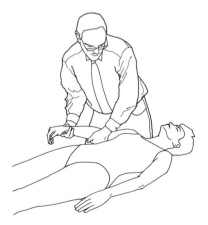

12.9C ULNT2 (radial): Elbow extension.

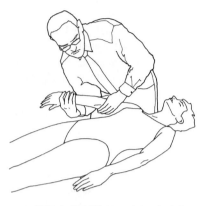

12.9D ULNT2 (radial): Whole arm internal rotation.

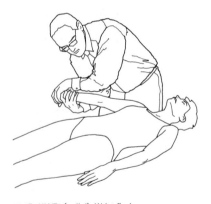

12.9E ULNT2 (radial): Wrist flexion.

ORDER OF MOVEMENT VARIATIONS

As for the ULNT1, the order of movement additions can be altered. In particular, the test can be performed "from the other end". This appears useful and quite sensitive for radial nerve based disorders below the elbow such as peripheral neurogenic contributions to de Quervain's tenosynovitis. An example is shown in figure 12.11. I have asked my patient to clench her fist around her thumb, then extended the elbow and now I am assessing the effects of shoulder girdle elevation and depression. Your patients may have quite specific hand positions which are symptomatic and which you could reproduce and then add other components of the test.

SENSITISING/STRUCTURAL DIFFERENTIATION ADDITIONS

Release of the shoulder girdle depression is the most useful structural differentiation movement. With skilled handling, only a small amount of pressure may need to be released to get a response change even in healthy individuals. I suggest that the pressure be released in a step wise manner to accurately judge responses. If evoked symptoms are more proximal, then the wrist position can be altered for structural differentiation.

This test for the radial nerve is not as sensitive as the median nerve test, that is, it is more difficult to reproduce symptoms. Perhaps this is due to the anatomy of the radial nerve including its smaller number of sensory fibres.

Many clinicians comment and it is quite clear clinically, that shoulder extension will place some more pressure along the radial nerve pathway. You could add this easily to the test. A test which is proposed to load the musculocutaneous nerve employs shoulder extension and is discussed later in this chapter.

Other sensitising additions could include the cervical spine, in particular lateral flexion away from the test side. You could also perform the test in some shoulder girdle protraction or retraction. The aggravating activities that you have identified for the problem would dictate which sensitising positions could be trialed.

This test can also be performed in prone (Fig. 12.12). Make sure you explain to your patient what you are doing as this position may be a bit threatening.

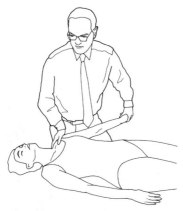

12.10 Technique variation for the ULNT2 (radial).

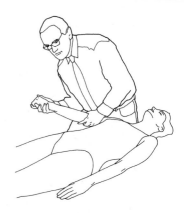

12.11 Technique for a distal to proximal ULNT2 (radial).

NORMAL RESPONSES

Yaxley and Jull (1991) after noting that this test was being used clinically without any normative data, performed a similar test to what has been described above on 50 asymptomatic 18-30 year old subjects. The most common sensory response was "....a strong painful stretch over the radial aspect of the proximal forearm (84% of all responses), often accompanied by a stretch pain in the lateral aspect of the upper arm (32%) or biceps brachii (14%) or the dorsal aspect of the hand (12%). See figure 12.13 for a summary. This symptom response area would make the radial nerve at the elbow a candidate for a source of the pain. Yaxley and Jull (1991) also found in their study that a range of 40⁰ of glenohumeral abduction was possible in the final test position. This was not gender or side dependent.

ULNT3 (ULNAR) - PERFORMANCE

INTRODUCTION

The neurodynamic tests described above place loading forces upon the brachial plexus and lower cervical nerve roots. However, as all the tests are performed with the elbow in extension, it does not permit a full examination of the ulnar nerve. Thus I believe it is worthwhile having a base test which includes elbow flexion. Bragard (1929) described an ulnar nerve test in 1929 and there have been a number of reports of suggested tests based on anatomical and clinical observations since (Pechan 1973; Buehler and Thayer 1988).

ULNT3 (ULNAR) - ACTIVE TEST

Ask your patient to either sit on the bed or stand. Demonstrate the position that you want her to try to mimic. My suggestion is similar to the elbow flexion test of Buehler (1988). Ask her to look at her hand and hold it up as though she was holding a tray of drinks. You can then add more loading by asking her to look away (Fig. 12.14), add more elbow flexion or depress the shoulder girdle. Cervical spine retraction is another worthwhile sensitising movement here.

Ask her to hold this position for up to a minute if symptoms are not reproduced. For people with a good range of movement, and especially younger flexible people, attempting the "mask" position may be worthwhile (Fig. 12.15).

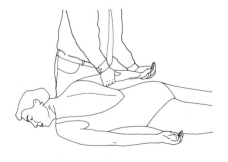

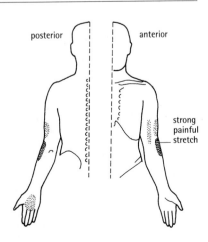

12.12 Technique for a ULNT2 (radial) in prone.

12.13 The normal responses to a ULNT2 (radial). See text for details. (Adapted from Yaxley G and Jull G (1991) A modified upper limb tension test: an investigation of responses in normal subjects. Australian Journal of Physiotherapy 37: 143-152).

ULNT3 (ULNAR) – PASSIVE TEST BEGINNING DISTALLY

The test is described here from the wrist first, and, for a bit of variety, using her left arm. This test usually presents the most handling difficulties of all the tests. Handling variations are described below.

A. STARTING POSITION

Start by positioning her close to the edge of the bed. Grasp her left hand with your right hand, my fingers are nearly parallel with hers and I can control all her fingers. Her left elbow is resting on my outer thigh and her elbow is in more than 90 degrees of extension (Fig. 12.16A). Her shoulder should be in as little abduction as possible. The illustration does not show it but I am standing in a stride-stand position. You can see this position in the reverse series (Fig. 12.17). This stride-stand position will allow a fluent body movement when I abduct her arm.

B. WRIST EXTENSION

Now extend her wrist. Make sure all her fingers extend, particularly those on the ulnar side (Fig. 12.16B). Check the responses to each phase of the test.

C. FOREARM PRONATION

Keeping all other components steady, pronate her forearm by pointing her fingers towards her face (Fig. 12.16C).

D. ELBOW FLEXION

Now flex her elbow, at the same time keeping all the other components still (Fig. 12.16D). Good stability will be possible if the arm is resting on the examiner's thigh as in the starting position. Note the responses, including whether the shoulder girdle elevates. This position will be sensitive enough to reproduce symptoms in many patients with medial epicondyle area symptoms.

E. LATERAL ROTATION

There will usually be some shoulder lateral rotation available here. Let her arm fall back and take up the movement (Fig. 12.16E).

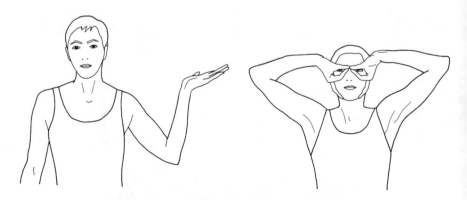

12.14 The ULNT3 performed actively.   12.15 The "mask" position for the ULNT3.

F. SHOULDER GIRDLE DEPRESSION

Make a fist, keep your wrist in a neutral position, and depress her shoulder girdle. You can then lean on the fist with your elbow straight as in figure 12.16F. This allows your arm to act as a pillar to control the depression and the abduction. Be very aware of symptoms. It is quite common for patients with peripheral neurogenic symptoms sourced in the ulnar nerve to report symptoms during this manoeuvre. In figure 12.16F, I have slipped my hand between her hand and shoulder. A hypermobile individual's wrist and elbow may be much more flexible than the model in figure 12.16F, and in this case, her hand may be flexed under my wrist.

G. SHOULDER ABDUCTION

Now carefully abduct the shoulder. Your left arm can act as a pillar and if you have that nice stride stand position I recommended earlier, you will be able to abduct the arm in a smooth and controlled action (Fig. 12.16G).

ULNT3 – PASSIVE TEST BEGINNING PROXIMALLY

I have just described the test from the wrist first. The ULNT3 can also be performed from the shoulder girdle. Some clinicians may prefer this for their base test. Here is a description for my patient's left arm.

A. STARTING POSITION AND SHOULDER GIRDLE DEPRESSION/ABDUCTION

Note the stride standing starting position. I place my left arm under her scapula and my fingers reach from under to grasp her shoulder. This is not just a shoulder stabilising position. Make sure that your arm is under the scapula and you will feel some of the weight of her shoulder girdle on your forearm. In this position you can depress the shoulder girdle (Fig. 12.17A) and then abduct the shoulder to about 110 degrees or to where you can appreciate changes in resistance or where symptoms are evoked.

B. LATERAL ROTATION OF THE ARM

Now laterally rotate the arm as in figure 12.17B. This can be a challenging position for patients in pain or patients who have had previous shoulder injuries. You may need to encourage them to let you move the shoulder. Check responses.

C. ELBOW FLEXION

Making sure you keep the above position held, flex her elbow (Fig. 12.17C).

D. WRIST AND FINGER EXTENSION/FOREARM PRONATION

This can be a bit tricky, but slide your right hand over her wrist and fingers and take her wrist and fingers into extension and the forearm into pronation (Fig. 12.17D). If forearm/hand symptoms are reproduced, you can carefully release the shoulder girdle position to see if it alters symptoms and thus suggest neurogenic involvement.

HANDLING COMMENTS/NORMAL RESPONSES/FURTHER SENSITISATION

Handling wise, this test is probably the most difficult of the upper limb neurodynamic tests. The distal to proximal sequencing that I described first is the only one where normal values have been attempted (Flanagan 1994). In this study, 82% of subjects reported responses in the hypothenar eminence and medial two fingers, and 64% reported pins and needles in the same area.

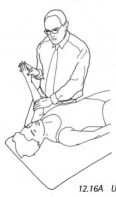

12.16A   ULNT3: Starting position.

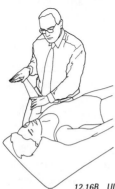

12.16B   ULNT3: Wrist extension.

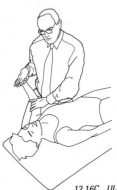

12.16C   ULNT3: Forearm pronation.

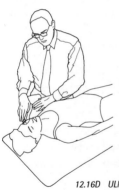

12.16D   ULNT3: Elbow flexion.

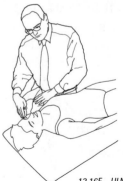

12.16E   ULNT3: Shoulder lateral rotation.

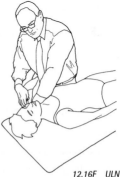

12.16F   ULNT3: Shoulder girdle depression.

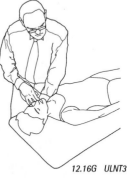

12.16G   ULNT3: Shoulder abduction.

I have described the ULNT3 test elsewhere (Butler 1991) with forearm supination rather than pronation. However it rapidly became clear that pronation is more sensitive than supination on a pure anatomical basis. For example, the distance between the pisiform bone and medial elbow is longer during pronation, hence the distance that the ulnar nerve must traverse is longer.

The main variations that clinicians are likely to use relate to order of movement additions. As in all the tests, variations to fit the patient's complaints are sought. For example, your patient may demonstrate a baseball pitching position as a problem. Watch and note the order of component recruitment and try to replicate it in the clinic. The proximal to distal technique is used by many clinicians. To maintain some standardisation in the base test system, to make all the tests start from the shoulder girdle, clinicians may wish to make this their base test. Clinicians with good handling skills may be able to perform techniques at the wrist and elbow during this position. If testing for obscure neuropathies in athletes, it may be worth redoing the test and taking up each component a little more firmly.

If the ulnar nerve always dislocates during elbow flexion, make sure that it has dislocated during the test. You may note that in different orders of movement the nerve may not dislocate. Dislocating ulnar nerves are common and occur in approximately 10% of the population (Childress 1975).

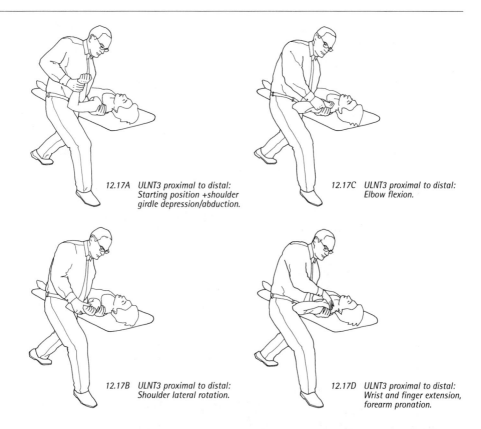

12.17A ULNT3 proximal to distal:
Starting position +shoulder
girdle depression/abduction.

12.17C ULNT3 proximal to distal:
Elbow flexion.

12.17B ULNT3 proximal to distal:
Shoulder lateral rotation.

12.17D ULNT3 proximal to distal:
Wrist and finger extension,
forearm pronation.

MUSCULOCUTANEOUS NERVE TEST

The musculocutaneous nerve is the fourth nerve that extends from the cervical spine to the fingers. It is smaller and less superficial than the ulnar, median and radial nerves and is not injured as much. However it should not be forgotten.

MUSCULOCUTANEOUS NERVE – ACTIVE TEST

Ask your patient to hold her thumb with her fingers, then ulnar deviate her wrist and then extend her elbow and shoulder (Fig. 12.18). Get them to watch the movement and then look away. The arm position is similar to the position a swimmer is in when she is about to dive into a pool to begin a race.

MUSCULOCUTANEOUS NERVE – PASSIVE TEST

A. STARTING POSITION

The suggested test is described for my patient's left arm. The starting position is similar to that for the ULNT 2 tests. That is, she lies on the bed with the shoulder of the arm to be tested over the side of the bed. The crossed arm starting position is used and you can see this clearly in figure 12.19A. Note also in the figure, that my right arm cradles her left elbow and my left hand holds her wrist.

B. SHOULDER GIRDLE DEPRESSION

Using my thigh, I carefully depress the shoulder girdle (Fig. 12.19B). Take the movement to where you feel the tissues tighten a little or to symptoms. You can also use the alternative shoulder girdle depression position discussed after the ULNT2 (radial), illustrated in figure 12.10.

C: ELBOW EXTENSION

With the shoulder girdle position held, guide the elbow into extension (Fig. 12.19C).

D: SHOULDER EXTENSION

Her shoulder girdle has to be off the bed far enough to allow shoulder extension to be added. With the above components held, ease the shoulder carefully into extension (Fig. 12.19D).

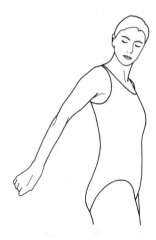

12.18 Musculocutaneous nerve test performed actively.

There may be about 30 degrees of extension. Be careful, because like the lateral rotation in the ULNT1, it might be a threatening manoeuvre for some patients.

E. WRIST ULNAR DEVIATION

The wrist is then ulnar deviated (Fig. 12. 19E,F). The handgrip that is shown in figure 12.19F facilitates this. Note how my index finger is in her palm, taking and controlling the thumb into flexion and opposition.

HANDLING COMMENTS/NORMAL RESPONSES/FURTHER SENSITISATION

A musculocutaneous nerve neurodynamic test has never been suggested before. The nerve is not often injured and the ULNT2 (radial) may replicate the symptoms of a musculocutaneous neuropathy. Wrist ulnar deviation strains the radial sensory nerve (Mackinnon and Dellon 1988) and as the lateral antebrachial nerve (continuation of the musculocutaneous nerve) overlaps the radial sensory nerve, a Finkelstein's test for tendinitis probably loads the terminal branches of the musculocutaneous nerve as well. I recall a patient with a failed decompression surgery for de Quervain's tenosynovitis and this test was the only one of the neural loading tests that reproduced symptoms. Maybe some "above elbow tennis elbows" will react to this test if the musculocutaneous nerve is injured or altered where it emerges between the brachialis and biceps muscles.

It may also be worth "exploring" from this point. To sensitise the test further, add lateral flexion of the neck away from the test side, a few degrees of arm abduction and lateral rotation of the whole arm. Structural differentiation will be convenient - elevate the shoulder girdle for below elbow symptoms and move the wrist for above elbow symptoms.

OTHER UPPER LIMB TESTS

Any peripheral nerve is capable of being injured and acquiring a capacity to generate impulses from the injury site. It does not have to be a large nerve either. Take for example, the tiny supraclavicular nerves. If you were to run your thumbnail back and forwards along your clavicle, you should feel two or maybe more of these nerves. They feel like thick fishing line and they will flick under your fingernail. One or more of these nerves may well be entrapped or injured after clavicular area trauma (Gelberman et al. 1975). However, the more commonly injured shorter nerves of the upper limb are the axillary and suprascapular nerves.

AXILLARY

The main physical threat to the axillary nerve is dislocation of the shoulder, particularly in an anterior direction, and fractures of the surgical neck of the humerus. Being so close to the most mobile joint of the body also means it must be well endowed with gliding and straining abilities that could be disrupted with trauma and the consequences of trauma.

In figure 12.20 is my suggestion to test the physical health of the nerve. I have held my patient's elbow and cradled her arm. The elbow does not necessarily have to be flexed. Internally rotate her arm, depress the shoulder girdle and then laterally flex the neck. Make sure it is a neck on thorax movement rather than a head on neck movement as the nerve arises from the lower cervical roots. A similar position would be easy to duplicate for an active movement examination.

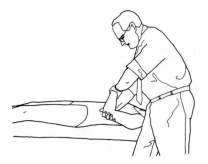

*12.19A   Musculocutaneous nerve test:
          starting position.*

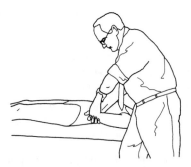

*12.19B   Musculocutaneous nerve test:
          shoulder depression.*

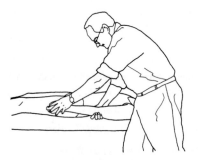

*12.19C   Musculocutaneoud nerve test:
          elbow extension.*

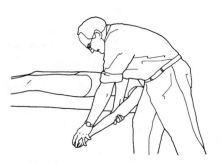

*12.19D   Musculocutaneous nerve test:
          shoulder extension.*

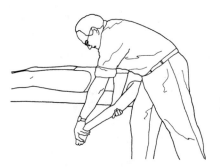

*12.19E   Musculocutaneous nerve test:
          wrist ulnar deviation.*

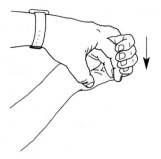

*12.19F   Musculocutaneous nerve test:
          ulnar deviation.*

SUPRASCAPULAR NERVE

This nerve is reasonably protected although there are reports that the nerve may be stretched where it passes through the suprascapular notch. Horizontal adduction and protraction/retraction would pull the nerve through the notch. This can be painful as noted by a number of clinicians (eg. Antoniadis et al. 1996).

My suggestion to test the physical health of the nerve is as follows. Stand on the opposite side to the side that you want to test. Pull your patient's arm into horizontal adduction and rest her elbow on your sternum (use padding for pointy elbows). Notice my control of her entire shoulder girdle in figure 12.21. Have her laterally flex her neck (on thorax) towards you, push with your chest down the shaft of her humerus to take her shoulder girdle away from her neck, depress her shoulder girdle and then with your hands, rotate her scapula. Medial rotation may be more sensitive.

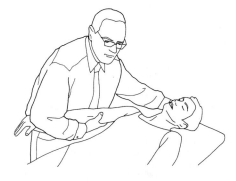

12.20 Axillary nerve test.

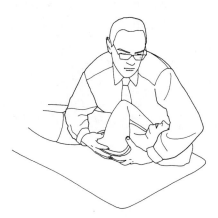

12.21 Suprascapular nerve test.

CHAPTER 12. REFERENCES

Adson AW (1951) Cervical ribs: symptoms, differential diagnosis and indication for the section of the insertion of the scalenus anticus muscles. Journal of the International College of Surgeons 16: 546-553.

Antoniadis G, Richter H, Rath S, et al. (1996) Suprascapular nerve entrapment: experience with 28 cases. Journal of Neurosurgery 85: 1020-1025.

Balster SM & Jull GA (1997) Upper trapezius muscle activity during the brachial plexus tension test in asymptomatic subjects. Manual Therapy 2: 144-149.

Bragard K (1929) Die nervendehnung als diagnostisches prinzip ergibt eine reihe neuer nervenph%oonomene. M₁nchener Medizinische Wochenschrift 76: 1999-2003.

Buehler MJ & Thayer DT (1988) The elbow flexion test. Clinical Orthopaedics and Related Research 233: 213-216.

Butler DS (1989) Adverse mechanical tension in the nervous system: a model for assessment and treatment. Australian Journal of Physiotherapy 35: 227-238.

Butler DS (1991) Mobilisation of the Nervous System, Churchill Livingstone, Melbourne.

Chavany JA (1934) A propos des neuralgies cervico-brachiales. Bulletin Medical (Paris) 48: 335-339.

Childress HM (1975) Recurrent ulnar-nerve dislocation at the elbow. Journal of Bone and Joint Surgery 38A: 978-984.

Cyriax J (1978) Textbook of Orthopaedic Medicine, 8th edn. Bailierre Tindall, London.

Edgar D, Jull G & Sutton S (1994) Relationship between upper trapezius muscle length and upper quadrant neural extensibility. Australian Journal of Physiotherapy 40: 99-103.

Elvey RL (1979) Brachial plexus tension tests and the pathoanatomical origin of arm pain. In: Idczak R (ed.) Aspects of Manipulative Therapy, Manipulative Physiotherapists Association of Australia, Melbourne.

Elvey RL (1986) Treatment of arm pain associated with abnormal brachial plexus tension. The Australian Journal of Physiotherapy 32: 225-230.

Elvey RL (1997) Physical evaluation of the peripheral nervous system in disorders of pain and dysfunction. Journal of Hand Therapy 10: 122-129.

Elvey RL & Hall T (1997) Neural tissue evaluation and treatment. In: Donatelli R (ed.) Physical Therapy of the Shoulder, Churchill Livingstone, New York.

Elvey RL, Quintner JL & Thomas AN (1986) A clinical study of RSI. Australian Family Physician 15: 1314-1322.

Gelberman RH, Verdeck WN & Brodhead WT (1975) Supraclavicular nerve-entrapment syndrome. Journal of Bone and Joint Surgery 57A: 119.

Ginn K (1989) An investigation of tension development in upper limb soft tissues during the upper limb tension test. International Federation of Orthopaedic Manipulative Therapists. Cambridge.

Kenneally M, Rubenach H & Elvey R (1988) The upper limb tension test: the SLR of the arm. In: Grant R (ed.) Physical Therapy of the Cervical and Thoracic Spine, Churchill Livingstone, New York.

Kleinrensink GJ, Stoeckart R, Mulder PGH, et al. (2000) Upper limb tension tests as tools in the diagnosis of nerve and plexus lesions. Clinical Biomechanics 15: 9-14.

Lord JW & Roseti LM (1971) Thoracic outlet syndrome. CIBA Clinical Symposia 23: 20-23.

Mackinnon SE & Dellon AL (1988) Surgery of the Peripheral Nerve, Thieme, New York.

Moses A & Carman J (1996) Anatomy of the cervical spine: implications for the upper limb tension test. Australian Journal of Physiotherapy 42: 31-35.

Novak CB, Lee GW, Mackinnon SE, et al. (1994) Provocative testing for cubital tunnel syndrome. Journal of Hand Surgery 19A: 817-820.

Omer GE & Bell-Krotoski J (1997) Sensibility testing. In: Omer GE, Spinner M & Van Beek AL (eds.) Management of Peripheral Nerve Problems, 2nd edn. WB Saunders Company, Philadelphia.

Pechan J (1973) Ulnar nerve manoeuvre as a diagnostic aid in pressure lesions in the cubital region. Ceskoslovenska Neurologie 36: 13-19.

Pullos J (1986) The upper limb tension test. Australian Journal of Physiotherapy 32: 258-259.

Rayan GM, Jensen C & Duke J (1992) Elbow flexion test in the normal population. Journal of Hand Surgery 17A: 86-89.

Reid S (1987) The measurement of tension changes in the brachial plexus. Manipulative Therapists Association of Australia, 5th biennial conference . Melbourne.

Selvaratnam PJ, Glasgow EF & Matyas TA (1988) Strain effects on the nerve roots of brachial plexus. Journal of Anatomy 161: 260-264.

Selvaratnam PJ, Matyas TA & Glasgow EF (1994) Noninvasive discrimination of brachial plexus involvement in upper limb pain. Spine 19: 26-33.

Shacklock M (1995) Neurodynamics. Physiotherapy 81: 9-16.

Smith CG (1956) Changes in length and position of the segments of the spinal cord with changes in posture in the monkey. Radiology 66: 259-265.

Wilson S, Selvaratnam PJ & Briggs C (1994) Strain at the subclavian artery during the upper limb tension test. Australian Journal of Physiotherapy 40: 243-248.

Wright IS (1945) The neurovascular syndrome produced by hyperabduction of the arms. American Heart Journal 29: 1-8.

Yaxley G & Jull G (1991) A modified upper limb tension test: an investigation of responses in normal subjects. Australian Journal of Physiotherapy 37: 143-152.

CHAPTER 13

RESEARCH AND NEURODYNAMICS –
Is neurodynamics
worthy of scientific merit?

JAMES W. MATHESON MS, PT, CSCS

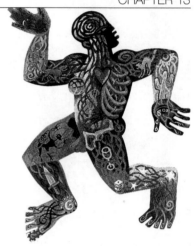

INTRODUCTION

A CRITICAL ANALYSIS OF NEURODYNAMICS

SUPPORT FROM ANATOMICAL AND PHYSIOLOGICAL EVIDENCE

THE EFFICACY OF NEURODYNAMIC TESTS

OPERATIONAL DEFINITIONS OF NEURODYNAMIC TESTS
RELIABILITY OF NEURODYNAMIC TESTS
VALIDITY OF NEURODYNAMIC TESTS

THE EMERGING NEW CONSTRUCT IN NEURODYNAMICS

RESEARCH RELATED TO TREATMENT EFFECTS

FUTURE RESEARCH INTO NEURODYNAMICS

APPENDIX A

REFERENCES CHAPTER 13

Problems can not be solved at the same level of awareness that created them.

Albert Einstein

INTRODUCTION

The demand for evidence based practice in physiotherapy has increased dramatically in the past decade. This increased demand for professional accountability has arisen from all third party payers, competition with other healthcare providers, and from within the profession itself (Jones 1992). A recent study using questionnaires, by Turner and Whitfield (1997) investigated English and Australian physiotherapists' reasons for the use of certain treatment techniques. Results revealed that more than 90% of the surveyed physiotherapists stated that their choice of treatment techniques directly reflected what they were taught as students. The results of the study also showed that empirical evidence from patient care and information gained from continuing education courses ranked high as reasons for choosing specific treatment techniques. Surprisingly, clinical research and review of the research literature ranked least important among the questioned physiotherapists as rationales for choosing treatment methods.

These findings are discouraging, yet challenging. They show the importance of quality continuing education, but they also illustrate how a new research-practice paradigm needs to become part of clinical practice. Knowledge of the current literature can help clinicians avoid the act of performing treatment techniques without exploring the rationale behind their treatment decisions. Numerous advocates of this type of evidence based clinical practice exist (eg. Sackett 1998; Di Fabio 1999; Rothstein 1999). However they are not proposing that clinicians become slaves to research data, demanding that only treatments supported by randomised controlled double blind studies be performed. Instead, they are suggesting that, as clinicians, we have an ethical responsibility to recognise and consider the current scientific evidence as it relates to the therapeutic techniques and interventions we are using on a daily basis.

Allied health professions, like physiotherapy, have reached the evidence based medicine era via concepts and systems based on the thoughts and clinical experiences of pioneering and often charismatic clinicians (review figure 1.1). These clinicians still dominate much continuing education, often presenting different methods of managing the same problem such as low back pain. Therefore, it becomes the responsibility of the practicing clinician to seek evidence supporting the efficacy of new and current treatment regimens. It is also the responsibility of instructors to provide evidence and encourage research. In this regard, neurodynamic assessment and management techniques are no different to any other. For survival and further development, the movement based professions must prove their value to patients and to the healthcare community. We must view this cry for evidence-based practice as an opportunity to validate our clinical skills through research. Payton (1994) has defined research as the goal-directed process of looking for a specific answer to a specific question in an organised, objective, and reliable way. He also reminds us that research is not just a search for what others have discovered, it is a rigorous search for new knowledge.

Most clinicians are hesitant to take on the time consuming requirement of a research study. Many clinicians are also in environments where research facilities and equipment are difficult to acquire, and support for a research culture is lacking. However, becoming a research based clinician does not have to equate with the act of publishing and performing clinical studies. Instead, it can equate with the concept of becoming a critical "user" of research. To be a successful user of research, you need to be aware of the current literature in your area of specialisation, be able to apply this literature to your clinical practice, and be able to balance your enthusiasm for new treatment techniques with a dose of healthy skepticism. Nowhere is this truer than in the field of manual therapy. The mobilisation techniques and "hands on" skills used in manual therapy will probably always remain somewhat of an art. Nevertheless, we must attempt to develop a common scientific canvas upon which to paint this manual art. This will help remove some of the uncertainty and variability that currently exists among clinicians. Having a common canvas will allow us to paint evidence instead of panacea.

A CRITICAL ANALYSIS OF NEURODYNAMICS

From dural tension (Cyriax 1978) to adverse mechanical tension (Breig 1978; Butler 1989) to neurodynamics (Shacklock 1995), the concept of manually examining the nervous system continues to change. The theory of considering the examination and rehabilitation of neural tissue disorders from both a biomechanical and physiological perspective is less than 20 years old. Now is the perfect time to ask ourselves the following two questions: "Is the neurodynamic approach worthy of scientific merit?" and "How can new evaluation and treatment techniques be critiqued for scientific merit?" Harris (1996) provides clinicians with some strategies to critically analyse the scientific merit of physiotherapy treatments. Harris presents five characteristics of nonstandard or alternative therapies followed by six criteria for evaluating the scientific merit of a new or existing therapy approach (table 13.1). In this chapter, these six criteria will be used to evaluate and discuss the current research literature in the area of neurodynamics. Another purpose of this chapter is to provide direction to both the student and current practitioner in evaluating the neurodynamics research literature and for integrating this literature into clinical practice. It is important to note that this chapter is not meant to serve as a comprehensive review of all the neurodynamics research. However, it should serve as a guide for clinicians and students who want to become critical users of the current and future neurodynamics literature.

SUPPORT FROM ANATOMICAL AND PHYSIOLOGICAL EVIDENCE

Having an understanding of the basic anatomical and physiological science underlying neurodynamics is a critical part of the clinical reasoning process. The following case report illustrates the importance of integrating basic neuroanatomy and neurophysiology research findings into clinical practice.

A patient, who was a physician, presented to a physiotherapist with a one-week history of neurological symptoms in her elbow and fourth and fifth fingers. During the subjective portion of the examination, the patient was unable to recall a mechanism of injury. Because this physiotherapist was a critical "user" of the neurodynamics research literature, he continued to ask the patient several specific questions. Subsequently, the patient revealed that she had been reading medical journals for 1-2 hours each night earlier in the week in preparation for a national conference. She stated that she often reads in bed lying on her side with the involved upper extremity positioned in extremes of wrist extension and elbow flexion to support her head. Already having a strong suspicion of the mechanism of injury, the physiotherapist performed a neuro-orthopaedic examination. This included clearing the cervical spine and ruling out potential soft tissue or musculoskeletal injuries with the relevant examination techniques and special tests. During the examination the physiotherapist was able to reproduce the patient's symptoms with palpation of the ulnar nerve distal to the medial epicondyle. The physiotherapist also found that the ULNT3 neurodynamic test was positive on the involved side. Further neurological examination revealed no abnormalities to tests of light touch, thermal sensation, or vibration. Integrating his research knowledge and examination findings together, the physiotherapist reasoned that the patient's symptoms were related to an intraneural inflammatory process that had occurred in the ulnar nerve in the cubital tunnel.

The patient, being a physician, was very interested in the physiotherapist's hypothesis and asked if she could review some literature that would support the diagnosis. Why did the physiotherapist think that the patient's reading position for several hours a week had been the mechanism of injury? What literature could the physiotherapist have used to defend his reasoning? To support his diagnosis the physiotherapist could have cited the recent literature review by Rempel et al. (1999). These researchers provide an excellent summary of the current literature on microscopic pathophysiological changes that occur in peripheral nerves when they are exposed to stretch, compression, or vibration. This literature review provides experimental support for the theory that low magnitude short duration extraneural pressures (ie. 30 mmHg for 2 hours) can cause long lasting pathological changes in the neural tissue. To support the hypothesis that the patient's reading position would have stressed the ulnar nerve, the physiotherapist could have used the results from several studies. Using cadavers, Pechan

CHARACTERISTICS OF NONSTANDARD THERAPIES	CRITERIA FOR EVALUATING SCIENTIFIC MERIT
1. Treatments are based on theories that are incongruent with anatomical or physiological function	1. Theories underlying the treatment approach are supported by valid anatomical and physiological evidence
2. Treatment is said to be effective for a broad range of diagnoses	2. Treatment approaches are designed for a specific type of the patient population
3. No adequately controlled studies in peer reviewed journals	3. Studies from peer-reviewed journals are provided that support the treatment's efficacy
4. Therapies that have an emotional appeal, and studies that fail to confirm their effectiveness are attacked	4. Peer-reviewed studies include well designed, randomized, controlled clinical trials or well designed single-subject experimental studies.
5. Treatments are incapable of causing harm	5. Potential side effects of the treatment are presented
	6. Proponents of the treatment approach are open and willing to discuss limitations

Table 13.1.   Characteristics of nonstandard therapies and criteria for evaluating the scientific merit of a treatment. Adapted from Golden (1980) by Harris (1996).

and Julis (1975) investigated the intraneural pressure of the ulnar nerve in the cubital tunnel. With custom instrumentation they monitored the intraneural pressure of the elbow in full extension as being 7 mmHg. They found that this intraneural pressure increased to 11-24 mmHg when the elbow was flexed to 90°. Finally, when they placed the cadaver elbow in a position of maximum flexion, wrist flexion, and shoulder abduction (similar to the position the patient was in when she was reading) the pressure increased to 3-6 times that of the resting values. Recently Gelberman et al. (1998) used magnetic resonance imaging (MRI) to show changes in the ulnar nerve during elbow flexion. These researchers performed MRI analyses of 20 elbow specimens from human cadavers. Cross-sectional images of the cubital tunnel and ulnar nerve were calculated and compared for different positions of elbow flexion. Results showed that as the elbow specimens were flexed, the cubital tunnel and ulnar nerve changed in area by as much as 50%. Pressure readings revealed that during elbow flexion there was an initial increase in intraneural pressure without a corresponding increase in extraneural pressure. The researchers suggested that this supported the theory that it was ulnar nerve traction rather than compression that caused increased intraneural pressure with elbow flexion.

These studies (Pechan and Julis 1975; Gelberman et al. 1998; Rempel et al. 1999) could have provided significant scientific support for the physiotherapist's hypothesis that the reading position of the patient was a probable contributing factor to the injury.

This case study illustrates that a basic knowledge of the microanatomy of peripheral nerves and their reactions to loading and compression is essential to evaluating, treating, and preventing neural tissue injury. As examiners of neural tissue, clinicians should integrate neuroanatomy and neurophysiology research into their clinical decision making skills. You will find additional molecular and biological support for understanding patient pain patterns and your clinical actions in chapters 2-5 of this text.

THE EFFICACY OF NEURODYNAMIC TESTS

In the last section a case study was utilised to help justify the importance of having a good understanding of the research underlying the anatomy and physiology of neurodynamics. In this section we are going to examine some of the past and present research literature in order to help determine if there is scientific support for the use of neurodynamic tests in the clinical setting.

Returning to the criteria from Harris (1996) listed in table 13.1; for neurodynamic tests to be worthy of scientific merit they must be designed for a specific population and be supported in well designed peer-reviewed studies. How does a reader judge the design of a test? First, one could examine the literature and decide if the study was detailed enough to allow it to be replicated by others. This would involve examining how clear the operational definitions were. A second method would involve examining the study to see if the neurodynamic techniques were reliable between subsequent tests carried out by a single examiner (intratester reliability) or between two or more examiners (intertester reliability). Finally, one could examine what support there was for the neurodynamic tests measuring the phenomena that they are believed to measure. In other words, are neurodynamic tests valid tests?

Operational definitions, reliability, validity, and randomised controlled clinical trials are some of the "buzzwords" of evidence based practice. Research often seems complicated, confusing, difficult to implement and difficult to judge. For example, how should we judge the value of

Phalen's test for diagnosing median nerve compression at the wrist, knowing that statements range from "it should no longer be used" (de Krom et al. 1990) to "demonstrates a real diagnostic and prognostic value" (Seror 1987). Therefore, we all need a basic understanding of research to make judgements on articles and to know which research findings should be implemented in practice. This section of the chapter will first define some of the terms used in research. Each term will then be used to critically examine relevant aspects of the current neurodynamics literature.

OPERATIONAL DEFINITIONS OF NEURODYNAMIC TESTS

An American task force (Rothstein et al. 1991) on standards and measurements in physical therapy (Appendix A) has defined an operational definition as follows:

"A set of procedures that guides the process of obtaining a measurement; includes descriptions of the attribute (a characteristic or quality that is measured) that is to be measured, the conditions under which the measurement is to be taken, and the actions that are to be taken in order to obtain the measurement."

In order to be meaningful, all measurements must be based on some type of operational definition. Operational definitions should be described in the methods section of all research reports. For example, an operational definition of a neurodynamic test would include the position of the subject, sequence of test movements, details of any instrumentation used during testing or treatment, a description of patient handling techniques, and quantification and direction of any test or mobilisation forces. Procedures describing when the test was stopped, what constituted a positive or negative test, and whether any additional sensitizing movements were added to the test should also be included in the operational definition of a neurodynamic test. Detailed operational definitions of testing methods and treatment protocols in neurodynamic research studies are necessary for future replication and reproduction of study results.

Determining the ideal operational definition of a neurodynamic test can be difficult given the large number of test variations that exist. All of the tests described by Butler (1991) and (Elvey 1986) involve multiple joint movements and handling techniques. This results in a large number of variables that are difficult to control. Several studies (eg. Selvaratnam et al. 1994; Coveney et al. 1997; Coppieters et al. 1999) examining neurodynamic tests have used specialised instrumentation to provide support for the involved extremity and standardisation of joint position. Custom built test frames and electrogoniometers and the accuracy of measurement which they allow may be ideal for research studies, however, they are not practical for use in the clinic. Some examiners of neural tissue have simply used only a sphygmomanometer cuff between the examiners thigh and subject's shoulder to maintain 40 mmHg of depressive force (Edgar et al. 1994), straps to stabilise the patient, and a standard goniometer to measure range of motion and have had good results when performing the ULNT2 (median) (Kelley and Jull 1998) and ULNT2 (radial) (Yaxley and Jull 1991; 1993) tests. These are devices that most clinicians have access to and could use when performing a case report on one patient. Regardless of what methods or equipment one uses to standardise neurodynamic tests in a clinical or research setting, it is more important that the test protocol be highly reproducible by the original examiner and by others.

A second concern that arises when operationally defining neurodynamic tests is that researchers must determine what criteria they will use to end the neurodynamic test. Some investigators (Jones 1989; Block et al. 1998), have used the onset of pain or symptoms (P1) as the end test condition of interest, whereas other researchers (Bell 1987; Kenneally et al. 1988; Yaxley and Jull 1991; Hines et al. 1993; Johnson and Chiarello 1997) have used the onset of resistance (R1) as an end test condition. Most recently, Coppetiers et al. (2000) used submaximal pain. Determining end test conditions such as P1, submaximal pain and R1 relies heavily on the perceptions and skill of the manual therapist. These variables inherently make the scientific examination of neurodynamic tests difficult. Some researchers (Edgar et al. 1994; Fidel et al. 1996; Hall and Quintner 1996; Balster and Jull 1997; Hall et al. 1998) have begun to question if these end test conditions truly reflect what is occurring when neurodynamic tests are performed. Hall et al. (1998) proposed that as an end test condition, the onset of reflex muscle activity (M1), might better reflect abnormal neural mechanics than either P1 or R1. Hall et al. (1998) monitored the electromyographic activity of the hamstring muscles during a straight leg raise (SLR) in healthy subjects and subjects with a history of lumbar radiculopathy. Hall and his colleagues found that the end test condition of M1 occurred significantly earlier in the radiculopathy group and suggested M1 as the indicator to end the test. The use of muscle responses to denote abnormal neural tissue sensitivity has been examined in the upper extremity as well (Hall and Quintner 1996; Balster and Jull 1997). Balster and Jull (1997) demonstrated increased reflexive muscle activity of the upper trapezius muscle in asymptomatic subjects with decreased neural tissue extensibility. Continued research is necessary to determine the best method to use the M1 end test condition reliably in a clinical setting. From a neurobiological perspective, the end test condition of interest will not only be related to perceptions and skills, but the operational state or mode of the central nervous system (see chapters 3 and 4).

In summary, when analyzing a research study containing neurodynamic tests, the reader should carefully examine how the neural tissue testing was operationally defined. How were the variables controlled? When was the test stopped? What end test condition was used? Did the examiners describe what was a normal test response? These questions will help the clinician determine if the operational definitions used by the researchers were good enough to allow reproduction of the study.

Table 13.2 provides the reader with a brief synopsis of several studies that investigated neurodynamic test results in healthy subjects. Although table 13.2 indicates that a substantial amount of normative data exists, only four of the studies depicted have appeared in peer reviewed publications. Clinicians need to continue to advance these studies or develop future studies with goals of publication in peer reviewed journals.

RELIABILITY OF NEURODYNAMIC TESTS

Good operational definitions allow clinicians to replicate and interpret clinical measurements. One way researchers determine if a clinical test is consistent and repeatable over several trials is to analyse the reliability. Depending the type of measurement that is performed, different types of reliability coefficients can be calculated. In all coefficients, the closer the value is to 1, the higher the reliability.

Commonly used procedures are Cohen's kappa, intraclass correlation, and Pearson's product moment correlation (Huck 2000). Percentage agreements and the t-test or analysis of variance (ANOVA) are also used.

STUDY	PUBLISHED IN:	N. TEST	N	AGE (YRS)	POINT TEST STOPPED	END ROM (°)	SXS TO BASE TEST REPORTED ON CHART	TEST ADDITIONS	SXS AFTER ADDITIONS	RELIABILITY INTRA– INTER–
Kenneally (1988)	Proceedings	ULTT1	50 50	18 – 30 50 – 67	(R1) wrist and finger extension	Not reported	Yes, similar in 77% R and 78% L	CCLF	↑ 91% R ↑ 94% L	Vague report of intra- and inter- being > 95%
Rubenach (1987)	Proceedings	ULTT1	116	18 – 30	(R1) wrist extension	Not reported	Yes, similar in 70% R and 71% L	ULTT1 other arm	↓ 62% R ↓ 61% L	Unavailable
Bell (1987)	Proceedings	ULTT1	100	18 – 30	(R1) wrist extension	Not reported	Unavailable	Bilateral SLR	↓ in 66%	Unavailable
Pullos (1986)	In journal as research notes	ULTT1	100	15 – 65	(R1? or P1?) elbow extension	Reported 95% C.I. (17° – 53°)	Not reported	CCLF	Not reported	Unavailable
Jones (1989)	Peer-reviewed	ULTT1	16	Not in report	(P1) during wrist/elbow extension	Not reported	Not reported	ICLF CCLF	Measured ROM at P1 after addition	0.49 0.74
Block (1998)	Abstract at conference	ULTT1	49	21 – 37	(P1 and R1) elbow extension	(P1) 46 +/- 14° R (R1) 15° +/- 10° R	Yes, similar in 65% of subjects	None	Not applicable	Only intra-rater 0.92 (P1) 0.76 (R1)
Hines (1993)	Peer-reviewed	ULTT1	25	19 – 50	(R1) elbow extension	Mean = 37° – 46° L depending on tester	Not reported	None	Authors found a significant difference (P < .05) among the 4 examiners	
Yaxley (1991)	Peer-reviewed	ULTT2b	50	18 – 30	(R1) shoulder abduction	41° +/- 4° R 42° +/- 4° L	Yes, similar in 84% of subjects	CCLF	↑ 78% R ↑ 80% L	High intra- and inter- based on ANOVAs
Flannagan (1993)	Unpublished Thesis	ULTT3	50	18 – 30	(P1) shoulder abduction	65° +/- 17° R	Yes	Release of shoulder depression	↓ 73%	Only intra-rater was reported as being 98%
Friberg (2000)	Abstract at conference	ULTTs 1, 2a, 2b, 3	88	Mean = 25 +/- 4	Not reported	Abstract did not report end ROM or reliability data. The examiners reported the location and type of Sxs (stretch, pain, paresthesia, anesthesia) for each test in detail.				
Johnson (1997)	Peer-reviewed	Slump	34	22 – 45	(R1) knee extension	11° +/- 9° R	Not reported	Examined effects of either ankle DF, ankle DF + medial hip rotation, and cervical spine extension on knee range of motion.		

Table 13.2 Normative neurodynamic test studies. ROM = range of motion. Sxs = Symptoms, R1 = point in range of motion where firm resistance is felt, R = right; L = left, CCLF = contralateral cervical spine lateral flexion, P1 = point in range of motion where symptoms are first felt, ICLF = ipsilateral cervical spine lateral flexion, DF = dorsiflexion. The goal of this table is to provide a brief synopsis of current research. The appropriateness of statistical methods and study design was not addressed.

Percent agreement is sometimes used to express the reliability of a study on, for example, the ability of two clinicians to agree on whether or not a neurodynamic test is positive in a group of patients with cervicobrachial pain. The percentage agreement is easily calculated as the ratio of the number of agreements between observers to the total number of comparisons made. However, the chief criticism of percentage agreement is that it does not take into account the agreement that is expected by chance alone (Haas 1991). Chance frequencies can often be rather high, and therefore, percentage agreement gives an overestimation of the reliability.

Cohen's kappa is used when researchers want to establish the reliability of nominal (categorical) data, such as in the above mentioned study. This may involve categorical data in which subjects described their neurological symptoms during the final position of a neurodynamic test. Potential symptom categories could be no symptoms present, a feeling of stretch, pins and needles, or numbness. Calculating a kappa coefficient would allow the researcher to determine how much agreement existed among the subjects in describing their symptoms. The advantage of the kappa statistic is that it is a measure of chance corrected concordance, that is, it corrects the observed agreement for agreement that is expected by chance alone. Kappa is somewhat more difficult to calculate, however, it is still easily computed by hand. A value greater than .75 indicates 'excellent' agreement, a value between .40 and .75 indicates 'fair to good' agreement, and a value less than .40 indicates 'poor' agreement (Fleiss 1986).

Different statistics have to be calculated when measurements are taken on an interval or ratio scale. Let's say we would like to know how much agreement there is between two clinicians on how high the leg has to be lifted during the SLR before symptoms are elicited. To answer this question, the **Pearson's product moment correlation** is a commonly used index. It evaluates how well the measurements of the first clinician can be predicted by a linear function from the measurements of the other clinician. However, this statistic has a major shortcoming as it does not account for systematic bias. If the first clinician systematically raises the leg higher than the other clinician, the reliability of the test will be overestimated. It is accepted that a Pearson's product moment correlation is no longer acceptable for assessing reliability (Roebroeck et al. 1993).

Another statistic, often used in neurodynamic research, but with shortcomings is the t-test or analysis of variance (ANOVA) to assess the reliability. A minor shortcoming is that these tests can only render a yes/no decision on reliability and can not quantitatively assess the strength of concordance. The major shortcoming however, is that the analysis can conceal large interexaminer disagreement. On the other hand, even trivial differences between clinicians can be highly significant if the sample size is large enough, leading to the presumption of poor reliability (Haas 1991).

The statistic of choice for the kind of studies where continuous data are involved, is the **intraclass correlation coefficient (ICC)**. The calculation of an ICC becomes more complicated and a statistical package will certainly help. As we would like to limit the discussion of the ICC to its understanding, it is important to know that ICCs come in different forms. Therefore, an ICC is always followed by two digits, for example ICC(2,1) or ICC(2,3). The first digit represents the type of ICC. As a discussion on the different types of ICCs is beyond the scope of this chapter, we refer for further information on this topic to Shrout and Fleis (1979). The second digit represents whether the unit of analysis is a single rating (or rater) or the mean of several ratings (or raters). In the latter case, the reliability of the mean of, for example, 3 ratings is of interest. This reliability will always be greater in magnitude than the reliability of the individual ratings. Therefore, researchers can decide to use a mean of several tests to increase the reliability of a test. We will illustrate this in the next paragraph.

Let's take reliability one step further and make it more clinically relevant. As mentioned above, a reliability coefficient ranges from 0 (or negative) to 1. The closer to 1, the better the reliability. In order to make reliability more meaningful, we need absolute estimates of reliability. Absolute reliability focuses on the amount of error to expect in a subject's recorded score. This measure is called the **standard error of measurement (SEM)**. An advantage of this measure is that it is no longer a rather abstract digit ranging from 0 (or negative) to 1, but it is expressed in the same unit of the measurement, for example, metres, degrees or seconds. The SEM can be used to form a band around an individual test result, making it possible to interpret a single measurement. Using a goniometric apparatus, Selvaratnam et al (1994) reported a reliability of 0.83 with a SEM of 16.8 degrees for a neurodynamic test (median nerve). These values yielded a 95% confidence interval of ± 33 degrees (1.96 * 16.8 degrees). This means that a patient's score ± 33 degrees would span the true score 95% of the time. Although the reliability was rather good, the large SEM questions the applicability of the test in daily practice. A more recent study (Coppieters et al 2000), demonstrated a high reliability when the neurodynamic test for the median nerve was consecutively performed in patients with neurogenic disorders. An ICC(2,1) of 0.98 with a SEM of 2.83 degrees was reported. When a mean of three scores was used, the ICC(2,3) augmented to 0.99 with a SEM of 1.64 degrees and a corresponding 95% confidence interval of only ± 3.2 degrees. Researchers should consider both correlation coefficients and the SEM when examining the reliability or consistency of their data.

To examine some of the reliability coefficients calculated by the authors of neurodynamic test normative studies, refer to table 13.2. It should be noted that the coefficients shown in Table 13.2 and in other studies investigating neurodynamic tests apply only to the data from measurements that were operationally defined in the study from which the data were obtained.

Because many researchers use different techniques to standardise their testing methods, researchers designing their own neurodynamic studies should conduct their own intra- and inter-reliability studies. Ideally, in the future all researchers will perform the base neurodynamic tests in the same way. This would increase the ability of researchers to share findings with one another. In summary, when performing neurodynamic tests in the clinic and as part of a research study, clinicians should do everything possible to minimise the influence of examiner, instrument, and patient error on their test results.

The reader who is considering research is referred to other texts, such as Huck (2000) and McEwan (1996) for case reports, Payton (1994) and Polit and Hungler (1999). Although Cohen's kappa and the intraclass correlation coefficient are the statistics of choice, it is important to realise that both have limitations. Refer to Haas (1991).

VALIDITY OF NEURODYNAMIC TESTS

Validity is defined as the degree to which a meaningful interpretation can be inferred from a measurement (Rothstein et al. 1991). Payton (1994) states that validity refers to the appropriateness, truthfulness, authenticity, or effectiveness of a study. In examining research studies and examination techniques, such as neurodynamic tests, clinicians need to become familiar with several different types of validity.

CONSTRUCT AND CONTENT VALIDITY.

Construct and content validity are two types of theoretical or conceptual validity. Generally, construct and concept validity are proven through logical argument rather than experimental study. Because of this fact, these two types of validity provide the least evidence based support for a clinical test or measure. Construct validity is the theoretical foundation on which all other types of validity depend. Construct validity attempts to answer the questions, "Can I use this measurement to make a specific inference?" and "What does the result of this test mean?" Rothstein (1985; 1993) has used the example of manual muscle testing (MMT), which today has lost its original construct validity. In 1916, Lovett developed MMT as a method to describe weakness in patients with damage to anterior horn cells in the spinal cord. The validity of Lovett's MMT was based on the theoretical construct that completely innervated muscles could generate greater tension than partially innervated muscles present in patients with anterior horn cell pathology. Today, some clinicians use MMT as a measure of strength or function. This construct is invalid and represents a gross deviation from Lovett's original goal of MMT. Clinicians and researchers should carefully consider if the constructs of their tests and measures are valid when conducting research or documenting patient progress in the clinic.

Closely related to construct validity, content validity deals with the concept of how well the measure reflects or samples the meaningful elements of the construct (Rothstein 1985; Rothstein et al. 1991; McEwen 1996). For example, based on an understanding of neuroanatomy and neuropathology, a test to measure proprioception could be constructed. A proprioceptive test demonstrating good content validity would sample only the proprioceptive elements of interest during testing. In contrast, if the test outcome was influenced by how well the subject could read directions or if taller subjects always seemed to do worse than shorter subjects, then the proprioception test would have poor content validity.

What is the "construct" of neurodynamic testing? What do the results of the neurodynamic test mean? When it was first created, neural tissue testing was based exclusively on a neuromechanical construct (Cyriax 1978; Breig and Troup 1979; Elvey 1986; Kenneally et al. 1988; Butler 1989). It was believed that the nervous system responded to mechanical induced stresses by distributing force throughout the spinal cord, meninges, nerve roots and peripheral nerves (Cyriax 1978; Breig and Troup 1979). Neurodynamic tests like the ULNT1 (Elvey 1979) and slump test (Maitland 1985; Philip et al. 1989) were designed to cause a build up of stress throughout certain sections of this continuous, innervated neuroanatomical pathway. Therefore, the original construct of neural tissue provocation testing was based on the theory that an ordered set of joint movements could be used to selectively increase tension within the neural tissue and their connective tissue sheaths (Elvey 1979). Furthermore, decreased mobility found upon testing was thought to imply fibrosis or neural tissue pathology in the nerve or nerves being tested (Cyriax 1978; Elvey 1979; Kenneally et al. 1988). To test the construct validity of these original hypotheses, researchers (Breig and Troup 1979; Lewis et al. 1998; Kleinrensink et al. 2000) have attempted to quantify the neural tension that occurs during neurodynamic tests.

Kleinrensink et al. (2000) applied buckle force transducers to the medial, lateral, and posterior cords of the brachial plexus of three embalmed human bodies. They also placed transducers on the radial, ulnar, and median nerves just distal to the plexus cords. These scientists recorded transducer output (nerve tension) during the ULNT1 (median nerve bias), ULNT2b (radial nerve bias), and ULNT3 (ulnar nerve bias) tests. They also assessed if tension was increased in each neurodynamic test with the addition of the combined motion of contralateral lateral cervical flexion and rotation (ULNT+). The results of this study demonstrated that only the ULNT1 and ULNT1+ had high sensitivity and specificity (see Appendix A). Although the radial and ulnar ULNTs increased tension in their corresponding nerves, this tension was not significantly greater or specific in the nerve named by the test. What does this mean clinically? The answer is illustrated with the following discussion. If a patient presented with isolated radial nerve pathology, the radial nerve test would most likely be positive. Although Kleinrensink et al. (2000) has shown that the ULNT2b increases tension more in the median nerve than the radial nerve, theoretically it may increase tension in the radial nerve to a point that an injured radial nerve would respond. On the other hand, if a patient presented with both radial and median nerve pathology, the ULNT2b could not selectively isolate one pathology over the other.

Based on the results of the above study, in this example, the ULNT1 could differentiate between the two nerves because it significantly increases tension in the median nerve without increasing tension in the radial nerve. A few questions could be raised regarding the operational definitions these authors used for the test positions. Did they block shoulder elevation during ULNT1 and ULNT3 or depress the shoulder during ULNT2b? How would this have changed the studies' results? A clinician may consider that the tests were sensitive and specific for tension in the tested nerves, whereas sometimes it appears the nerve movement is sensitive. Lewis et al (1998) demonstrated that shoulder depression did not significantly increase tension during the ULNT1 test. However, this was only analysed in a stepwise manner and it is unknown what influence shoulder depression had on median nerve tension in the final position of the test. Further investigation of ULNTs in which test order is varied need to be investigated to determine whether certain test sequences may cause a greater linear build up of tension. Regardless of these questions, these studies (Lewis et al. 1998; Kleinrensink et al. 2000) should be recognised as useful attempts to assess the mechanical aspects of the construct validity of the ULNTs.

A basic belief of neurodynamic tests is their ability to selectively differentiate or "sample" neural tissue from other non-neural structures in the neighbouring area. This belief, which represents the content validity of neurodynamic tests, has been investigated in anatomical studies. Moses and Carman (1996), in a precise histological and gross analysis, examined the anatomy of the lower cervical nerves. Their anatomical findings revealed that the lower cervical nerves have several connections to other innervated structures as they exit the spinal cord and travel to the periphery. These structures include the zygapophyseal joints and intervertebral discs, sites of other common musculoskeletal disorders. If inflamed, these structures could interfere with the selective testing of neural tissues during upper extremity neurodynamic tests. In another study, Wilson et al. (1994) examined two embalmed cadavers in order to determine the effects of ULNT1 on the subclavian artery. These researchers found that the sensitising manoeuvre of contralateral lateral cervical flexion to the base ULNT1 position did indeed produce arterial strain. These cadaver studies bring into question the content validity of the original theory that neurodynamic tests selectively isolate neural tissue.

CONVERGENT AND DISCRIMINANT VALIDITY

Up to this point, our discussion of validity has focused on research in support of the original theoretical hypotheses of neural tissue testing. Clinically, experimenters often use additional methods to provide support for construct validity for the specific tests they use in their studies. One method involves the researcher providing correlational evidence that shows that a strong relationship exists between the test and some predetermined variable while simultaneously a corresponding weak relationship exists between the test and other variables. This strong/weak relationship must be logically related to the theory of the construct behind the test or measure (Huck 2000). Convergent validity exists when the test, as predicted, demonstrates a strong correlation between two variables. Discriminate validity exists when the test, as predicted, demonstrates a low correlation between two variables.

The convergent and discriminate validity of the ULNT1 was first examined in a study by Selvaratnam et al. (1994). They examined the response to the ULNT1 in 25 patients reporting unilateral shoulder and upper arm pain following open-heart surgery and 25 athletes with similar pain from throwing injuries. The subjects in the cardiac group were considered to have a high probability of brachial plexus pain secondary to their surgical procedure. Thus, it was predicted that a high number of positive ULNT1 tests would be present in this group. The sports injury group was thought to represent pain originating only from the shoulder. Therefore, it was predicted that a low number of positive ULNT1 tests would be found in this group. Finally, 25 asymptomatic subjects were used as a control group. Their results demonstrated that the cardiac group had significantly greater positive results (loss of elbow range of motion with contralateral cervical flexion) than those of the other two groups. This illustrates the convergent validity of the ULNT1. The discriminative validity of the ULNT1 was shown in this study by its ability to find a low number of positive test results in the sports and control groups. This supported their hypothesis that neurodynamic testing could discriminate between local and referred pain.

Studies, like the one described above, that examine whether neurodynamic tests can discriminate between neural and non-neural tissue pathology, contribute to the evidence available to clinicians that support the validity of neurodynamic tests. Table 13.3 provides a brief summary of several studies that examine the presence of positive neurodynamic tests in suspected disorders of neural origin.

CONCURRENT AND PREDICTIVE VALIDITY

The final two types of validity I am going to discuss are types of criterion based validity. Criterion based validity refers to a test's ability to infer similar results when compared to a comparable test that has established validity. When this comparison is performed at approximately the same time, the researcher is examining the concurrent validity of the test. A second form of criterion based validity is called predictive validity. Predictive validity is assessed by comparing a test to supporting evidence that is obtained at a later date. The concurrent validity of the ULNT1 was examined in patients with carpal tunnel syndrome by Coveney et al. (1997). This investigator compared neurodynamic testing to a "gold standard" confirmation diagnosis using nerve conduction testing. The use of nerve conduction studies (NCS) as a gold standard is arguable because false positive or negative findings may exist (Rosenbaum and Ochoa, 1993). In Coveney als. study, the ULNT1 was positive in 14 of the 17 subjects who had positive nerve conduction tests for carpal tunnel syndrome. This

STUDY	PUBLISHED IN:	NTPT	DIAGNOSIS	CONTROL N	STUDY N	FINDINGS OF NEURAL TISSUE PROVOCATION TESTING	INTRA-RATER RELIABILITY	INTER-RATER RELIABILITY
Coveney (1997)	Proceedings	ULTT1	Carpal Tunnel Syndrome	None	11	Test assessed as positive when it reproduced patient's Sxs. Neurodynamic test results compared to nerve conductions studies.		Only intra-reliability was reported. The authors stated 82% – 100% for sx response
Grant (1995)	Peer-reviewed	ULTT2b	Repetitive task workers	10	15	Compared the end ROM for shoulder abduction between the repetitive task and non-repetitive task workers. They found a significant ↓ in shoulder abduction ROM in the SBK workers.	RMSE = 1°	P = 0.004
Quintner (1989)	Peer-reviewed	ULTT	Upper limb pain and paraesthesiae	20 (40 arms)	37 (61 arms)	In 36 of the control group arms, the author found a full range of extensibility. The ULTT was positive in 55 of the symptomatic arms. The author found no false positive tests.	No reliability statistics were calculated	
Kelley (1998)	Peer-reviewed	ULTT2a	Status post breast cancer surgery	5 20	14	A significant ↓ in shoulder abduction end ROM was found on both the surgical side (11°) and non-surgical side (7°) when comparing pre- and post-operative ULT2a NTPTs.	RMSE = 3° for abduction ROM	RMSE = 3° for abduction ROM
Young (1991)	Proceedings	ULTT1	Colle's fracture	20	20	Author found that the ULTT reproduced symptoms of post fracture pain in the symptomatic group.	Unknown	
Yaxley (1993)	Peer-reviewed	ULTT2b	Tennis elbow	None	20	Shoulder abduction ROM was on average 12° less in the involved arm. Patient's Sxs were reproduced in 55% of cases.	See earlier study (65)	
Wright (1994)	Peer-reviewed	ULTT1 ULTT2b	Chronic tennis elbow	None	16	Significant differences (P < 0.05) between involved and non-involved arms were found when comparing elbow ROM for the ULTT1 and ULTT2b in patients with tennis elbow.	No reliability statistics were calculated	
Turl (1998)	Peer-reviewed	Slump	Hamstring strain	14	14	Although no flexibility differences existed between groups, the slump test was + in 57% of the injured group and 0% of controls. Controls were well matched to injured group	No reliability statistics were calculated	
Yeung (1997)	Peer-reviewed	Slump	Patients with post-accident "whiplash"	40	20	They reported an ↑ in cervical Sxs in 17 of the test subjects with the addition of left ankle DF.	r = 0.85 r = 0.94	
Pahor (1996)	Peer-reviewed	Slump	Inversion ankle sprains	None	18	They diagrammed Sx response and location. The slump test with the addition of ankle PFI demonstrated the greatest ↓ in knee extension ROM.	RMSE = 2° RMSE = 4°	

Table 13.3 Results of neurodynamic tests in subjects with neural tissue pathology. ROM = range of motion; Sx(s) = Symptom(s); SBK = screen based keyboard; R = right; ROM = range of motion; RMSE = root mean square error; DF = dorsiflexion; PFI = plantar flexion with inversion.The goal of this table is to provide a brief synopsis of current research. The appropriateness of statistical methods and study design was not addressed.

represents a sensitivity of 82%, implying a high degree of accuracy. Specificity was calculated to be 75%, with the ULNT1 being negative in three of the four subjects who had negative nerve conduction studies. A more detailed explanation of clinically useful measures, such as sensitivity and specificity are presented below.

Shacklock (1996) examined the diagnostic validity of the ULNT3 in a case study of a patient with a surgically proven ulnar neuropathy. Initially the patient presented to physiotherapy with left medial elbow pain that she described as intermittent, deep and burning in quality. There was also as cold tingling feeling extending from the medial elbow to the little finger. Ultrasound scans of the involved region and patient's cervical spine X-rays were negative. On neurodynamic testing, the patient was found to have a positive ULNT3 and ULNT1. The patient eventually underwent exploratory surgery and it was discovered the ulnar nerve was entrapped. This study illustrates how the ULNT3 test may be more sensitive than a routine neurological examination and ultrasound scanning for neuropathy. Although, the ULNT1 and ULNT3 tests were both positive before surgery, the ULNT3 was more specific in reproducing the patient's symptoms. Furthermore, following surgical release the ULNT1 produced only the normal response defined by Kenneally et al. (1988). This case report raises several interesting questions and additional studies involving more than one subject are required to determine the diagnostic validity of neurodynamic tests.

DESCRIBING THE ACCURACY OF A DIAGNOSTIC TEST

The accuracy of a diagnostic test is usually determined by examining the ability of the test to assist clinicians in making a correct diagnosis. A good diagnostic test is one that minimises the probability of the clinician finding a positive response in healthy people and negative test results in people with pathology. In other words, a good diagnostic test is one that minimises the probability of an occurrence of either a false positive or a false negative result. The accuracy of a diagnostic test is assigned a probability value between 0.0 and 1.0 by calculating two different conditional probabilities called the sensitivity and specificity. The closer the probability value is to 1, the more accurate the test is in determining the correct response. The sensitivity of the test is defined as the probability that people who truly should have the positive response receive a positive response when the test is performed. The specificity of the test is defined as the probability that people who should truly have a negative response correctly receive a negative response when the test is performed. Using the data from Coveney et al's (1997) study of the ULNT1 response in subjects with a clinical presentation of carpal tunnel syndrome, table 13.4 illustrates how sensitivity and specificity are calculated.

In clinical practice, it is often impossible to calculate the sensitivity and specificity of a clinical test. This is because sensitivity and specificity assume that the researcher or clinician already has the true answer. Sensitivity assumes that one has somehow first identified people with a true positive response, and then determines what percentage the desired test is correct in identifying these people. Likewise, specificity assumes that one has somehow first identified people with a true negative response, and then determines what percentage the diagnostic test is correct in identifying these people. However, in the clinical setting the opposite happens. First the test is performed and then the clinician asks, "Given that the test is positive, what is the probability that my patient truly has a positive response?" Or, "Given that the test is negative, what is the probability that my patient truly has a negative response?" These questions are answered by calculating the positive predictive value and negative predictive value of the test respectively. The positive predictive value of a test is defined as the probability that a person who receives a positive test result will truly have a positive response. The negative predictive value of a test is defined as the probability that a person who receives a negative test result will truly have a negative response. Like sensitivity and specificity, positive and negative predictive values will always fall between 0 and 1. Table 13.4 illustrates how positive and negative predictive values are calculated.

THE EMERGING NEW CONSTRUCT IN NEURODYNAMICS

In order to examine the scientific merit of the neurodynamic tests, we have critically discussed the importance of operational definitions, reliability and validity in neurodynamic research. The original construct of neurodynamic testing was that it determined neural tissue involvement by specifically stressing neural tissue, in particular, peripheral nerve and the meninges. There was always a difficulty here because it is self evident that other structures will have physical forces placed upon them during a neurodynamic test. Hence the tests required other clinical data to assume positivity.

A challenge to the original construct of neurodynamics has emerged recently with the increasing awareness that the responses to the tests are not solely due to mechanical effects on neural tissues, but also coexisting inputs and the processing state of the CNS (chapter 3). The response of the CNS to inputs is not fixed. Responses may be due to varying contributions of primary (tissue based) and secondary (CNS based) hyperalgesia. We are now aware of the importance of psychosocial factors in determining aspects of movement, including range of movement (chapter 7). To be valid, a neurodynamic test would have to reliably sample components of both the central and peripheral nervous systems and be performed in the context of a new conceptual pain model, perhaps as suggested in this text. Admittedly, we don't have a sufficiently sophisticated construct for neurodynamic testing that integrates bio-psycho-social theory with "neurodynamic" theory. However, we can attempt this clinically under a clinical decision making framework (eg. Gifford and Butler 1997; Butler 1998; Gifford 1998) and now hopefully link it into research.

RESEARCH RELATED TO TREATMENT EFFECTS

A review of the literature revealed that only a small number of published research studies on neural tissue mobilisation exist in the peer reviewed literature. These are briefly discussed below.

		GOLD STANDARD NERVE CONDUCTION TEST		
		disorder present	disorder absent	
diagnostic test	positive	A true positive 14	B false positive 1	positive predictive value $\frac{A}{A+B} = \frac{14}{15} = 93\%$
ULNT 1	negative	C false negative 3	D true negative 3	negative predictive value $\frac{D}{C+D} = \frac{3}{6} = 75\%$
		sensitivity $\frac{A}{A+C} = \frac{14}{17} = 82\%$	specifity $\frac{D}{B+D} = \frac{3}{4} = 75\%$	

Table 13.4   Results of the ULNT1 in subjects with c.t.s. as determined by nerve conduction tests. Data taken from Coveney et al. (1997).

Kornberg and Lew (1989) analysed the effects of slump stretching in a group of patients with a grade 1 hamstring strain, without a history of lumbar spine pathology. This study involved setting up a double blind survey in 8 professional Australian Rules football clubs. Four of the clubs treated subjects with a traditional physiotherapy protocol including R.I.C.E. (rest, ice, compression and elevation), ultrasound, electrical stimulation, and hamstring stretches. In the remaining four clubs, the experimental group received similar treatments with the addition of slump stretching. Results revealed that the number of games missed was significantly lower in the experimental group receiving the slump stretching. The authors concluded that slump stretching, when combined with traditional therapy for grade I hamstring injuries, is more effective than traditional therapy alone.

Dreschler et al. (1997) compared two groups of subjects who met their inclusion criteria of lateral epicondylitis. Eight subjects were assigned to a group that received ULNT2b neural mobilisation techniques and anterior/posterior mobilisations of the radial head. Subjects in this group also performed a home mobilisation program of exercises involving the ULNT2b test position. The standard treatment group of ten subjects received continuous ultrasound and transverse friction massage to the common extensor tendon. Stretching of the wrist extensors and a dumbbell resistance program was carried out after the modality treatment. All subjects were treated twice per week for 6-8 weeks. Follow up data was obtained at three months following cessation of treatment. The results demonstrated that the combination treatment of radial head and ULNT2b mobilisation techniques was superior to the traditional treatment of modalities, stretching, and strengthening. Unfortunately, the researchers were unable to separate the effects of the radial head and neural tissue mobilisations.

Vicenzino et al. (1996) examined the effects of cervical spine manipulative therapy on pain and dysfunction in lateral epicondylalgia. The technique used was a grade III passive contralateral lateral glide technique at the C5-6 motion segment, with the arm in a position that involved ULNT2 (radial) components. This study was a randomised, double blind, placebo controlled, repeated measures design involving 15 subjects with a history of lateral epicondylalgia symptoms. The ULNT2b was used to assess neural tissue mobility before and after treatment. Significant improvements in ULNT2b response, pressure pain threshold, pain score, and pain free grip strength were found. This study is paramount because it demonstrated that mobilization of accessory structures such as the cervical spine might influence the mobility of the nervous system. Hall et al. (1997) demonstrated significant improvements in 12 subjects' pain, functional capacity and neck and shoulder mobility after a 4 week treatment period utilising a similar technique. Improvements were maintained at 3 months.

Coppieters and Stappaerts (2000) also analysed the immediate effects of the lateral glide technique in a randomised controlled trial, where 14 patients with cervicobrachial neurogenic disorders were included, using similar criteria to Hall (1997). Ultrasound was used in the control condition. The range of motion, pain intensity and symptom provocation during ULNT1 were used as outcome measures. Results indicated that the experimental group demonstrated a significant increase of approximately 19.5 degrees, whereas the control condition demonstrated no improvement. Immediate increases in ULNT1 range of motion for the experimental group ranged from approximately 6 to 46 degrees. Elicited pain responses also deceased for the experimental group. The large variability in improvement might demonstrate that the inclusion criteria might require refinement.

Two studies found in the literature examined the effects of neural tissue mobilisation either without a comparison to a control group or without randomization. Sweeney and Harms (1996) examined the relationship between hand mechanical allodynia and the ULNT1. Twenty-nine subjects with mechanical allodynia after nerve injury were examined before and after a two-week neural mobilisation program using a ULNT1 home mobilisation program. All subjects were non-responsive to a standard physiotherapy programme including tactile and vibratory stimulation treatment. To assess improvement, pre- and post- ULNT1 tests were recorded. At the initial assessment, 19 of the affected extremities had limitations greater than 20(of elbow extension with the ULNT1. Pain symptoms were reproduced or increased in 25 of the 29 subjects during the initial ULNT1. Following the two-week mobilisation program, 26 subjects were able to reach full elbow extension during the post ULNT1 test. Furthermore, 19 of the subjects felt that their symptoms had improved.

A study by Rozmaryn et al. (1998) investigated the effects of nerve and tendon gliding exercises in patients with carpal tunnel syndrome. One hundred and ninety-seven patients (240 hands) were treated by standard conservative methods (splinting, anti-inflammatory medications) and placed into two groups, an experimental group of 93 patients that performed nerve and tendon gliding exercises and a control group of 104 patients who did not perform the gliding exercises. The results revealed that significantly more patients in the control group had surgery compared to the experimental group (71% vs. 43%). This study is significant because it demonstrates that effective, non-surgical treatment can affect the number of patients undergoing carpal tunnel release surgery.

Maher and Scrimshaw (1999) analysed whether the addition of neural mobilisation to standard physiotherapy rehabilitation affected the outcome of patients who had undergone spinal surgery. Eighty-one patients were randomly assigned to a control and experimental group. Results demonstrated that at discharge, both groups had large improvements in their pre-operative pain status and a small reduction in their pre-operative SLR range. At 6 weeks, both groups had improved their pre-operative status in terms of SLR, pain and disability. As there were no differences between the experimental and control group, the authors concluded that the addition of neural mobilisation to standard physiotherapy did not affect the patients' condition in the short term. Six and twelve months follow ups were not available yet.

Another post-operative study was performed by Weirich et al. (1999). They compared the effects of immediate (20 patients) and delayed (16 patients) mobilisation in patients who underwent anterior subcutaneous transposition of the ulnar nerve. The authors believed that early neural excursion affected the establishment of an enhanced epineural soft tissue gliding mechanism. Both groups demonstrated significant relief of primary symptoms. Between the two groups, there was no significant difference in relief of pain, paresthesia, weakness or overall level of satisfaction. However, in the immediate mobilisation group, patients returned to work and resumed activities of daily living earlier than in the delayed mobilisation group (1 versus 2.75 months).

To provide the strongest cause and effect argument for the use of neural tissue mobilisation techniques, randomised controlled clinical trials and systematic reviews are essential. Although these studies are required to document a cause-effect relationship between treatment and outcome, they are often not practical projects for the practising clinician. This is frustrating because it is the clinician that depends on proof that these techniques work. One alternative that is gaining popularity is the case report. Case reports cannot establish that an intervention caused a specific result, however they can describe practice (McEwen 1996). By describing in detail certain patient examination and treatment techniques, clinicians can enhance the learning of others, stimulate new hypotheses, and provide the clinical researcher with a proposed research project. In addition, most of the peer-reviewed physiotherapy journals accept case reports for publication. More case reports are needed in the field of neurodynamics. Three excellent examples of neurodynamic case reports involving neurodynamics are the use of neurodynamics in a patient with chronic de Quervain's tenosynovitis by Anderson and Tichenor (1994), use of slump and prone knee bend neural tissue mobilisation in three subjects by Wise (1994), and a recent study by George (2000). This case report involved the use of slump stretching neural mobilisation in a 38 year old patient with a four year history of deep posterior thigh pain and intermittent lateral foot pain. These three case studies exemplify how the practising clinician can help narrow the gap between practice and research. Although, case reports can not prove a treatment's effectiveness, they can describe the performance of techniques in such a way as to initiate a topic for a future randomised controlled trial.

This section demonstrates a critical need for research examining the effects of neural tissue mobilisation. This is the area of neurodynamics lacking the most evidence and thus would be an excellent area for future research. Without evidence from well designed controlled studies or the sharing of successful techniques from publishing case reports, treatment of neural tissue via mobilisation will remain a nonstandard therapy technique (table 13.1).

FUTURE RESEARCH INTO NEURODYNAMICS

The last two criteria in table 13.1 from Harris (1996) that determine if a technique is worthy of scientific merit are that potential contraindications of the treatment are presented and that the proponents of the treatment approach are open and willing to discuss its limitations. It is not the purpose of this chapter to go into detail regarding the contraindications of neurodynamic treatment. The reader is referred to other resources (chapter 7 this text and Butler 1991) that list and describe the limitations of neurodynamic treatment. The final criteria from table 13.1 does require some discussion. Do the proponents of neurodynamics appear to be open and willing to discuss its limitations? This question is easily answered by reviewing several of the commentaries (Butler 1998; Elvey 1998; Wright 1998) that appeared in a recent physiotherapy journal monograph. These commentaries are from acknowledged pioneers and experts in the field of neurodynamics. They also openly discussed how neurodynamics has changed markedly in the past decade and they admitted that their initial concepts based on a simple mechanical evaluation of neural mobility have errors.

Hopefully this chapter has stimulated your desire to review the current neurodynamic literature and become an effective user of and contributor to neurodynamic research. Clinicians and researchers in the area of neurodynamics need to continue to develop a common language in which to examine and share ideas and treatment techniques. Throughout this chapter we attempted to answer the question, "is neurodynamics worthy of scientific merit?" The answer to this question is left for the clinician or researcher reading this book. You must ask yourself if there exists substantial information to evaluate and treat a patient using neurodynamic tests and mobilisations. You should also consider whether you can envisage incorporating neural mobilisation techniques into the broad evidence guidelines in chapter 14. By basing your decision on the current available research, considering the criteria of nonstandard and standard treatments by Harris, and carefully considering the empirical evidence from patient treatment, you may arrive at an answer. By even attempting this endeavour, you have demonstrated some of the qualities of an evidence-based practitioner.

In the last twenty years, we have become more aware of the nervous system. This awareness has allowed us to evaluate the patient more fully from a neuro-orthopaedic approach. This neuro-orthopedic approach to evaluation continues to be updated on a regular basis with new and exciting research. Recently, we have begun to carefully consider and integrate pain into this model of evaluation as well. In order to apply this new information, all clinicians must become critical "users" of the research literature. At a minimum, this means staying up to date with the current literature, gaining experience in the clinic, and sharing ideas and case reports with others. Much of the evaluation and treatment of patients using neurodynamics remains and will always remain an art. However, we must provide these artistic endeavours with a solid scientific foundation. We must consider whether these new evaluation and treatment techniques are worthy of scientific merit. This can be accomplished by making clinical decisions in rehabilitation using the integration of basic research, clinical research, empirically based clinical experience, expert opinion, and outcome studies. This task is formidable and we as a profession must rise to the challenge. We not only owe it to ourselves, we owe it to the patients who have turned to us for help.

APPENDIX A

STANDARDS FOR TESTS AND MEASUREMENTS IN PHYSIOTHERAPY PRACTICE

Reprinted from Rothstein JM, Campbell, SK, Echternach JL et al. Standards for tests and measurements in physiotherapy practice. Physiotherapy 71: 589-622, with permission from the APTA.

Construct: a concept developed for the purpose of measurement; support for the construct is through logical argumentation based on theoretical and research evidence *(see construct validity)*

Operational definition: a set of procedures that guides the process of obtaining a measurement; includes descriptions of the attribute that is to be measured, the conditions under which the measurement is to be taken, and the actions that are to be taken in order to obtain the measurement

Reliability: the consistency or repeatability of measurements; the degree to which measurements are error-free and the degree to which repeated measurements will agree

Intertester reliability: the consistency or equivalence of measurements when more than one person takes the measurements; indicates agreement of measurements taken by different examiners

Intratester reliability: the consistency or equivalence of measurements when one person takes repeated measurements separated in time; indicates agreement in measurements over time

Validity: the degree to which a useful (meaningful) interpretation can be inferred from a measurement

Construct validity: the conceptual (theoretical) basis for using a measurement to make an inferred interpretation; evidence for construct validity is through logical argumentation based on theoretical and research evidence (see construct)

Content validity: a form of validity that deals with the extent to which a measurement is judged to reflect the meaningful elements of a construct and not any extraneous elements

Criterion-Based (criterion-related) validity: three forms of criterion-based validity exist: concurrent validity, predictive validity, and prescriptive validity; the common element is that, with each of these forms of validity, the correctness of an inferred interpretation can be tested by comparing a measurement with either a different measurement or data obtained by other forms of testing

Concurrent validity: a form of criterion-based validity in which an inferred interpretation is justified by comparing a measurement with supporting evidence that was obtained at approximately the same time as the measurement being validated

Predictive validity: a form of criterion-based validity in which an inferred interpretation is justified by comparing a measurement with supporting evidence that is obtained at a later point in time; examines the justification of using a measurement to say something about future events or conditions

Sensitivity of a test: an indication of how well a diagnostic test identifies people who should have a positive finding; the numerical representation of sensitivity is a ratio formed by dividing the number of persons with a true-positive response on a test by the number of persons who should have had a positive response (ie, the number of persons who are known to have properties that would indicate that they should test positive)

Specificity of a test: an indication of how well a diagnostic test identifies people who should have a negative finding; the numerical representation of specificity is a ratio formed by dividing the number of persons with a true-negative response on a test by the number of persons who should have had a negative response (ie, the number of persons who are known to have properties that would indicate that should test negative)

REFERENCES CHAPTER 13

Anderson M & Tichenor CJ (1994) A patient with de Quervain's tenosynovitis: a case report using an Australian approach to manual therapy. Physiotherapy 74: 314-326.

Balster SM & Jull GA (1997) Upper trapezius muscle activity during the brachial plexus tension test in asymptomatic subjects. Manual Therapy 2: 144-149.

Bell A (1987) The upper limb tension test - bilateral straight leg raising - a validating manoeuvre for the upper limb tension test. Proceedings Fifth Biennial Conference , Manipulative Therapists Association of Australia, Melbourne.

Block CA, Cantrall CE & Threlkeld AJ (1998) Responses of asymptomatic subjects to the upper limb tension test with a median nerve bias. Physical Therapy 78: Abstract PL-RR-228 S76.

Breig A (1978) Adverse Mechanical Tension in the Central Nervous System, Almqvist and Wiksell, Stockholm.

Breig A & Troup J (1979) Biomechanical considerations in the straight leg raising test. Spine 4: 242-250.

Butler DS (1989) Adverse mechanical tension in the nervous system: a model for assessment and treatment. Australian Journal of Physiotherapy 35: 227-238.

Butler DS (1991) Mobilisation of the Nervous System, Churchill Livingstone, Melbourne.

Butler DS (1998) Commentary - Adverse mechanical tension in the nervous system: a model for assessment and treatment. In: Maher C (ed.) "Adverse Neural Tension Reconsidered", Australian Physiotherapy Association, Melbourne.

Butler DS (1998) Integrating pain awareness into physiotherapy - wise action for the future. In: Gifford LS (ed.) Topical Issues in Pain, NOI Press, Falmouth.

Coppieters MW & Stappaerts KH (2000) The immediate effects of manual therapy in patients with cervicobrachial pain of neural origin: a pilot study. In: Proceedings: International Federation of Orthopaedic Manipulative Therapists Conference, Perth.

Coppieters MW, Stappaerts KH & Staes FF (1999) A qualitative assessment of shoulder girdle elevation during the upper limb tension test 1. Manual Therapy 4: 33-38.

Coppieters MW, Stappaerts KH, Staes FF, et al. (2000) Shoulder girdle elevation during neurodynamic testing: an assessable sign? Manual Therapy 5(3): in press.

Coveney B, Trott P, Grimmer KA, et al. (1997) The upper limb tension test in a group of subjects with a clinical presentation of carpal tunnel syndrome. In Proceedings: Tenth Biennial Conference: Manipulative Physiotherapists Association of Australia , Melbourne.

Cyriax J (1978) Mechanisms of symptoms: Dural pain. Lancet: 919-921.

de Krom MC, Kester AD, Knipschild PG, et al. (1990) Efficacy of provocative tests for diagnosis of carpal tunnel syndrome. Lancet 335: 393-395.

Di Fabio RP (1999) Myth of evidence based medicine. Journal of Orthopedic and Sports Physical Therapy 29: 632-633.

Drechsler WI, Knarr JF & Snyder-Mackler L (1997) A comparison of two treatment regimens for lateral epicondylitis. Journal of Sport Rehabilitation 6: 226-234.

Edgar D, Jull G & Sutton S (1994) Relationship between upper trapezius muscle length and upper quadrant neural extensibility. Australian Journal of Physiotherapy 40: 99-103.

Elvey RL (1979) Brachial plexus tension tests and the pathoanatomical origin of arm pain. In: Idczak R (ed.) Aspects of Manipulative Therapy, Manipulative Physiotherapists Association of Australia, Melbourne.

Elvey RL (1986) Treatment of arm pain associated with abnormal brachial plexus tension. The Australian Journal of Physiotherapy 32: 225-230.

Elvey RL (1998) Commentary - treatment of arm pain associated with abnormal brachial plexus tension. In: Maher C (ed.) Australian Journal of Physiotherapy Monograph No. 3, Australian Physiotherapy Association, Melbourne.

Fidel C, Martin E, Dankaerts W, et al. (1996) Cervical spine sensitising manoeuvres during the slump test. Journal of Manual and Manipulative Therapy 4: 16-21.

Flanagan M (1993) Normative responses to the ulnar nerve bias tension test. Thesis, University of South Australia, Adelaide .

Fleiss JL (1986) The Design and Analysis of Clinical Experiments, John Wiley & Sons, New York.

Friberg R, Reeder M, Tally D, et al. (2000) Symptom distribution for upper limb tension tests 1, 2A, 2B, 3 (Abstract P015. Journal of Orthopedic and Sports Physical Therapy 30: A6.

Gelberman RH, Yamaguchi K & Hollstein SB (1998) Changes in interstitial pressure and cross-sectional area of the cubital tunnel and of the ulnar nerve with flexion of the elbow. Journal of Bone and Joint Surgery 80A: 492-501.

Gifford L & Butler D (1997) The integration of pain sciences into clinical practice. The Journal of Hand Therapy 10: 86-95.

Gifford LS (1998) Pain, the tissues and the nervous system. Physiotherapy 84: 27-33.

Golden GS (1980) Nonstandard therapies in developmental disabilities. American Journal of Diseases in Childhood 134: 487-491.

Grant R, Forrester C & Hides J (1995) Screen based keyboard operation: the adverse effects on the neural system. Australian Journal of Physiotherapy 41: 99-107.

Haas M (1991) Statistical methodology for reliability studies. Journal of Manipulative and Physiological Therapeutics 14: 119-132.

Hall T, Elvey RL, Davies N, et al. (1997) Efficacy of manipulative physiotherapy for the treatment of cervicobrachial pain. In proceedings: Tenth Biennial Conference: Manipulative Physiotherapist's Association of Australia , Melbourne, Australia.

Hall T & Quintner JL (1996) Responses to mechanical stimulation of the upper limb in painful cervical radiculopathy. Australian Journal of Physiotherapy 42: 277-285.

Hall T, Zusman M & Elvey R (1998) Adverse mechanical tension in the nervous system? Analysis of straight leg raise. Manual Therapy 3: 140-146.

Harris S (1996) How should treatments be critiqued for scientific merit? Physical Therapy 76: 175-181.

Hines T, Noakes R & Manners B (1993) The upper limb tension test; inter-tester reliability for assessing the onset of passive resistance R1. Journal of Manual and Manipulative Therapy 1: 95-98.

Huck S (2000) Reading Statistics and Research, Addison Wesley Longman, New York.

Johnson EK & Chiarello CM (1997) The slump test: the effects of head and lower extremity position on knee extension. Journal of Orthopedic and Sports Physical Therapy 26: 310-317.

Jones D (1989) The inter-therapist reliability of the brachial plexus tension test. Australian Journal of Physiotherapy 35: 60.

Kelley S & Jull G (1998) Breast surgery and neural tissue mechanosensitivity. Australian Journal of Physiotherapy 44: 31-37.

Kenneally M (1985) The upper limb tension test. In Proceedings. Fourth Biennial Conference, Manipulative Therapists Association of Australia , Manipulative Therapists Association of Australia, Brisbane.

Kenneally M, Rubenach H & Elvey R (1988) The upper limb tension test: the SLR of the arm. In: Grant R (ed.) Physical Therapy of the Cervical and Thoracic Spine, Churchill Livingstone, New York.

Kleinrensink GJ, Stoeckart R, Mulder PGH, et al. (2000) Upper limb tension tests as tools in the diagnosis of nerve and plexus lesions. Clinical Biomechanics 15: 9-14.

Kornberg C & Lew P (1989) The effect of stretching neural structures on grade one hamstring injuries. Journal of Orthopaedic and Sports Physical Therapy June: 481-487.

Lewis J, Ramot R & Green A (1998) Changes in mechanical tension in the median nerve: possible implications for the upper limb tension test. Physiotherapy 84: 254-261.

Lovett RW & Masten EG (1916) Certain aspects of infantile paralysis and a descriptive method of manual testing. Journal of the American Medical Association 66: 729.

Maher C & Scrimshaw S (1999) Does neural mobilisation influence the outcome of spinal surgery. 13th World Conference of Physical Therapy , Yokahama, Japan.

Maitland G (1985) The slump test: examination and treatment. Australian Journal of Physiotherapy 31: 215-219.

McEwen I ed. (1996) Writing Case Reports: A How To Manual for Clinicians, American Physical Therapy Association, Alexandria VA.

Moses A & Carman J (1996) Anatomy of the cervical spine: implications for the upper limb tension test. Australian Journal of Physiotherapy 42: 31-35.

Pahor S & Toppenberg R (1996) An investigation of neural tissue involvement in ankle inversion sprains. Manual Therapy 1: 192-197.

Payton OD (1994) Research: The Validation of Clinical Experience, FA Davis, Philadelphia.

Pechan J & Julis F (1975) The pressure measurement in the ulnar nerve: a contribution to the pathophysiology of cubital tunnel syndrome. Journal of Biomechanics 8: 75-79.

Philip K, Lew P & Matyas T (1989) The inter-therapist reliability of the slump test. Australian Journal of Physiotherapy 35: 89-94.

Polit DF & Hungler BP (1999) Nursing Research: Principles and Methods, 6th edn. Lippincott, Philadelphia.

Pullos J (1986) The upper limb tension test. Australian Journal of Physiotherapy 42: 258-259.

Quintner JL (1989) A study of upper limb pain and paraesthesiae following neck injury in motor vehicle accidents: assessment of the brachial plexus tension test of Elvey. British Journal of Rheumatology 28: 528-533.

Rempel D, Dahlin L & Lundborg G (1999) Pathophysiology of nerve compression syndromes: response of peripheral nerves to loading. Journal of Bone and Joint Surgery 81A: 1600-1610.

Roebroeck ME, Harlaar J & Lankhorst GJ (1993) The application of generalizability theory to reliability assessment: an illustration using isometric force measurements. Physical Therapy 73: 386-395.

Rothstein JM (1985) Measurement in Physical Therapy, Churchill Livingstone, New York.

Rothstein JM (1993) Reliability and validity: implications for research. In: Bork CE (ed.) Research in Physical Therapy, JB Lippincott, Philadelphia.

Rothstein JM (1999) Immelmann's indignation. Physical Therapy 79: 1024-1025.

Rothstein JM, Campbell SK, Echternach JL, et al. (1991) Standards for tests and measurements in physical therapy practice. Physical Therapy 71: 589-622.

Rozmaryn LM, Dovelle S, Rothman ER, et al. (1998) Nerve and tendon gliding exercises and the conservative management of carpal tunnel syndrom. Journal of Hand Surgery 11: 171-179.

Rubenach H (1985) The upper limb tension test: the effect of the position and movement of the contralateral arm. In: Proceedings, Manipulative Physiotherapists Association of Australia, 4th biennial conference, Brisbane.

Sackett DL (1998) Editorial: evidence based medicine. Spine 23: 1085-1096.

Selvaratnam PJ, Matyas TA & Glasgow EF (1994) Noninvasive discrimination of brachial plexus involvement in upper limb pain. Spine 19: 26-33.

Seror P (1987) Tinel's sign in the diagnosis of carpal tunnel syndrome. Journal of Hand Surgery 12B: 364-365.

Shacklock M (1995) Neurodynamics. Physiotherapy 81: 9-16.

Shacklock MO (1996) Positive upper limb tension test in a case of surgically proven neuropathy. Manual Therapy 1: 154-161.

Sweeney J & Harms A (1996) Persistent mechanical allodynia following injury of the hand. Journal of Hand Therapy 9: 328-338.

Turl SE & George KP (1998) Adverse neural tension: a factor in repetitive hamstring strain? Journal of Orthopedic and Sports Physical Therapy 27: 16-21.

Turner P & Whitfield TW (1997) Physiotherapists' use of evidence based practice: a cross national study. Physiotherapy Research International 2: 17-29.

Weirich SD, Gelberman RH, Best SA, et al. (1999) Rehabilitation after subcutaneous transposition of the ulnar nerve: immediate versus delayed mobilization. Journal of Shoulder and Elbow Surgery 7: 244-249.

Wilson S, Selvaratnam PJ & Briggs C (1994) Strain at the subclavian artery during the upper limb tension test. Australian Journal of Physiotherapy 40: 243-248.

Wright A (1998) Foreword - a reappraisal of the "adverse neural tension" phenomenon. In: Maher C (ed.) Australian Journal of Physiotherapy Monograph No 3, Australian Journal of Physiotherapy, Melbourne.

Yaxley G & Jull G (1991) A modified upper limb tension test: an investigation of responses in normal subjects. Australian Journal of Physiotherapy 37: 143-152.

Yaxley G & Jull G (1993) Adverse tension in the neural system: a preliminary study of tennis elbow. Australian Journal of Physiotherapy 39: 15-22.

Yeung E (1996) The response to the slump test in a group of female whiplash patients. Australian Journal of Physiotherapy 43: 245-252.

Young L & Bell A (1991) The upper limb tension test response in a group of post colles' fracture patients. Manipulative Physiotherapists Association of Australia, 7th biennial conference, Sydney.

CHAPTER 14

MANAGEMENT STRATEGIES –
INTEGRATION OF NEURODYNAMICS

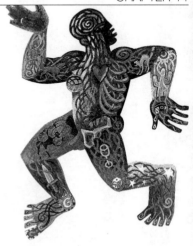

INTRODUCTION

"BIG PICTURE" EVIDENCE BASED APPROACH

INCORPORATION OF NEURODYNAMICS INTO MANAGEMENT

USE AS A REASSESSMENT TOOL

EXPLANATION

INTRODUCTION
EXPLAINING NEURODYNAMIC TEST FINDINGS AND PERIPHERAL NEUROGENIC PAIN
EXPLAINING NEURODYNAMIC TEST FINDINGS AND CENTRAL SENSITIVITY
NERVE IMAGES CAN BE SCARY

NEURODYNAMICS AND PASSIVE MOBILISATION

GENERAL COMMENTS
GUIDELINES FOR TECHNIQUES FOR MORE PERIPHERAL NEUROGENIC/NOCICEPTIVE
MECHANISMS
PASSIVE MOVEMENT TECHNIQUES FOR MORE CENTRAL DISORDERS
PASSIVE TECHNIQUE CONCEPTUALISATION
NEUROGENIC MASSAGE

ACTIVE MOBILISATION AND NEURODYNAMIC TESTS

INTRODUCTION
MOVEMENT BREAKDOWNS
ORDER OF MOVEMENT VARIATIONS AND "TRICK MOVEMENTS"
SLIDER/TENSIONER
ACTIVE MOVEMENTS – USE OF MEANINGFUL ACTIVITY
PACING
WARM UP/WARM DOWN MANOEUVRES WITH A FOCUS ON THE NERVOUS SYSTEM

POSTURAL ADVICE AND NEURODYNAMICS

SUMMARY

REFERENCES CHAPTER 14

INTRODUCTION

In the final two chapters I discuss the integration of neurodynamics into management strategies. I am hoping that information in the previous chapters can be merged into any existing management strategies. Perhaps the material has altered your management framework already. Clinical reasoning approaches are very adaptable and they thrive on change.

If you were asked the question, "why are you doing that?" of any of your management strategies, you should have a defensible answer. Skilled and uncorrupted clinical reasoning should allow answers based on evidence, basic sciences and logic. The answer "because I was taught to do it" exposes a shaky professionalism.

"BIG PICTURE" EVIDENCE BASED APPROACH

What you and I do as clinicians will always be different - our personalities, interactional skills, needs and education see to that even before we implement some management strategy. The atmosphere and environment of management will always vary. However, there is a basic blueprint for evidence based management strategies that every practitioner can use.

"Big picture" management strategies that have been shown to help patients in acute and chronic musculoskeletal pain, can be identified. This list is constructed from diverse sources (Frank 1973; Gerteis et al. 1993; Achterberg 1996; Kendall et al. 1997; Linton 1998; Waddell 1998). It is also taken from various national clinical guidelines for the management of low back pain (AHCPR 1994; Waddell et al. 1996; NHMRC 1998). For specific details, reference to these guidelines is recommended. This list is aimed at all professions who deal with musculoskeletal pain and is in no particular order.

1. Identify patients with "red flags" (chapter 7) and manage accordingly.

2. Educate the patient and relevant associates about the nature of the whole problem including health status of the tissues, role of the nervous system, and results of investigative tests. Such information and any new information must make sense to the patient and be continually updated during management.

3. Provide prognostication and with the patient, make realistic goals, which include clear recommendations about activities and progression of activities. Regular reviews are necessary with attention to the interests of all stakeholders.

4. Closely related to 2 and 3 is the promotion of self care, control and motivation.

5. Decrease unnecessary fear related to the injury and its effects on movements, leisure and work activities. Manage catastrophisation. This may mean challenging some beliefs and superstitions. It also requires that clinicians understand peripheral and central mechanisms of pain.

6. Get patients active and moving as early as is possible and appropriate after injury, by any safe active and passive means possible. In chronic pain, utilise patient favoured activities, but also address feared activities.

7. Help the patient identify and experience success and a sense of mastery of the problem or parts of the problem. Provide positive feedback for all "well" behaviours. This is important for compliance to programmes and to change behaviour.

8. Perform a skilled physical evaluation which is likely to be more "low tech" and functional in more chronic pain states and more specific in acute and tissue based problems. Results should be communicated immediately to the patient.

9. Acknowledge that combinations of biological, psychological and social inputs combine with existing neural architecture to produce pain and disability. Manage all inputs where possible and appropriate.

10. Use any measures possible to reduce pain, especially in the acute stage and use patient controlled analgesia where possible.

11. Minimise number of treatments and contacts with all medical personnel.

12. In chronic pain states, and pain states where there is a failure to improve, multidisciplinary management may be necessary.

13. Manage identified and relevant physical dysfunctions/impairments.

14. Assess and assist recovery or improvement of general physical fitness.

15. Assess effects of injury on patient's creative outlets and assist patient with regaining creativity and discovering new creative outlets.

These are very broad and general points. Any clinician operating under this framework could be said to be working under best evidence. To some degree, it may not matter what the therapy is, as long the above is followed. However, this broad perspective provides a framework for the reasoned use of specific techniques such as the neurodynamic tests, manipulation, muscle strengthening and graduated activity. It allows a place for the clinical creativity necessary for individual patients, especially the "grey zone" patients (chapter 6) where the pathobiology of the pain state is unknown and can only be reasoned. In some pain and disability states, specific techniques for specific population groups may help, for example, specific exercises for joint instability from spondylolisthesis (O'Sullivan et al. 1997) or nerve and tendon mobilisation for carpal tunnel syndrome (Rozmaryn et al. 1998). Obviously the population group needs urgent identification and the proposal in this book is that categorisation could be based on pathobiology using current neurobiological knowledge.

There is an important aspect of pain in society that is often forgotten. Most people with pain do not seek attention and they presumably self treat or carry on as usual. Only one quarter of people who suffer an acute episode of low back pain seek assistance (McKinnon et al. 1997) and therefore go through the process of turning into a patient. The messages of evidence, in particular early activation post injury, anxiety reducing education and the availability of useful techniques, need to reach the public as well.

INCORPORATION OF NEURODYNAMICS INTO MANAGEMENT

The first step is to make a reasoned judgement that the test or movement is related to a physically unhealthy/sensitive nervous system. The second step is to make the judgement that the test or movement is reflective of part of the patient's problem and worthy of improvement or use as an indicator of progression. Then there are a number of ways in which the physical finding can be used in management:

• Use as a reassessment tool

• Explanation

• Passive mobilisation

• Active movement, including movement breakdowns, order of movement variations, sliders and tensioners and integration into meaningful and purposeful activity

• Use in posture and ergonomic interventions.

Assessment has been described in a general sense in chapter 7 and more specifically related to neurodynamic tests in chapter 10.

USE AS A REASSESSMENT TOOL

Most clinicians and scientists will use tests such as the SLR as a form of reassessment of a management strategy. Presuming that you have established that the test is relevant to their disorder, the reassessment should include range of movement, pain responses and other movement behaviours (eg. neck movement, hip hiking and various spontaneous manoeuvres such as muscle spasm, even sympathetic activation). If an SLR has improved and function has improved, then you will have established a possible relationship between the physical finding and the test. Remember that insurance companies, researchers and some medical people will not share your delight at a vastly improved SLR unless it translates into productivity. The movement must therefore be one of a number of parameters which are indicative of change in the condition.

I hope that you feel comfortable about testing either "ends" of the body and testing the other or "good" side as part of validation of your management. For example, if you note a sensitive passive neck flexion for lumbar pain and your patient is undergoing any form of management for their lumbar spine, passive neck flexion is worth reassessing. Changes, especially if maintained, can be very positive feedback for your patient. Remember the continuum of the nervous system. Your patient's reassessment position should be the same as for the original assessment. For example a reassessment of SLR should be performed with the head and neck in the same position as before.

I also hope that you can take on the concept that changes may have occurred because of alterations in the physical health and sensitivity of local structures and/or the sensitivity setting of the central nervous system. Large changes in range are probably due to changes in motor control rather than a pure physical change. The changes may have occurred because of you. It is still all part of manual therapy. It could be an education session, a skilled and careful physical assessment and making some contacts with the patient's workplace which alter sensitivity and thus ranges of movement such as the straight leg raise. If you can take on the bio-psycho-social model (chapter 7) and the concept of distributed processing in the brain (chapter 2), this should be clear.

Some manual therapy approaches encourage an instant reassessment after a technique. This is fine but take care with the relevance of the immediate reassessment. You may be simply playing with impulses in a healing environment. Such assessment plays a part, but real improvement must be both functional and stakeholder orientated (chapter 7).

Sensitivity to palpation and neurological findings such as changes in reflexes can also be used as reassessment tools.

EXPLANATION

INTRODUCTION

A physical evaluation which pays due attention to neurodynamics can be extremely useful for educating patients about the nature of their disorders. The knowledge can be part of a useful management process. We, the clinicians, who touch and move patients and who have time with patients, are ideally positioned to be the mediators between the image of pain and disability that the patient has and the reality of the biology. We must aim to replace or adapt maladaptive beliefs, superstitions and attitudes and to decrease anxiety, fear and catastrophising, with the ultimate goal of improving physical confidence and abilities. There are a number of areas for discussion here.

If you have read the initial chapters, there will be many questions related to neuropathic pain that you could now begin to answer for patients, although we all need practice at this new skill. Questions about pain spreading, influences of stress, an understanding of why antalgic postures occur, why treatment works sometimes and not others, why nerve root problem can be agonising and set up chronic pains states, why certain drugs work while others don't. We have all had patients in the past whose pain and disability could not be understood. I used to think privately of them as "the pain everywhere kind." The various groups in pain related sciences are now handing us explanations for patients' pain states on a plate. The next step is to take this material to patients.

The majority of back pain educational classes still focus on structures. This is fine to a point. However many people who end up in back education classes are probably past a dominance of peripheral sensitivity. Their pain state will probably now have components of central sensitivity and perturbed output and homeostatic systems. High levels of catastrophising (Sullivan et al. 1998), depression, anxiety and fear are likely (eg. Gatchel et al. 1995). There is some recent promising research which shows that provision of neuroscience education, in comparison to a traditional structural education will reduce worry and probably distress in chronic low back pain sufferers. Those provided with a neuroscience education were less inclined to think that pain is an indicator of harm and more inclined to think it has emotional influences (Moseley 2000).

The comment "educate the patient" is very often misused and misunderstood. What may be quite simple for an acute injury becomes increasingly difficult for a patient in severe and unremitting pain. General guidelines are produced by many professional associations, but each patient will have specific requirements. Education, like a passive movement technique, has to be linked to improved function. That is, the next step to activity and exercise has to be taken at the same time as the education. There are some aspects of education in relation to neurodynamic test findings that are worth discussing.

EXPLAINING NEURODYNAMIC TEST FINDINGS AND PERIPHERAL NEUROGENIC PAIN

In the slump test, neck extension commonly relieves evoked lumbar, pelvic and hamstring area pain. Passive neck flexion will evoke lumbar symptoms in approximately 25% of patients with low back pain (Troup 1986). If we were patients, we may find these responses odd, perhaps distressing and would want them to be explained. These symptoms can be explained in terms of transmission of load through a continuous and sensitive structure. For some patients it may link what they thought were two or more problems, so there may be less concern about a worrying new problem. It is not difficult to explain the sensitive continuum if you do it at the same time as performing neurodynamic tests. For some, the anatomy book can be helpful and, if your patients don't mind pictures of cadavers, I have often used the pictures in Breig's book (1978), some of which are also reproduced in Butler (1991) and Gifford (1998).

While a mechanical explanation will satisfy some patients, the discussion should go further. Findings can also be explained in terms of stimuli as well as mechanics. Abnormal impulse generating sites can be reactive to various stimuli such mechanical, temperature, metabolic, adrenaline and immune. Inflamed connective tissue will also be responsive to various stimuli. A combination of inputs may be ultimately responsible for an action potential (chapters 2 and 3). It may be helpful for patients to realise that (nor)adrenaline can make a nerve sensitive or put the nerve close to firing so that only small, seemingly inconsequential movement can hurt. Or that their level of positivity may be linked in to the sensitivity of neural structures. There is nothing wrong with a discussion of "happy and sad hormones" when it can be linked to the benefits of positivity and health of tissues. The action potential drawing (Fig. 2.4) may be useful to discuss how close a neurone can be to firing and some of the stimuli which can contribute to the firing. Metaphors may be useful. For example, the metaphor of the car just running smoothly or revving and about to take off (close to threshold) may help some people grasp the concept of variable thresholds of nerve firing. There may be various other stimuli (eg. temperature, metabolic) keeping neurones close to spike and perhaps these stimuli can be identified.

You may find your explanations of tests useful for compliance and understanding when there are a number of components to a problem. For example, your patient may have persistent ankle pain which was positive in a slump test. The slump test also evoked back pain. What you have found may help patients make the link between the foot and the back and provide part of the rationale for proposing that total spinal mobilising exercises may also be necessary for the ultimate health of the foot.

No peripheral neurogenic pain can be explained without reference to the central nervous system. In particular, ongoing peripheral neurogenic pain and nerve root disorders require the inclusion of the CNS in any educational discussion.

EXPLAINING NEURODYNAMIC TEST FINDINGS AND CENTRAL SENSITIVITY

Primary hyperalgesia is much easier to explain than secondary hyperalgesia. We have an old and practised language for it and patients find it instantly acceptable. Central sensitivity can be extremely difficult to explain to a person who has had a series of tissue based explanations. It can go instantly against the reality of their sensory experiences. In central sensitivity, the upper limb neurodynamic test (or any physical test) may involve minimally unhealthy tissues, even quite normal tissues, yet can still be sensitive. The neurodynamic test now takes its place as one of many inputs which may be perceived as pain. The general concept of central sensitivity will need to be explained first.

Imagine a patient who has had a whiplash injury one year ago and now has persistent pain in her neck which has spread to most of the spine and both arms. She may well have a diagnosis of fibromyalgia or myofascial syndrome. She is sensitive to most inputs including palpation, noise and the ULNT1. I think the key messages for successful management and explanation of the sensitive ULNT1 can be brought down to 4 general components. You can follow these in figure 14.1. Note that this is just a personal way of explaining. You will hopefully have your own variations on this:

1. Relevant specific physical dysfunctions, including those which may involve nerves or meninges need to be acknowledged, however this information should also be presented with the fact that the tissues have had time to heal. After one year, they have been through the normal process that an injured tissue goes through. The tissues may still be unhealthy, sensitive, unfit, crying out for movement, but they have had all the time to heal. They are sensitive, due to their ill health, and perhaps because the brain thinks they need to be sensitive.

2. In the central nervous system, a very real biological process has occurred which has the ability to magnify inputs. This may mean inputs which don't normally hurt now hurt, or painful inputs now hurt a lot more. Your patient must be aware that the symptoms she is experiencing are no longer true indications of the health status of the tissues (This is not necessarily easy). Thus conscious and subconscious processing has been based on faulty data which is her own natural interpretation perhaps aided by iatrogenic contributions (discussed below). Noise as an aggravating factor could be used as an example in this patient. Normally noise is not bothersome, however, with the changes in the neural tissues, the input can now be amplified into excessive noise. Metaphors can be useful here and there are some mentioned below. It all comes down to pain not necessarily serving as an accurate guide to tissue health and level of activity.

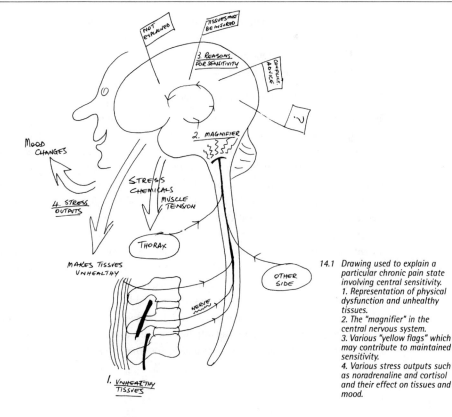

14.1 Drawing used to explain a particular chronic pain state involving central sensitivity.
1. Representation of physical dysfunction and unhealthy tissues.
2. The "magnifier" in the central nervous system.
3. Various "yellow flags" which may contribute to maintained sensitivity.
4. Various stress outputs such as noradrenaline and cortisol and their effect on tissues and mood.

3. There are probably a number of reasons why the nervous system is extra sensitive. You may have identified some of these, the patient may be aware of others. Many of these are psychosocial yellow flags. Some patients may have one or two major ones, another patient may have numerous flags (chapter 7). An aware therapist could manage some of these, such as beliefs and fears about reinjury, even carefully apologising for the failed management of professional colleagues. Other contributing factors may require multidisciplinary help.

4. A sensitive nervous system produces chemicals which keep the system sensitive. This includes adrenaline and cortisol and also chemicals from the immune system. These generally make tissues more sensitive and slow to heal. The stress chemicals can also make you a bit depressed and down. You may be able to show the patient that when she is in a good mood, her ranges of movement and functional abilities are better.

This is admittedly simplistic, but it provides a framework which could be expanded to suit individual patients. The description is a clinical variation on the educational model proposed by Gifford (1998). Popular press reports and articles written for the public may help. Perhaps write your own explanation to give to patients and to provide a form of discussion. Narratives about other patients and metaphors may be helpful. Make sure that all health providers are giving a similar message. Somehow, the message that this is a real injury in neural tissues, not only muscles and joints, needs to be delivered in a positive way.

Some metaphors may help here with the concept of upregulation. I mentioned back in chapter 2, the concept of a car motor just ticking over and running smoothly or one which is revving and about to go with the slightest acceleration. The kettle just about to boil is another.

Some colleagues use the metaphor of a phone ringing to an empty house. There is a message going to the house but noone to receive it. However a phonecall to a house which is full of people waiting for an important call is the opposite and the news will spread around very quickly. The latter example is more like central sensitivity.

PATIENTS WILL ALWAYS DEFINE YOUR PROGRESSION

Particular patients can sometimes mark your own clinical progression. In 1996, I was teaching a post-graduate course with Louis Gifford. We had a number of patients suffering chronic pain on the course and we were seeing if we could alter their pain behaviours over a week of education, skilled assessment and change of movement patterns in relation to pain. One patient stands out. I listened to a group of therapists assess and examine a young woman who had had two spinal surgeries. She was still suffering chronic back and leg pain and was quite disabled and unfit. On physical examination she seemed fine; that is, she moved well, her neurodynamic and other physical tests were a bit sensitive but did not appear relevant to her current pain experience and her reflexes and muscle power were good and equal on both sides. The group decided that there was a significant central sensitivity component and (after much practice and discussion the previous day) began to explain it . They were discussing point 2 above, about how the system becomes sensitive and how it can exaggerate pain, and yet how real a problem that was. There was a beautiful drawing, something resembling figure 14.1 on the table. She listened quietly and intently. Then she asked the students to stop talking, she picked up the drawing and looked at it quietly for what seemed like a long time. Finally she said "so I really don't need all my pain do I?"

Of course, it is not always like this and there was still a lot of work to go for this particular patient, but a significant start had been made to recovery of more productive movement behaviours.

NERVE IMAGES CAN BE SCARY

Through much of his life, Gustav Mahler, the Austrian composer had a fear of death and a hope of resurrection which was expressed strongly in his music. Early in life, he was found to have a heart murmur from a harmless, congenital valve defect. His wife reported that his doctor had said, "Well this heart is nothing to be proud of". This had a profound effect on him - for Mahler, it signified the beginning of the end. He avoided strenuous walks, swimming and cycling and always checked his pulse (Sandblom 1996). For most of us the outputs of pain and injury affect us and those close to us. For someone as creative as Mahler, such outputs have impacts on millions of people. (You might wonder what kind of music, if any, Mahler would have otherwise produced).

So be careful with your explanations. The terms "trapped and compressed nerves" convey strong images. They are in the same class as "disc prolapse" or "degenerated joint" or "next step will be a cortisone needle into the painful spot". I think the commonly available red plastic models of disc compression can sometimes be too exaggerated. A red piece of plastic disc usually squeezes onto a nerve. The plastic of its construction is nothing like the plasticity of the nervous system. Most people associate the word meninges with meningitis and an association with a nasty disorder and prognosis, so be careful here. The "tough ligamentous covering" on the nervous system may be better. We all surely have examples of patients operating on unhelpful belief systems. The more serious a person believes their illness to be, the more they will hang onto the words of the expert. And the more exaggerated descriptions become over time as patients reconstruct their clinical experience.

Care is needed with a description of central sensitisation. Patients, despite best efforts, may take it as their problem is "all in their head". The seemingly simple message that their system is firing a little higher than most can be difficult to convey. Patients must know that it's quite normal, we all get it, and it's how the nervous system learns. The delivery of education can be paced and you will have to make a judgement about this process (Vlaeyen et al. 1995; Turner et al. 1998). I believe we need a number of ways to explain central sensitivity and a series of different metaphors adaptable to each patient's life framework. I also think we need to know our neurobiology and keep up with advances in the area. We are fortunate too that the hands on license allows explanation during and after physical assessment.

Information delivery must be contextual, and if it reflects the truth then there should be little problem. It shouldn't be hard to deliver because the truth in most musculoskeletal pain states is usually good news. We all have crumbling discs and are degenerating slowly into the earth, but it doesn't have to hurt. Many people have compressed nerves and scar in nerves but experience minimal or no pain. However, what actually makes something continue to hurt is not really known, but a reasonable biologically based judgement can be made based on the information in chapters 2-5, together with the knowledge that peripheral and central contributions will usually coexist.

Not all patients want to know what is going on - the passive copers will just want you to get them better and the active copers may want so much that it can become a problem. Handing out information comes with the same individual variations as a passive mobilisation technique. For further reading and support for the uses for education, refer to Indahl et al (1995), Turner (1996) and Hawley (1995), among many others.

NEURODYNAMICS AND PASSIVE MOBILISATION

A number of professions offer various forms of passive mobilisation therapy. With the current environment of emphasis on self care, the value of passive movement therapies, especially for long term management, have been questioned. If passive mobilisation is combined with, or replaced by active educational based approaches, then this may be a better approach, especially for chronic pain sufferers. For some patients this may be very unfortunate if they miss out on an effective therapy. Passive movement in its various forms may assist restoration of tissue health and the movements may provide for a more acute patient memory of the prescription for an active treatment. Good hands, a supportive treatment environment and appropriate passive movement are a collection of inputs into the CNS. This collection of inputs signals that it is possible to perform a certain movement and perhaps experience a little pain without evoking a stress response. Remember too, when education becomes a critical aspect of management the person who has skillfully touched and examined the sore areas may be the one whose advice is taken.

There is nothing wrong with skilled passive movement and techniques. It is the selection of patient, selection of technique, links with co-existing treatments, timing and limitations of the technique which are the issue.

A list of broad management guidelines related to mobilisation via neurodynamic tests follows. Some of these guidelines will overlap with suggested guidelines for active exercise.

GENERAL COMMENTS

1. Reject notions of "neural stretches" or "sciatic stretches" and the crudity of assessment which usually precedes such a management strategy.

2. Passive mobilisation should form part of a management strategy which is likely to include other elements such as active movements, education, fitness enhancement and work adjustments. Passive mobilisation is unlikely to form a treatment by itself. It can be helpful to consider that you are mobilising a sensitive movement which happens to include a physically unhealthy or sensitive nervous system.

3. Be open about the reasons for the responses you get. It may be dispersal of fluids around and in neurones, stretching scar, enhancing vascularity, freeing mechanical forces on nerves, altering central nervous system threshold settings etc. But it may also be associated with you. That is, your personality, empathy, skills, interactional abilities and the practice environment, all mediated through the hardware, wetware and distributed processing of your patient's CNS.

4. Passive movement and mobilisation could be seen as part of the patient's self education about what their body is capable of. The patient's nervous system is actually testing you and the environment which you have provided.

5. Judgements about efficacy of technique should also consider whether the technique contributed to the evidence based features listed at the start of this chapter. For example, passive mobilisation might lead to an increase in range of motion, which may then decrease

anxiety and lift expectations and mood. Skilled therapists should be able to find functional expressions for improved ranges of motion.

6. Early movement after injury appears best. This has been demonstrated post peripheral nerve surgery (eg. Hunter 1991; Nathan et al. 1995; Seradge 1997) and with spinal pain (discussed below).

GUIDELINES FOR TECHNIQUES FOR MORE PERIPHERAL NEUROGENIC/NOCICEPTIVE MECHANISMS

The following can be used as guidelines only. Clinical data leading to the selection of an appropriate patient may come from any of the reasoning categories (chapters 6 and 7). For example, as a very broad comment, patients will be subacute, more likely to have primary hyperalgesia, have physical dysfunctions related to the overall presentation, no red flags and minimal yellow flags and be quite responsive to physical evaluation. Guidelines have also been proposed by Hall and Elvey (1999) and Elvey and Hall (1997).

DIRECT NERVE MOBILISATION - SOME GUIDELINES

1. Start movements away from a presumed site of pathology. This was probably taken to extremes in the past (Butler 1989; Butler 1991), but the concept is still useful. It should be a bit safer and may allow less focusing on the painful area. For example with a sprained ankle, as part of management, extending the knee while the hip is held in flexion will provide movement of peripheral neural structures at the foot. Wrist and elbow movements will mobilise the brachial plexus from a distance. Movements from the non or less painful side, which are likely to have more processing rather than mechanical effects are suggested. I propose that if a neurone with a bilateral receptive field can be "fed" non painful inputs from a movement which is a familiar pain provocative movement, then the contribution of that neurone to a processing output of pain perception should be reduced.

2. For some acute pain states, having your "knowing hands" on the painful area and mobilising may be very reassuring to your patient. Consider having the rest of the body in a neurally unloaded position while performing techniques in such cases.

3. Consider the starting position. In sensitive acute states, movement can be performed with the rest of the body "unloaded." So for example, shoulder girdle oscillations could be performed in some elbow flexion and cervical lateral flexion to the test side. Or, if you have found what appears to be a successful technique, consider performing it again with the body in a more loaded position. So, for example, if a hip flexion/knee extension technique appears helpful, consider performing it again with the spine in contralateral lateral flexion.

4. Where there is a number of positive tests, you may consider mobilising the less provocative test. For example, where a SLR and a PKB is responsive, try mobilising the less sensitive test first. In a patient with a thoracic outlet syndrome, all the upper limb neurodynamic tests may be positive, so select one which is the least provocative.

5. Application of order of movement. This principle may have use to allow better or different access to a neuropathy (chapter 5). Use the broad principle that the movement taken up first allows a better challenge of neural tissue at that site. Note that this does not always hold, particularly when there are multiple sites of injury along the nerve. However, a suggested examination technique for the median nerve in the carpal tunnel would include a ULNT1

taken from the wrist first, as described in chapter 12. From this position, the wrist could be mobilised and would provide a vigorous mobilisation.

6. If passive movements are successful and relevant to the pain state, then integrate active mobilisation as soon as possible. Try to integrate the improvement into work, leisure or creative activity. For example, if the range and sensitivity of the SLR is improved, try to get your patient to work out how this could be translated to better function.

7. You may be able to make a clinical judgement to aim for a large range, out of tension movement, or a movement in some tension. Large movements seem better for gliding nerves through tunnels, providing a gentle "milking" of venous congestion or "inflammatory soup" in the epineurium and mesoneurium as well as decreasing fear of movement and motor responses. Movement in some tension may be better for challenging stiffness in neural tissues, organising scar and intraneural oedema.

8. Progression of technique may mean increasing the number of repetitions of the technique, the strength of the technique, mobilising the joint component which "houses" pathology while loaded (eg. mobilising the hip joint in SLR). It also means a shift to active and functional activities and progressive supply of information where possible and relevant.

9. Prognosis is a reasoning category. As a broad guide, beneficial responses to passive mobilisation should be evident within two or three treatment sessions to warrant continuing treatment. For frank tethering, surgical options need consideration. Any passive mobilisation should a graduated and monitored event.

ROLE OF THE "NEURAL CONTAINER"

Where the nervous system is physically unhealthy, neighbouring structures are likely to be also. For example, physically based management for a patient with a carpal tunnel syndrome could involve (if assessed and deemed to be appropriate), active and passive mobilisation of the carpal bones, massage of the skin across the carpal tunnel, attention to a tight pectoris minor muscle and the postures which have lead to it, some scapular stabilisation work and attention to the cervical or thoracic spines. This "along the tract" thinking may allow identification of contributing sites to a pain state. Contributions may be seen in the form of physical forces on neural structures, but also additional sites of input into the CNS. It also makes you realise how general physical fitness is important for isolated lesions such as carpal tunnel syndrome as Nathan and Keniston (1993) found.

Movement of the anatomical structures surrounding sensitive neural tissue have been advocated (Elvey 1986; Hall and Elvey 1999). A cervical lateral glide technique proposed by Elvey (1986) for C6 nerve root involvement, involves positioning the arm and then gliding the C5-C6 motion segment to the contralateral side in a slow and oscillating manner. In skilled hands and with subacute conditions, this seems a useful technique.

Where there appears to be a significant container component, as a broad guideline, try addressing the container first, and assessing responses to the neurodynamic test.

PAIN AS A GUIDELINE?

Pain per se should not be universally used as guide to a passive or active mobilisation technique. It depends on the **mechanisms** of pain. Refer to chapters 3 and 4. Pain can be a guide in acute, more nociceptive and peripheral neurogenic pain states. However it loses its useful warning role in more chronic states, and hence its guidance role for the therapist will also be lost. So while nudging and teasing at pain or techniques short of pain may be appropriate in the more acute pain states, movement and techniques will have to "go into" the patient's pain in more chronic states. What is important though, is that your patient understands the reason for exercise into some pain and thus limits the possibility of a stress response.

If we are frightened of pain and don't understand it, this will be carried to the patient.

Equally, physiotherapists should have no fear of techniques that elongate the neural structures in appropriate patients. After all, this is what we do with every movement of our bodies and every muscle mobilising technique. Therefore, in situations such as the failed carpal tunnel surgery at 6 weeks and the slowly responding but stable nerve root lesion at 2 months, I have no problems making a reasoned judgement based on data collection as in chapter 7 and 10, which leads to using graduated movements which I know will elongate the nervous system. It doesn't have to be forceful. These tissues are designed for strain, it's part of their normal function and their physical health depends on this ability to strain. There may well be a little "no pain, no gain" as long as both therapist and patient fully understand the meaning of the pain and the techniques are graduated and monitored.

The aim of a manual therapy approach should always be to have the best effect for the most minimal force. Where more vigorous mobilisations are performed, also consider addressing the health of surrounding tissues, the order of movements that allows less forceful input to access pathological change and have the patient perform the mobilisation themselves.

Motor responses during tests are inevitable as part of the CNS value judgement about the importance of the injury, you and the level of threat your technique poses. Elvey and Hall (1997; 1999) have drawn our attention to this and suggest techniques should be performed in relation to the initial motor response (M1), or techniques constructed to avoid them. Gifford (1998) suggests in cases where there is a significant motor response, to perform the technique addressing more of a muscle stretch sensation. For example, instead of performing a SLR, perform a hip flexion/knee extension manoeuvre. The M1 is a useful cue and it serves a reminder that restrictions to movement are due to sensitivity and not necessarily a physical tethering. Motor responses will change when your patient understands her pain state better and feels that the movements are less of a threat. However, a motor response is a processed response, like pain or an endocrine or autonomic responses. It does not necessarily come before or after pain and like pain is not necessarily an indication of tissue health status, especially in more chronic and central pain states. Its use as a guide to technique strength would appear more appropriate in peripheral neurogenic pain, especially that with a source at nerve root level.

The motor responses could be used in treatment. For example, you may perform a ULNT1, evoking a motor response in the trapezius muscle, or your patient may laterally flex her lumbar spine during an SLR. Ask the patient to be aware of the response and see if she can consciously change it next time you perform the technique.

PASSIVE MOVEMENT TECHNIQUES FOR MORE CENTRAL DISORDERS

When sensitivity appears more central, as it is likely to be in more chronic disorders, the importance of passive mobilisation diminishes. A more active, educational based programme is more efficacious. However, this does not preclude a skilled physical examination. Central sensitivity states usually need inputs to keep the sensitivity going and there may well be multiple sites of altered afferent input, especially post trauma which are worth treatment. The real key though is that passive treatment is not offered up as the main management option or presented as the cure.

Passive and active movements will inevitably mobilise the meninges, spinal cord and brainstem (chapter 5). On the basis that moving body parts require movement for their health, a physically healthy cord and brainstem is clearly ideal, not only for meningeal health, but also for vascular perfusion, CSF flow, lymph drainage and distribution of transmitters and modulators some of which perfuse through the extracellular fluid (Zoli et al. 1998). Of course this is speculative, but the thoughts arise from the clinic. Movements encouraged by yoga, Feldenkrais, ball and matwork, even correction of forward head postures must mobilise cord and brainstem neurones and glia. Presumably, in most cases, this provides therapeutic movement. However techniques like the slump test are also going to mobilise cord and brainstem, especially if upper cervical flexion is used. The suggestion is that techniques such as the slump slider/tensioner movements described below and lumbar rotations with thorax, neck and arms moving in the opposite directions may be beneficial to the CNS in a physical sense as well as in an electrochemical sense. A case study by Zvulun (1998) is worthy of contemplation. It describes beneficial effects for neural mobilising in a case of cervical cord compression. The concept is instantly challenging, but it must be balanced by the fact that cord and brainstem movements are unavoidable parts of any spinal motion. With skilled assessment and progressive monitored mobilisation, balanced by reasoned prognoses, CNS mobilisation may contribute to improvement of CNS pain states. Here is an area for research.

Passive stretch and movements can also be achieved to some degree via balls and water and slings and gravity and if this provides a way of offering novel, non-painful, functionally relevant input to the central nervous system, and healthy nervous system movement, then great.

PASSIVE TECHNIQUE CONCEPTUALISATION

Physical techniques can be performed with different applications of body parts. This conceptualisation may allow access to pathology or allow a varietal and novel presentation to the central nervous system.

TISSUE MOBILISATION WITH THE NERVOUS SYSTEM POSITIONED

You could perform passive mobilisation of any structure, with the nervous system positioned. Examples are carpal bone mobilisations with the arm in an upper limb neurodynamic test position, or mobilisation of the head of the radius with the arm in an ULNT2 (radial) position. Rib mobilisations could be performed with the body in a slump position. You could perform muscle techniques with the nervous system on load eg. hamstring "hold/ relax" techniques, or you could perform upper cervical extensor stretches in varying degrees of SLR. You could do a myofascial skin release technique around cutaneous nerves in the interscapular area. Breathing exercises for rib mobilisation could be performed in slump positions. Some of these techniques are described in chapter 15.

NERVOUS SYSTEM MOBILISATION WITH THE TISSUES POSITIONED

If your reasoning suggested that the median nerve would benefit from movement in the carpal tunnel, the most gentle way to treat this would be to perform wrist flexion and extension with the elbow flexed, arm by the side and with the patient looking at her hand, ie. with the whole median nerve complex on slack. As a progression the same hand movements could be performed in increasing elbow extension and then increasing shoulder elevation or depression.

Lumbar rotations may be a beneficial way to encourage nerve root and dural movements. As a progression it could be performed in some straight leg raise.

Randomised controlled trials have shown that not much benefit can be gained by traction for non-specific low back pain (eg. Beurskens et al. 1997) and there is no real biological reason why there should be. However, before disregarding traction, you might ask how the traction could be made better. There could be better selection of patients (perhaps subacute nerve root disorders), and the traction technique could be made more dynamic. Traction will alter the shape of the intervertebral foramina. You could move the nervous system while the traction is on. For example, during intermittent lumbar traction with her knees on a stool, the patient's knee could then be extended. During cervical traction, part of the upper limb neurodynamic tests could be added. For example, while the traction is on, have your patient extend her elbow(s). You can be quite creative here and still defend your management decisions on the basis of biology or evidence if there is a useful improvement. Don't forget to reassess reflexes after such a technique.

NEUROGENIC MASSAGE

Neurogenic massage is not usually discussed in textbooks, although it would be impossible to use techniques such as massage and deep frictioning without physically influencing nerves. Although crude, it does seem a biologically reasonable thing to do where there is swelling around nerves, venous stasis and organising scar in the peripheral nerve connective tissue sheath. Neurogenic massage would not appear appropriate for elevated CNS sensitivity in disorders such as fibromyalgia or acute and active abnormal impulse generation sites. Any neurogenic massage techniques would be best included as part of an active or passive mobilisation programme. That patients can usually perform it themselves is an advantage as it may be a useful self help pain treatment, especially if the problem wakes them at night.

Theoretically, any segment of nerve, or the tissues next to the nerve may be massaged. Areas where massage may be worth trying include areas where swelling pools around nerves (eg. sural nerve lateral to the Achilles tendon), in tunnels (eg. carpal tunnel, posterior tibial tunnel, Guyon's canal), and where nerves travel through potentially tight fascia (cutaneous branches of the thoracic spinal nerves in the interscapular region). Any areas of post traumatic or surgical swelling which included peripheral nerve could be considered. I can't say what the best technique for massage is, but go carefully, and try massaging next to the nerve first.

Jabre (1994) presented 20 male patients with ulnar neuropathy at the elbow, diagnosed by EMG/nerve conduction studies. They were taught a "nerve rubbing" technique where the ulnar nerve was rubbed up and down its longitudinal axis at the cubital tunnel for 5 minutes. "Most had improved by the end of one month, reporting a general reduction in symptoms by at least 50%". Most patients also obtained relief by nerve rubbing if they were woken at night. Jabre

(1994) noted that nerve rubbing would initially increase symptoms, but after a couple of minutes, patients would experience significant relief.

ACTIVE MOBILISATION AND NEURODYNAMIC TESTS

INTRODUCTION

Rest is a wonderful analgesic. Unfortunately, it is often too easy to take it for too long, particularly if people are compensated (Those who are not compensated may replace it with medication). In the last decade there has been a movement against rest for low back pain, since the Quebec Task Force recommendations (Spitzer et al. 1987) and an influential article by Deyo et al. (1986). This article reported no increase in back pain morbidity if prescribed best rest was reduced from 7 days to 2 days. Meanwhile numerous studies continue to show that early activity post injury/surgery is best (eg. Malmivaara et al. 1995; Waddell 1998; Abenhaim et al. 2000; Rosenfeld et al. 2000).

There is still much work needed to decide which activity is best for which patients and at which time. Individual bio-psycho-social based judgements are needed here. Rest may have an analgesic effect due to tissue unloading but also because of rest from the workplace and associated pressures and responsibilities. Task forces are currently unable to recommend specific techniques and propose activity of any form, combining strength, stretching and fitness (eg. Abenhaim et al. 2000). It seems that it is the movement in general which is important and gratefully received by the brain.

There are two main aspects here to consider in activity prescription. First, all healing tissues, especially those with large amounts of connective tissue, enjoy appropriate movement to assist healing and best restoration of mechanical abilities. In this regard, the nervous system is probably no different to other connective tissues. Secondly, activity should be a mode of managing maladaptive central nervous system responses. Therefore activity should be set in relation to tissue health and to sensitivity and it can be used to treat both. It therefore aims to assist the two categories of pathobiology in the clinical reasoning model.

The movement based therapists have a number of ways in which physically unhealthy and sensitive nervous systems can be integrated into active programmes. I prefer the word

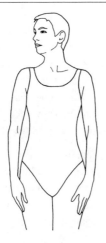
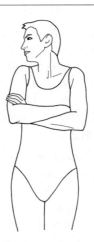

14.2 In A. the patient has a painful neck on rotation.
B. There may be less pain and more range in rotation, if the shoulders were elevated and elbows flexed.

"activity" to "exercise." The term "exercise" instantly evokes negativity in many people, particularly those in pain. In particular, neurodynamic based concepts such as movement breakdowns, order of movement variations and the slider/tensioner concept could be integrated into therapeutic activity.

MOVEMENT BREAKDOWNS

The movement breakdown concept can be utilised for tissue health and to present painless aspects of a painful movement to the CNS. Consideration of neurodynamics allows a movement, especially one involving mechanosensitivity of the nervous system, to be performed in a gentler less aggressive way. For a patient with a sensitive neck including neural structures, to exercise her neck, say in rotation or retraction/protraction, make sure she has her arms folded and perhaps shoulder girdles elevated (Fig. 14.2 A,B). You could encourage cervical movement by getting your patient into a sitting position, or supine with knees flexed to take off more load from the nervous system. Subsequent neck exercises can be performed with the arms by the side or in a progressively more neurally loaded position. The concept is simple - perform the activity with the system off load. For example, breathing exercises for a person in acute pain could be performed with the knees flexed and arms folded. There are patients in chronic pain who will say that every movement they do on the planet hurts. You may find that you can demonstrate some painless movements in a neurally unloaded position.

While a useful way to assist recovery of tissue health, the movement breakdown concept is a useful way to gradually expose a person to a feared activity. For example, a patient may have a fear of lifting and bending due to a previous horrible nerve root disorder. To start her off, you could get her bending forward while sitting in a chair. A progression could be bending forward with a knee extended. This could be done on a ball for example (Figs. 14.3 A,B,C). Have her relearn the lost art of pelvic tilting while she is there. Various homonculi are waiting to be "nourished". A patient who is frightened of weight bearing could be gradually exposed to weight bearing via sitting, then standing using a scale, or even graduating the hardness of the material under the foot. Everyone will be empowered if the progression is a combined therapist/patient decision.

The link between tissue health and decreasing pain and anxiety is somewhat arbitrary. They can be linked into paced activities nicely. For example, your patient may have chronic

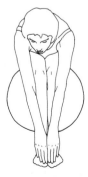
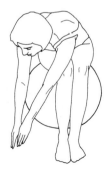
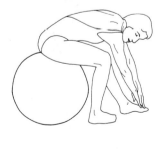

14.3A,B,C   Example of movement breakdowns using a ball.

abdominal/hip area pain. She may not have extended her spine or hips for a long time and she can no longer lie on her stomach. There is no use performing slump/knee bend techniques as in chapter 12. Leave those for the more athletic. In this situation, the test will have to be broken down. The postures could go in a sequence from the patient lying on her stomach with pillow(s) to lying on the stomach without pillows to lying on the stomach with some knee flexion then to some spine extension. (Figs. 14.4 A,B,C,D,E). You could even add some neck flexion. This process does not only need pacing by posture but also by time. It should also be performed short of pain provocation. Pacing is discussed in further detail below.

ORDER OF MOVEMENT VARIATIONS AND "TRICK MOVEMENTS"

This principle has a number of applications. Broadly speaking, the movement and gliding features of the nervous system are best tested at a joint component by loading the system at that component first (chapter 5). So if you were to push a door closed with your wrist flexed, the movement would probably begin at the wrist first. However, if you reach up and wipe the ceiling or change a light bulb, it will be more likely that the shoulder and elbow will have been extended first. In chapter 15 there are some exercises suggested for carpal tunnel syndrome which either challenge the median nerve at the tunnel first or challenge it via shoulder and elbow movements.

Consider order of movement variations in the gross sense. Take the movement of getting out of a chair. Most people do it from hip flexion and put their dominant foot first. This pattern of input could comprise a cue which initiates brain processing with the final result being the

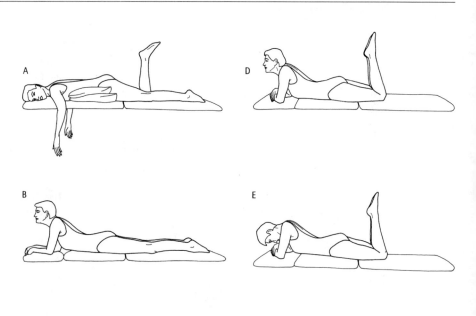

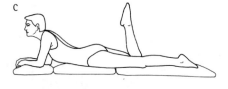

14.4 A,B,C,D,E *Progressive breakdown of movements involving prone knee bend and slump. See text for details.*

perception of pain and adjustments in homeostatic systems. Perhaps you could break the movement up, and get them to use the opposite leg or initiate the activity with the head first. Most people dry their back one way, do up shoelaces one way, pick things up off the floor in a particular pattern. Chronic pain sufferers in particular have a poorer quality and selection of movement available. Where possible, make an attempt to present movement to the CNS in a novel and different way which can be accepted with less output activation.

"Trick" movements are closely related here. Elimination of, or reduction of gravity can be useful. The most commonly used examples are swinging the arm in a pendulum fashion while bent over, or in supine, pushing the arms up as though performing a benchpress. Again, this may be useful for tissue health but the various homonculi in the brain are also going to enjoy some shoulder movement which may have been denied them for some months. Another good example is where your patient has a painful neck and may be frightened to move it. Perhaps even the initiation of cervical rotation with lateral gaze of the eye may be a cue to initiate processing related to pain perception. In this case ask her to keep looking forward at a fixed spot and then to rotate her body. This can also be done on a swivel chair.

Different environments may also be useful. For example, in water, if your patient had her arms in front of her, walking into deeper water or squatting would mobilise shoulder elevation.

SLIDER/TENSIONER

The slider/tensioner principle was developed when working with Shacklock and Slater (Butler et al. 1994; Shacklock et al. 1994; Slater et al. 1994), on the simple basis of designing techniques to encourage patients to move more. If you were to hold behind your knee as in figure 14.5 and then extend your knee at the same time as flexing your neck, we considered this a tensioner - it places a load on the nervous system from "both ends" at the same time. If you were to extend your neck and extend your knee at the same time, this would be more of a slider. A slider will allow better movement and less challenge and presumably allows nervous system movement rather than the generation of tension. In most situations, the generation of tension as in a tensioner is also more likely to induce symptoms and induce protective muscle responses.

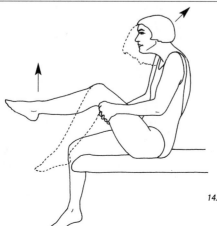

14.5 *If the knee is extended at the same time as the neck is extended this is regarded as a slider. If the neck is flexed at the same time as the knee is extended, this is a tensioner.*

You can be very clinically creative here. The concept can engender novel movements and activity and can be fun. You could use the other side of the body as well. One arm could be taken into a tensioning position while the other is on slack. If you put your hands over your ears and then extend each elbow turn at the same time as looking at your hand, you have some nice sliding movements. If you lie supine and depress your shoulder girdle on the same side as extending your knee, then you have a tensioner. An exercise used by Lewit (1985) and shown in figure 14.6A and 14.6B engages similar principles. You could use the water or exercise balls (Fig. 14.7A and 14.7B). Figure 14.4D and 14.4E are also examples of sliders and tensioners. The slump longsitting position provides many opportunities for tension/slider combinations and these are discussed in chapter 15.

When we were originally using the concept in the clinic, it was performed on a very physical basis, and we acknowledged that the mechanical component was very simplistic. However the concept can be taken further and it fits nicely with the evidence based direction described earlier in the chapter. This could be a useful way to reduce fear of movement, as the sliders usually allow a little more movement. More importantly perhaps, it includes distraction. Picture a patient sitting in a chair, wary of movement, and say, post lumbar surgery or disc trauma. While she is extending her knee, if she were to extend her neck at the same time, her focus on the knee movement would be diluted. And it seems clear that large normal movement are not only good for tissue healing, but in a nonstressful environment are rather nourishing for the homonculi. Presumably you may be able to disengage the anterior cingulate cortex or other key contributing areas out of the pain processing circuit to some degree.

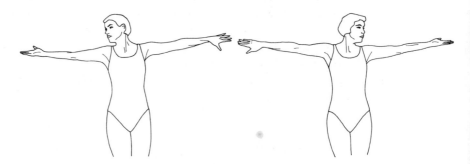

14.6 A,B Variations on the tensioner/slider concept.

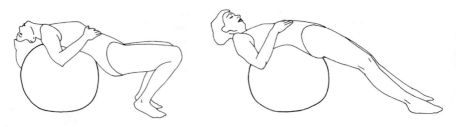

14.7 A,B Variations on the tensioner/slider concept.

With the slider/tensioner, use of vision will also be helpful. It's a way of adding another input to the processing. So for example, a person extending her arm out and looking at her hand is performing more of a slider. If the action is painless the vision may reinforce the fact that the movement can be achieved painlessly. Vision is a powerful stimulus to the brain about the reality of the body (Ramachandran and Rogers—Ramachandran 1996; Ramachandran and Blakeslee 1998).

ACTIVE MOVEMENTS – USE OF MEANINGFUL ACTIVITY

While exercises and activity serve their purposes, as far as possible it is best to have the patient perform activity which challenges the nervous system in meaningful, functional and creative ways. The patient must be able to see that they need a particular activity for their best function. In the upper limb especially, it is possible to think of numerous activities which link to movement. A meaningful, functionally important activity, should be accepted by the CNS better than a structured and perhaps less relevant exercise.

Activities such as wall and floor pushups (Fig. 14.8A), and lifting imaginary and real weights on the palm of the hand (Fig. 14.8B) are examples of challenges for the median nerve. These movements can be graduated. For example, pushups could be graduated from wall pushups, to standing and leaning over a table and pushing up on the extended wrist, to a half pushups lying supine to a full pushup. Throwing a ball also utilises the median nerve and this can be easily graduated, for example, see figures 14.8C and 14.8D. I suspect that all computer operators would be benefit from learning how to juggle – the action requires supination

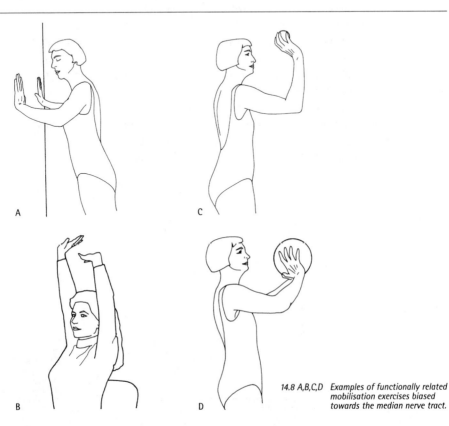

14.8 A,B,C,D   *Examples of functionally related mobilisation exercises biased towards the median nerve tract.*

instead of the persistent pronation which computers demand, and there is use of elbows, shoulders, eyes and neck. And its fun.

When drying your back after a shower, straightening a collar or combing your hair, you are using the physical abilities of the ulnar nerve to achieve the positions (Fig. 14.9). Drumming actions, pouring fluids and the "baksheesh" position are examples of movements which challenge the radial nerve. If you hold your thumb in the palm of your hand with your fingers and then push the extended arm backwards, this must provide a physical challenge on the musculocutanous nerve. Most forms of dancing provide excellent upper limb neural mobilisation. For example, flamenco dance has superb combinations of radial and median nerve in a creative, yet distractive environment (Fig. 14.10). So does yoga, Tai Chi and most dance activities.

The lower limb and trunk usually require a more specific active prescription. Walking, of course challenges the sciatic/tibial tract. Those who watched the comedian John Cleese's "Ministry of Funny Walks" may get some good ideas. Kneeling activities load the femoral tract. The slump can be integrated in sitting activities. Many muscle tests also challenge neural pathways, for example stretch tests for the iliopsoas group also elongate the femoral and genitofemoral nerves.

Maitland (1986) once said memorably, "technique is the brainchild of ingenuity".

PACING

Pacing means prescribing activity, exercise, technique and exposure to stimuli at a rate which is accepted by the person and beneficial for their health. The concept of pacing has been inherent in the above discussions. There is nothing magical about pacing. Cardiac rehabilitation is an example of pacing based on restoration of tissue health. Pacing is inherent in Maitland's concept (1986) where the prescription of a passive movement is paced, based on a decision of severity, nature and irritability of the disorder. Any technique is then altered on the basis of response. However pacing can also be linked to active movements, psychosocial influences on pain and disability and be used as form of CNS retraining. You can pace by posture, time, number, environment, gravity, tissue healing and psychosocial inputs. The patient must be intimately involved in the prescription.

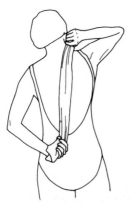

14.9 Drying the back with a towel is an example of a ulnar nerve mobilisation.

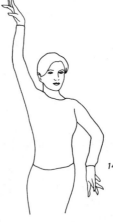

14.10 A flamenco dance posture. Dance, yoga, Tai Chi all engage the nervous system in a physical sense as well as providing input in a creative environment.

The overall guide to activity prescription is to set the activity to a level dependent on the pathobiological mechanisms. That is, you make a judgement about sensitivity related to the health of tissues and on processing related to pain. This does not mean that you necessarily ask your patients to stop at pain, but you make a judgement about the mechanisms of pain, and perhaps encourage people to work into pain or to gain control of the pain by knowingly stopping an activity before the pain.

A pacing prescription involves determining a level of realistic pain-free activities followed by a gradual increase in activity, guided by joint patient/clinician agreements. In those with more chronic pain, there is a need for a written exercise timetable and guidance over time and flare-up contingency plans. It is important that patients use time or number and not pain level as their guide to stopping and changing activity or posture (Harding and Williams 1995). Altering activity at 80% of the time, number or distance which usually evokes pain has been suggested (Shorland 1998). Tissue beneficial effects may initially be minimal, but the central nervous system has a chance to retrain. Movements that have always been painful and perhaps learnt to be painful even by association to other inputs, will automatically cause a stress response. One aim of pacing is to teach the CNS that activities which it had learnt are painful do not necessarily have to be painful. Many things can be paced, for example, taking a cervical collar off, going for a walk, doing the ironing, a particular exercise, exposure to noise, even to psychosocial forces. Activity could be paced in regard to pain, sweating, nausea or any other symptoms. Paced exposure to painful movements and stimuli goes nicely with paced and continued provision of education (Vlaeyen et al. 1995).

Neurodynamics exercises or tests as described above could be included into a pacing programme. A difficulty occurs when there seems to be a conflict of pacing and trying to get a patient to tease and nudge movements into pain. Both are needed. It may be that certain activities are paced and then others are allowed to be teased and edged into pain. The key thing though, is that the patient must be in control of their pain. Activities causing pain must be processed as non-dangerous and not deserving of a stress response. For activities paced short of pain, that person should be aware of why she is doing it otherwise it may seem a useless process. Link it to the education session discussed earlier.

The patient with ongoing pain often loses movements and fitness and gets stiffer, all of which leads to tissue ill health, probably altered CNS representations of tissues and movements, psychological distress at work and leisure and sometimes social pursuits become curtailed. This can lead to a cycle of breakout over activity attempts followed by under activity, which has been well described as a feature of the chronic pain sufferer, (eg. (Sternbach 1987). These are ideal patients for a pacing programme.

The descriptions in this text form just one part of the management strategies for chronic pain. For further details and practical examples on pacing and associated education, there is highly recommended literature by Shorland (1998), Harding (1995; 1998; 1998), Wittink (1997), Strong (1996) and Caudill (1995).

WARM UP/WARM DOWN MANOEUVRES WITH A FOCUS ON THE NERVOUS SYSTEM

If you watch a professional sporting team warm up and if you have a knowledge of neurodynamics, there will be some very familiar techniques demonstrated. Many athletes may have evolved to a mobilisation which involves neurodynamics. The best warm up is not known, however if the athlete feels better and is confident then that is a good outcome. Warm ups help prevent injury at least in netballers (Hopper 1986) and it helps prevent hamstring injuries in Australian Rules football players (Seward and Patrick 1992), although no relationship between youth indoor and outdoor soccer injuries and warm up could be shown (Hoff and Martin 1986).

The aim of a warm up is to best prepare the tissues and central nervous system for the activity ahead. It should involve some light aerobic activity which may induce mild sweating, that is, the stress system is mildly activated, some activity which is related or similar to the activity about to be performed and a series of stretches should be involved (Vincenzino and Vincenzino 1995). A beneficial sports or activity warm up should result in a heating of muscle to approximately 103 degrees F or 39 degrees C, with core temperatures raised a degree or so (Shellock 1983; Malone et al. 1996). It is inevitable that the nervous system is also warmed, perhaps the stretch releases some peptides in the tissues sensitising nerve endings and bringing a bit more blood to the area. Also the connective tissues of nerve should deform better and it may well conduct a little faster. Recently used synapses may function better, just as short term memory is better than long term. The warmth in muscle appears to last about 10 to 15 minutes (Asmussen and Boeje 1945) so it would be prudent to do any manoeuvres in this time (Malone et al. 1996).

Various techniques have been demonstrated in the self treatment chapter in Butler (1991). They can easily be adapted with knowledge of the neurodynamic base tests (chapters 11 and 12) and integrating the above suggestions such as tensioner/slider and order of movement.

POSTURAL ADVICE AND NEURODYNAMICS

We don't always have to be movers. Sensitivity can be decreased with advice or postural changes. For example, a patient in a wheelchair who is resting her arms on the wheelchair table may have the ulnar nerve in her cubital tunnels repeatedly compressed. Forward head postures in the presence of degenerative changes in the neck may pinch lower cervical nerve roots. The postural changes involved with nerve root disorders may allow a few days for an AIGS to settle and may not necessarily need to be corrected with urgency.

Some advice could be offered with regard to sleeping positions. For example, patients with non-resolving cubital tunnel syndrome may alter their nocturnal elbow flexion patterns by sleeping with a bean bag cushion in the cubital fossa (Seror 1993) with good results. Some people sleep on their sides with their wrists forced into flexion. A night wrist splint may help. Any arms above the head sleeping postures should be avoided. In acute lumbar pain states, it may be as simple as keeping the knees flexed to enhance sleeping. For sensitive necks a "sleeping collar" is often beneficial. This can be made out of thin foam, approximately 5 cm wide. Tight sheets can sometimes force the feet into plantar flexion and inversion, so be careful with elderly or bed ridden patients.

In table 14.1, there is a list of the individual nerves and known mechanical forces which could lead to neuropathy. On review of this literature, repetitious movement and persistent extremes of range in either direction have potential for injury. For example hip flexion pinches the femoral nerve and extension elongates it. Knowledge of neurodynamics and the forces which the nervous system has to contend with should be a part of ergonomic assessment and design Refer to the major peripheral nerve entrapment textbooks for further details regarding

NERVE	AUTHOR	INJURING MOVEMENT
Sciatic nerve	(Mumenthaler and Schliack 1991)	Sitting for long periods, or on a hard edge
Common peroneal nerve at the fibula head	(Nobel 1966) (Koller and Blank 1980) (Stewart 1993) (Mumenthaler and Schliack 1991)	Ankle sprains Squatting, eg. strawberry picking Repeated leg crossing Tight garters, splints, casts
Superficial peroneal nerve at the foot	(Johnston and Howell 1999) (Mumenthaler and Schliack 1991)	Repeated ankle sprains Shoes too tight, metal capped boots
Deep peroneal nerve at foot	(Borges et al. 1981) (Akyuz et al. 2000)	Tight shoes or boots, esp. high heels Sitting on ankles with flexed knees (Namaz prayer position)
Tibial	(Goldner and Hall 1997) (Schon and Baxter 1990)	Excessive exercise – compartment syndrome Running in shoes lacking arch support
Sural	(Reisin et al. 1994)	Tight ankle bracelet, sustained compression
Femoral	(Sammarco and Stephens 1991) (Sinclair and Pratt 1972)	Repetitive combined lumbar extension and hip flexion in a dancer Surgery - prolonged periods in the lithotomy position (hip flexion, abduction, ext rotat.)
Lateral femoral cutaneous	(Scharli and Ayer 1984) (Mumenthaler and Schliack 1991)	Wearing tight jeans Weight gain
Saphenous	(Fabian et al. 1987)	Sitting on surfboard gripping the sides
Pudendal	(Hershfield 1983)	Long bicycle ride
Brachial plexus	(Drye and Zachazewski 1996)	Head and neck contralateral lateral flexion with shoulder depression (football stingers)
Ulnar At wrist	(Mellion 1991) (Dawson et al. 1983) (Friedland and St John 1984)	Cycling (wrist extension plus compression) Using wrist as a hammer (eg. mechanics) Prolonged playing video games
Ulnar At elbow	(Sunderland 1978)	Full elbow flexion plus compression, eg. taxi driver, chair bound invalids
Radial Upper arm	(Mumenthaler and Schliack 1991) (Sunderland 1978)	Crutch palsy (weight of the crutch in the axilla) Saturday night palsy
Radial At the elbow	(Roles and Maudsley 1972)	Repetitive supination and pronation
Radial sensory	(Massey and Pleet 1978) (Mackinnon et al. 1986)	Tight handcuffs, bracelets Repetitive pronation/supination
Median Upper arm	(Marinacci 1967)	Sleeping with an arm over a chair ("Saturday night palsy") could effect all upper limb nerves
Median	(Silverstein et al. 1986) At the wrist (Savage et al. 1990)	Repetitive and forceful flexion/extension of the wrist Vibration
Musculocutaneous	(Braddom and Wolfe 1978) (Young et al. 1990)	Heavy biceps exercise Strap of a heavy bag at the elbow
Axillary	(Mumenthaler and Schliack 1991) (Aita 1984)	Anterior inferior shoulder dislocation Sleeping with arm above head
Suprascapular	(Ringel et al. 1990)	Repetitive overhead motions, eg. volleyball, swimming
Accessory (XI)	(Mumenthaler and Schliack 1991) (Paljarvi and Partenen 1980)	Comatose surgical patient head down with shoulder supports "love bite"
Long thoracic nerve	(Mumenthaler and Schliack 1991) (Mendoza and Main 1990) (Sunderland 1978)	Tight bandages, forcefull shoulder movements, eg. sledge hammer use Overuse injury eg., golf, archery, bowling, basketball, grenade throwing practice

Table 14.1 Reported mechanical (compressive or elongative) injuries of peripheral nerve other than blunt trauma, fractures, neuromas, surgical intervention, anomalies and disease. Only one report of a similar injury is included.

specific nerve tracts (eg. Sunderland 1978; Szabo 1989; Mumenthaler and Schliack 1991; Dawson et al. 1999; Stewart 1999).

SUMMARY

There is limited evidence based work which suggests that the inclusion of specific neurodynamics work will improve outcomes (although see chapter 13). However, there is plenty of broad contextual evidence which suggests that patients who can get tissues as fit and as healthy as possible, who improve cardiovascular fitness and who can positively alter health hindering beliefs, superstitions and environmental forces can benefit.

Under this framework, concepts of neurodynamics have a place if they can be applied using uncorrupted clinical reasoning science. Meanwhile, the clinicians and researchers must continue refining the specifics of individual tissue diagnosis and mobilisation skills including those for the nervous system. This will only occur if we can better define the actual pathobiological processes which are behind the creation of pain and disability.

CHAPTER 14 REFERENCES

Abenhaim L, Rossignol M, Valat JP, et al. (2000) The role of activity in the therapeutic management of back pain. Spine 25: 1S-33S.

Achterberg J (1996) What is medicine? Alternative Therapies 2: 58-61.

AHCPR (1994) Clinical Practice Guideline Number 14. Acute low back problems in adults. Agency for Health Care Problems and Research. US Department of Health and Human Services. Rockville, MD.

Aita JF (1984) An unusual compressive neuropathy. Archives of Neurology 41: 341-343.

Akyuz G, Us O, Turan B, et al. (2000) Anterior tarsal tunnel syndrome. Electromyography and Clinical Neurophysiology 40: 123-128.

Asmussen E & Boeje OVE (1945) Body temperature and capacity for work. Acta Physiologica Scandinavica 10: 1-22.

Beurskens AJ, de Vet HC, Koke AJ, et al. (1997) Efficacy of traction for nonspecific low back pain. 12- week and 6-month results of a randomised clinical trial. Spine 23: 2756-2672.

Borges LF, Hallett M, Selkoe DJ, et al. (1981) The anterior tarsal tunnel syndrome. Journal of Neurosurgery 54: 89-92.

Braddom RL & Wolfe C (1978) Musculocutaneous nerve injury after heavy exercise. Archives of Physical Medicine and Rehabilitation 59: 290-292.

Breig A (1978) Adverse Mechanical Tension in the Central Nervous System, Almqvist and Wiksell, Stockholm.

Butler DS (1989) Adverse mechanical tension in the nervous system: a model for assessment and treatment. Australian Journal of Physiotherapy 35: 227-238.

Butler DS (1991) Mobilisation of the Nervous System, Churchill Livingstone, Melbourne.

Butler DS, Shacklock MO & Slater H (1994) Treatment of altered nervous system mechanics. In: Boyling JD & Palastanga N (eds.) Grieve's Modern Manual Therapy, 2nd edn. Churchill Livingstone, Edinburgh.

Caudill MA (1995) Managing Pain before it Manages You, Guildford Press, New York.

Dawson DM, Hallett M & Wilbourn AJ (1999) Entrapment neuropathies, 3rd edn. Lippincott, Williams and Wilkins, Philadelphia.

Deyo RA, Diehl AK & Rosenthal M (1986) How many days of bed rest for acute low back pain? A randomised clinical trial. New England Journal of Medicine 315: 1064-1070.

Drye C & Zachazewski JE (1996) Peripheral nerve injuries. In: Zachazewski JE, Magee DJ & Quillen WS (eds.) Athletic Injuries and Rehabilitation, WB Saunders, Philadelphia.

Elvey RL (1986) Treatment of arm pain associated with abnormal brachial plexus tension. The Australian Journal of Physiotherapy 32: 225-230.

Elvey RL & Hall T (1997) Neural tissue evaluation and treatment. In: Donatelli R (ed.) Physical Therapy of the Shoulder, Churchill Livingstone, New York.

Fabian RH, Norcross KA & Hancock MB (1987) Surfer's neuropathy. New England Journal of Medicine 316: 555.

Frank JD (1973) Persuasion and Healing, John Hopkins University Press, Baltimore.

Friedland RP & St John JN (1984) Video-game palsy: distal ulnar neuropathy in a video-game enthusiast. New England Journal of Medicine 319: 450.

Gatchel RJ, Polatin PB & Kinney RK (1995) Predicting outcome of chronic back pain using clinical predictors of psychopathology. Health Psychology 14: 415-420.

Gerteis M, Edgman-Levitan S & Daley J eds. (1993) Understanding and Promoting Patient-Centred Care: Through Patient's Eyes, Jossey Bass, San Francisco.

Gifford LS (1998) Factors influencing movement - neurodynamics. In: Pitt-Brooke J, Reid H, Lockwood J et al. (eds.) Rehabilitation of Movement, WB Saunders, London.

Gifford LS (1998) Pain, the tissues and the nervous system. Physiotherapy 84: 27-33.

Goldner JL & Hall RL (1997) Nerve entrapment syndromes of the lower back and lower extremities. In: Omer GE, Spinner M & Van Beek AL (eds.) Management of Peripheral Nerve Problems, 2nd edn. W.B. Saunders, Philadelphia.

Hall TM & Elvey RL (1999) Nerve trunk pain: physical diagnosis and treatment. Manual Therapy 4: 63-73.

Harding V (1998) Application of the cognitive-behavioural approach. In: Pitt-Brooke J (ed.) Rehabilitation of Movement, Saunders, London.

Harding V (1998) Cognitive-behavioural approach to fear and avoidance. In: Gifford LS (ed.) Topical Issues in Pain, NOI Press, Falmouth.

Harding V & Williams A (1995) Extending physiotherapy skills using a psychological approach: cognitive behavioural management of chronic pain. Physiotherapy 81: 681-688.

Hawley DJ (1995) Psychoeducational interventions in the treatment of arthritis. Baillieres Clinical Rheumatology 9: 803-823.

Hershfield HB (1983) Pedaller's penis. Canadian Medical Association Journal 128: 366-367.

Hoff GL & Martin TA (1986) Outdoor and indoor soccer: injuries among youth players. American Journal of Sports Medicine 14: 231-233.

Hopper D (1986) A survey of netball injuries and conditions related to those injuries. Australian Journal of Physiotherapy 32: 231-239.

Hunter JM (1991) Recurrent carpal tunnel syndrome, epineural fibrous fixation, and traction neuropathy. Hand Clinics 7: 491-503.

Indahl A, Velund L & Reikeraas O (1995) Good prognosis for low back pain when left untampered: a randomized clinical trial. Spine 20: 473-477.

Jabre JF (1994) "Nerve rubbing" in the symptomatic treatment of ulnar nerve paraesthesiae. Muscle & Nerve 17: 1237.

Johnston EC & Howell SJ (1999) Tension neuropathy of the superficial peroneal nerve: associated conditions and results of release. Foot & Ankle International 20: 576-580.

Kendall NAS, Linton SJ & Main CJ (1997) Guide to assessing psychosocial yellow flags in acute low back pain: risk factors for long term disability and work loss, Accident Rehabilitation & Compensation Insurance Corporation of New Zealand and the National Health Committee, Wellington.

Koller RL & Blank NK (1980) Strawberry pickers' palsy. Archives of Neurology 37: 320-321.

Lewit K (1985) Manipulative Therapy in Rehabilitation of the Motor System, Butterworths, London.

Linton SJ (1998) The socioeconomic impact of chronic back pain: is anyone benefiting? Pain 75: 163-168.

Mackinnon SE, Dellon AL, Hudson AR, et al. (1986) Histopathology of compression of the superficial radial nerve in the forearm. Journal of Hand Surgery 11A: 206-209.

Maitland GD (1986) Vertebral Manipulation, 6th edn. Butterworths, London.

Malmivaara A, Hakkinen U & Aro T, et al (1995) The treatment of acute low back pain - bed-rest, exercises, or ordinary activity? The New England Journal of Medicine 332: 351-355.

Malone TR, Garrett WE & Zachazewski JE (1996) Muscle: Deformation, injury, repair. In: Zachazewski JE, Magee DJ & Quillen WS (eds.) Athletic Injuries and Rehabilitation, WB Saunders, Philadelphia.

Marinacci AA (1967) The value of the electromyogram in the diagnosis of pressure neuropathy from "hanging arm". Electromyography 7: 5-15.

Massey EW & Pleet AB (1978) Handcuffs and cheiralgia parasthetica. Neurology 28: 1312-1313.

McKinnon ME, Vickers MR, Ruddock VM, et al. (1997) Community studies of the health service implications for low back pain. Spine 22: 2161-2166.

Mellion MB (1991) Common cycling injuries: management and prevention. Sports Medicine 11: 52-57.

Mendoza FX & Main K (1990) Peripheral nerve injuries of the shoulder in the athlete. Clinics in Sports Medicine 9: 331-342.

Moseley L (2000) The effect of neuroscience education on pain attitudes, somatic perception and catastrophising in perople with chronic low back pain. Australian Pain Society Annual Conference. The Progress of Pain , Melbourne.

Mumenthaler M & Schliack H (1991) Peripheral Nerve Lesions, Thieme, New York.

Nathan PA & Keniston RC (1993) Carpal tunnel syndrome and its relation to general physical condition. Hand Clinics 9: 253-261.

Nathan PA, Keniston RC & Meadows KD (1995) Outcome study of ulnar nerve decompression at the elbow treated with simple secompression and an early programme of physical therapy. Journal of Hand Surgery 20B: 628-637.

NHMRC (1998) Acute pain management: scientific evidence, National Health and Medical Research Council, Canberra.

Nobel W (1966) Peroneal palsy due to hematoma in the common peroneal nerve sheath after distal torsional fractures and inversion ankle sprains: report of two cases. Journal of Bone and Joint Surgery 48A: 1184-1195.

O'Sullivan PB, Twomey LT & Allison GT (1997) Evaluation of specific stabilizing exercise in the treatment of chronic low back pain with radiologic diagnosis of spondylolysis or spondylolisthesis. Spine 22: 2959-2967.

Paljarvi L & Partenen J (1980) Biting palsy of the acccessory nerve. Journal of Neurology, Neurosurgery and Psychiatry 43: 744-746.

Ramachandran VS & Blakeslee S (1998) Phantoms in the Brain, William Morrow, New York.

Ramachandran VS & Rogers–Ramachandran D (1996) Synaesthesia in phantom limbs induced with mirrors. Proceedings of the Royal Society of London B. 236: 377-386.

Reisin R, Pardal A, Ruggieri V, et al. (1994) Sural neuropathy due to external pressure: report of three cases. Neurology 44: 2408-2409.

Ringel SP, Treihaft M, Carry M, et al. (1990) Suprascapular neuropathy in pitchers. American Journal of Sports Medicine 18: 80-86.

Roles NC & Maudsley RH (1972) Radial tunnel syndrome: resistant tennis elbow as a nerve entrapment. Journal of Bone and Joint Surgery 54B: 499-508.

Rosenfeld M, Gunnarsson R & Borenstein P (2000) Early intervention in whiplash-associated disorders. Spine 25: 1782-1787.

Rozmaryn LM, Dovelle S, Rothman ER, et al. (1998) Nerve and tendon gliding exercises and the conservative management of carpal tunnel syndrome. Journal of Hand Therapy 11: 171-179.

Sammarco GJ & Stephens MM (1991) Neuropraxia of the femoral nerve in a modern dancer. American Journal of Sports Medicine 19: 413-414.

Sandblom P (1996) Creativity and Disease, Marion Boyars, New York.

Savage R, Burke FD, Smith NJ, et al. (1990) Carpal tunnel syndrome in association with vibration white finger. Journal of Hand Surgery 15B: 100-103.

Scharli AF & Ayer G (1984) Meralgia paraesthetica in kindersalter. Jeans krankheit. Kinderarzt 15: 9-12.

Schon LC & Baxter DE (1990) Neuropathies of the foot and ankle in athletes. Clinics in Sports Medicine 9: 489-509.

Seradge H (1997) Cubital tunnel release and medial epicondylectomy. Journal of Hand Surgery 22A: 863-866.

Seror P (1993) Treatment of ulnar nerve palsy at the elbow with a night splint. Journal of Bone and Joint Surgery 75B: 322-327.

Seward HG & Patrick J (1992) A three year survey of Victorian football league injuries. Australian Journal of Medicine and Science in Sport 24: 51-54.

Shacklock MO, Butler DS & Slater H (1994) The dynamic nervous system: structure and clinical neurobiomechanics. In: Boyling JD & Palastanga N (eds.) Grieve's Modern Manual Therapy, 2nd edn. Churchill Livingstone, Edinburgh.

Shellock FG (1983) Physiological benefits of warm-up. Physician and Sports Medicine 11: 134-139.

Shorland S (1998) Management of chronic pain following whiplash injuries. In: Gifford LS (ed.) Topical issues in pain, NOI Press, Falmouth.

Silverstein BA, Fine LJ & Armstrong TJ (1986) Hand and wrist cumulative trauma disorders in industry. British Journal of Industrial Medicine 43: 779-784.

Sinclair RH & Pratt JH (1972) Femoral neuropathy after pelvic operation. American Journal of Obstetrics and Gynaecology 112: 404-408.

Slater H, Butler DS & Shacklock MO (1994) The dynamic nervous system: examination and assessment using tension tests. In: Boyling JD & Palastanga N (eds.) Grieve's Modern Manual Therapy, 2nd edn. Churchill Livingstone, Edinburgh.

Spitzer WO, Le Blanc FE & Dupuis M (1987) Scientific approach to the assessment and management of activity-related spinal disorders: a monograph for clinicians. Report of the Quebec Task Force on Spinal Disorders. Spine 12: 1-59.

Sternbach RA (1987) Mastering Pain, Ballantine Books, New York.

Stewart JD (1999) Focal Peripheral Neuropathies, 3nd edn. Lippincott, Williams and Wilkins, Philadelphia.

Strong J (1996) Chronic Pain: The Occupational Therapist's Perspective, Churchill Livingstone, New York.

Sullivan MJL, Stanish W, Waite H, et al. (1998) Catastrophizing, pain and disability in patients with soft tissue injuries. Pain 77: 253-260.

Sunderland S (1978) Nerves and Nerve Injuries, 3rd edn. Churchill Livingstone, Melbourne.

Szabo RM (1989) Nerve Compression Syndromes, Slack, Thorofare NJ.

Troup JDG (1986) Biomechanics of the lumbar spinal canal. Clinical Biomechanics 1: 31-43.

Turner JA (1996) Educational and behavioural interventions for back pain in primary care. Spine 21: 2851-2859.

Turner JA, LeResche L, Von Korff M, et al. (1998) Back pain in primary care. Spine 23: 463-469.

Vincenzino B & Vincenzino D (1995) Considerations in injury prevention. In: Zuluaga M, Briggs C & Carlisle J (eds.) Sports Physiotherapy, Churchill Livingstone, Melbourne.

Vlaeyen JWS, Kole-Snijders AMJ, Boeren RGB, et al. (1995) Fear of movement/(re)injury in chronic low back pain and its relation to behavioural performance. Pain 62: 363-372.

Waddell G (1998) The Back Pain Revolution, Churchill Livingstone, Edinburgh.

Waddell G, Feder G, McIntosh A, et al. (1996) Low back pain evidence review, Royal College of General Practitioners, London.

Wittink H & Michel TH (1997) Chronic Pain Management for Physical Therapists, Butterworth-Heinemann, Boston.

Young AW, Redmond AD & Belandres PV (1990) Isolated lesions of the lateral cutaneous nerve of the forearm. Archives of Physical Medicine and Rehabilitation 71: 251-252.

Zoli M, Torri C & Ferrari R (1998) The emergence of the volume transmission concept. Brain Research Reviews 26: 136-147.

Zvulun I (1998) Mobilizing the nervous system in cervical cord compression. Manual Therapy 3: 42-47.

CHAPTER 15

CLINICAL ASPECTS
OF NEURODYNAMICS

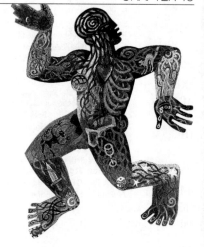

INTRODUCTION

In this chapter, I have selected some commonly encountered clinical syndromes for discussion. The syndromes provide a vehicle for discussion of the integration of aspects of neurodynamics into management, particularly manual techniques. Neurodynamic features are not specific for the disorder discussed, and should be adaptable to other pain states. This chapter also provides a chance to speculate, share clinical findings and make links back to earlier chapters.

When a patient has a neurodynamic test related to his/her pain state (chapter 10), the concept of conservative decompression of the nervous system should be helpful.

CONSERVATIVE DECOMPRESSION OF THE NERVOUS SYSTEM

In a basic but clinically realistic format, your thoughts about disorders involving the nervous system will often focus around "turning nerves off", decreasing the general sensitivity and making sure the problem doesn't happen again. Surgical decompression of peripheral nerves and roots is an accepted procedure. Conservation decompression should also be considered as a procedure. This will encourage a closer look at the variety of techniques to stop nerves firing ectopically and to make them healthier.

Specific guidelines are found in chapter 14, but a general list for conservative decompression would be:

• Decrease the sensitivity of the entrapped or irritated tissue, by removing relevant stimuli (eg. adrenaline, temperature, mechanical, psychological stress) and decreasing the threshold of the CNS (eg. better understanding, goal setting, description of the natural course of the entrapment, yellow flag management).

• Improve the health of the container tissues (eg. remove fluid around nerve, mobilise and exercise muscles, joints and fascia around neural tissues).

• Improve the ability of the whole nerve tract to absorb traction forces, thus assessing and ensuring nerve/container health elsewhere in the limb and/or body if required.

• Assess and improve nerve/container health in a dynamic sense. For example the nerve/container relationship must be healthy through all desired movements.

• Assess and modify any adverse ergonomic or environmental forces.

CARPAL TUNNEL SYNDROME

The example of carpal tunnel syndrome (CTS) is used to demonstrate how the basic science of neurodynamics should encourage a more extended evaluation. Examples of tensioners and sliders and the use of order of movement variations in management are provided. CTS is also a useful syndrome to reflect on the possible local neurobiological effects of mobilisation.

Carpal tunnel syndrome has more written about it than any other entrapment neuropathy, despite being described for little more than 40 years. The reading on sensitivity and specificity of tests for carpal tunnel syndrome is confusing, making optimal management difficult. I hope that this text, particularly the patterns of peripheral neurogenic pain (chapter 3) and the skilled neurodynamics evaluation (chapters 7,10,12) can assist you in picking the true carpal tunnel syndromes. Physical evaluation can be performed much better and should form the basis of diagnosis (Gunnarsson et al. 1997). There are some difficulties with sensitivity and specificity in electrodiagnosis (Rosenbaum 1999). Maybe skilled analytical physical examination could become the gold standard one day?

EXTENDED PHYSICAL EVALUATION

Preliminary studies (Coveney et al. 1997) have already shown the ULNT1 to have high sensitivity and specificity for electrically diagnosed carpal tunnel syndrome. Existing tests like Phalen's tests and the tethered median nerve stress test (hyperextending the index finger at the distal interphalangeal joint with the wrist in supination) (LaBan et al. 1989) can be taken further. To make tests more sensitive, the elbow and shoulder could be added, specific finger movements included and compression could be added to the elongation. This will certainly make the tests more sensitive, hopefully not at the expense of specificity.

I have suggested some tests for an extended physical evaluation of the neurodynamics of the median nerve in the carpal tunnel, based on neurobiology, neurodynamics and existing studies.

• ULNT1 (chapter 12).

• ULNT1 (reversed): should allow the test to focus more on the tunnel and its contents (chapter 12).

• ULNT2 median: shoulder depression components may be more potent than shoulder abduction (chapter 12).

• ULNT2 median (reversed): if the base ULNT2 (median) shows some positivity.

• Compression: (Durkan 1991) (Fig.15.1).

• Compression plus ULNT position.

• Phalen's test (Fig 15.2).

• Reversed Phalen's test (wrist extension).

• Phalen's test in ULNT1 or ULNT2 position.

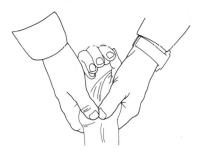

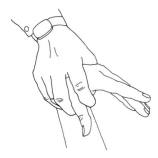

15.1 Carpal tunnel compression test.

15.2 Phalen's test. The test as described by Phalen was to hold the forearms vertically and allow both hands to drop into complete flexion for one minute. In this figure compression has been placed onto the flexed wrist.

Focusing load on individual fingers and the thumb appears clinically worthwhile and is the basis of LaBan's (1989) tethered median nerve stress test. It presumably allows a more specific loading on fascicles and facilitates interfascicular movements. In figure 15.3, I have begun a ULNT1 from the wrist first, focusing on the index finger, thumb and ulnar deviation, all aiming for a better challenge of the median nerve. Variations are also shown in figure 15.4 (reverse Phalen's plus thumb abduction extension plus carpal tunnel compression) and figure 15.5 (wrist extension plus index finger extension plus compression). A further extension could be to sustain a test. Phalen (1966) suggested maintaining wrist flexion for up to one minute. This may be required to replicate a clinical situation dependent on slow ischaemosensitivity. Reproduction of symptoms is the goal. You would expect the ease of eliciting symptoms to equate with the level of symptoms and general physical dysfunction. Thus the test you use should be relevant (chapter 10).

ACTIVE CTS MOBILISATION BASED ON SLIDERS, TENSIONERS AND ALTERED ORDER OF MOVEMENT

As Rozmaryn et al. (1998) acknowledged, conservative management of carpal tunnel syndrome has not been adequately explored. Splinting and anti-inflammatory medications are the mainstay of conservative management. These authors showed that an active exercise programme, including nerve and tendon gliding exercises, was useful in preventing significant numbers of patients with carpal tunnel syndrome progressing to surgery (further details in chapter 13).

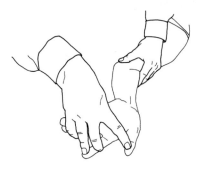

15.3   In a reversed ULNT1, a focus has been placed on the thumb and index finger and wrist ulnar deviation to allow more load and gliding to be placed on the median nerve at the wrist and hand.

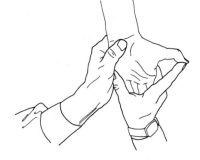

15.4   Reverse Phalen's test, thumb extension plus carpal tunnel compression. This position could be sustained and/or further loading could be placed on the median nerve by adding elbow extension and shoulder elevation/extension.

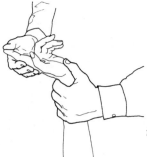

15.5   Wrist extension and supination plus index finger extension plus carpal tunnel compression - an extension on the tethered median nerve stress test.

You can be very creative here, yet still base and adapt any exercises to the reasoned status of tissue health and general sensitivity. Note figure 15.6 and try the manoeuvre yourself. With the wrist in a neutral position, a series of "air slicing" movements will mobilise lots of structures, including the median nerve, without placing too much strain on the nerve in the carpal tunnel or compression by tunnel contents. "Slicing" can be done in pronation or supination. However, if the wrists were held firmly together and then a diving, twisting motion performed (I call it the "busy bee" for want of a better name), then the movement will be more powerfully directed at the wrist and its contents first (Fig. 15.7).

Another more structured exercise is shown in figure 15.8A and 15.8B. In 15.8A, the model has her right wrist and fingers held flexed by her left hand and then in figure 15.8B, this hand position is maintained and then the arm is elevated. In more sensitive patients, you may wish to start with wrist extension/elbow flexion, then extend the elbow and as a progression, elevate the arm. This exercise can also be done for individual fingers, appears clinically worthwhile and has a neuroanatomical base. Many patients with carpal tunnel syndrome perform work involving intense and repetitive hand movements. The rest of the arm needs inclusion in exercises, not only for neural and nonneural arm tissue health but to "feed the homonculi" as well (chapter 2).

In the previous chapter, the concept of slider and tensioner was discussed and some median nerve based functional activities are illustrated (chapter 14, Figs. 14.8A,B,C,D). An example of a slider for the median nerve using shoulder girdle depression, would be to have the patient's arm by her side and as she extends her wrist, she elevates her shoulder. With the basic concept you can become quite innovative.

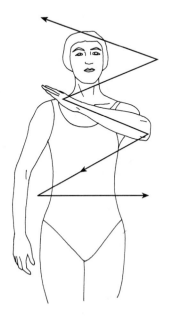

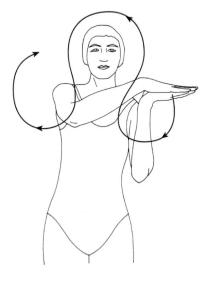

15.6 A mobilisation exercise for the median nerve, limiting the neurodynamics at the wrist.

15.7 Compared to figure 15.6, the mobilisation exercise now emphasises working the median nerve at the wrist.

If I was prescribing active nerve mobilisation for the median nerve I would probably add some ulnar and radial nerve based mobilisation as well. After all, connections between the nerves are common (chapter 8) and the brachial plexus could well be involved in the carpal tunnel syndrome. It wouldn't take much alteration to provide a focus on the ulnar nerve. Some starting positions are shown in chapter 12 (Figs. 12.14 and 12.15). Think of the radial nerve. The active examination techniques described in chapter 12, (Fig. 12.8) provides nice slider movements. Another exercise which could be used for the radial nerve is illustrated in figures 15.9A and 15.9B. The model has internally rotated both hands and locked fingers and then elevated her arms. If she moved to the left, then the right side would be loaded more. These movements could also be incorporated into exercises during pauses in intense hand activity.

THOUGHTS ON THE LOCAL BIOLOGICAL EFFECTS OF THESE EXERCISES?

This is always a healthy thing to contemplate. We are well aware that movement helps many patients with carpal tunnel syndrome (eg. Nathan et al. 1993; Garfinkel et al. 1998; Rozmaryn et al. 1998). But what does the movement do to tissues in relation to their particular stage of healing. And what does it do to the central nervous system in relation to its particular stage of coping. Have a go at reasoning the nature of pathobiological changes that you are trying to alter. It may make you realise the crudity of technique compared to the complexity of the pathobiology. But it will make you think of refining and targeting treatment to reasoned pathobiology.

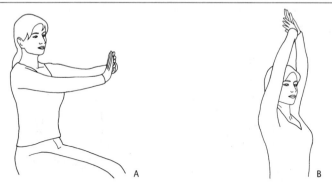

15.8A,B   An easy to perform median nerve mobilisation. A. starting position (or with elbow flexed if sensitive) B. elevation. This test could be performed with individual fingers. See text for further details.

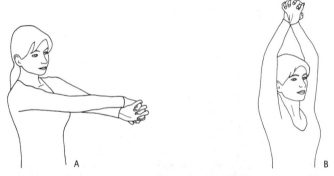

15.9A,B   An easy to perform radial nerve mobilisation. See text for details.

Readers should take any opportunities to view a diagnostic ultrasound of the median nerve and marvel at how it moves and slides during movements. Phalen (1972) was often impressed by the venous engorgement, swollen tissues and congestion in operated carpal tunnels and commented that venous stasis would add further pressure. You can visualise the "milking of the nerve" (Rozmaryn et al. 1998) with movement. There are pressure gradients in tunnels such as the carpal tunnel and the intervertebral foramina (Figs. 15.10 A,B). Neurones in tunnels need nourishment. A pressure gradient exists between the artery and vein so that blood is forced into the tunnel, across blood nerve barriers, and then it must flow out of the tunnel (Sunderland 1978, reviewed in Butler 1991). It is easy to see that tunnel pressure changes (eg. container changes, swollen nerves, scar in the tunnel) will affect venous blood flow and that in some states that gentle mobilisation may be very helpful. Normalising this pressure gradient should remove some of the mechanical and metabolic stimuli influencing ion channels. Movement would presumably also disperse inflammatory soup collected in the connective tissues of nerve, and mechanical constraints on axonal transport systems (chapter 5).

Oedema provides a fertile ground for fibroblast activity. Inflammation and swelling in nerves, especially when intrafascicular, is not easily dispersed as there are no lymphatic channels crossing the perineurium (Lundborg 1988). Movement will naturally help fluid dispersal and it should be beneficial to minimise scar formation. Fibrosis in the mesoneurium (chapter 5, figure 5.5) and consequent loss of the gliding function will mean that the fascicles inside may have to glide more to compensate and thus risk damage. Pathological attachments to surrounding tissues will create foci of mechanical pressure and with intraneural fibrosis, the ability of the nerve to accommodate strain will be affected. A fibrotic area is likely to have consequences for neurodynamics elsewhere along the nerve track. This may be part of the double crush syndrome (discussed later in this chapter. Neural scarring and movement are discussed by Millesi (1995), Sunderland (1978), Lundborg (1988) and Butler (1991). Attention to early movement post injury seems biologically ideal. This can be provided in a spectrum of gentle nerve movements in the tunnel without moving the tunnel to vigorous mobilisation, in an attempt to return the nervous system to its usual physical abilities.

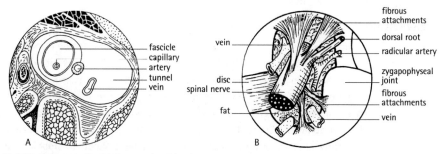

15.10A,B Pressure gradients exist around peripheral nerves.
A. transverse section of the carpal tunnel. The pressure gradient must be artery>capillary>fascicle>vein>tunnel. From Butler DS (1991) Mobilisation of the Nervous System. Churchill Livingstone, Melbourne, with permission.

B. Lateral view of a lumbar intervertebral foramen and an emerging spinal nerve. A similar pressure gradient to the carpal tunnel will exist. From de Peretti F, Micalef, JP, Bourgeon, A. et al. (1989) Biomechanics of the lumbar spinal nerve roots and the first sacral root within the intervertebral foramina. Surgical and Radiological Anatomy 11: 221-225, with permission.

NERVE ROOT COMPLEX

I used to fear patients with severe nerve root disorders, but on reflection it was my lack of understanding of the basic neuroscience underpinning neurogenic disorders which led to the fear. For patients it must be much worse. The features of neurodynamics I wish to highlight here are the importance of evaluation of the container of the nervous system, the value of neurobiological explanations and some thoughts on the neurodynamic evaluation of the more minor nerve root injuries.

IMPORTANCE OF THE CONTAINER AND PINCHING FORCES

Elongation and gliding of the nervous system has been a focus of the physical evaluation of the nervous system in this book. While tests such as the straight leg raise and the upper limb neurodynamic tests are appropriate for nerve root disorders, pinching forces on nerve roots should also be considered. There are what could be called "container dependent " nerve root syndrome presentations ie. the syndrome need changes in surrounding tissues to evoke symptoms. There are also more "neural dependent" presentations, that is placing elongative forces on neural structures will evoke symptoms. Cervical extension evoking cervical neurogenic pain from a nerve root source would be an example of a container dependent presentation while a ULNT or PNF evoking pain would be an example of a neural dependent presentation.

Intervertebral foramina are smaller in extension and ipsilateral lateral flexion (eg. Panjabi et al. 1983; Schonstrom et al. 1989; Yoo et al. 1992). There is space around emerging nerve roots and so spinal extension movements should not be problematic. We can usually star gaze for some time. However, a combination of events may lead to problems in extension. With degenerative changes such as vertebral approximation, disc pathology and facet changes, the likelihood of pinching in extension increases (Panjabi et al. 1983; Penning 1992). Nerve pinching must be quite common as we all get a bit arthritic and it would appear that the contained neural structures require altered sensitivity for the pinching force to evoke pain. Thus an active abnormal impulse generating site (chapter 3) must be present. Ischaemic, mechanical, adrenergic and inflammatory stimuli may combine to form the basis of the pain state. Nerve roots in particular have been shown to be highly sensitive to byproducts of disc inflammation (Saal et al. 1990; Olmarker et al. 1993). Cervical and lumbar containers are discussed in the next section.

CERVICAL ROOTS

In the cervical spine, extension activities will often aggravate nerve root pain. For example, Stitik et al. (1999) refer to a "salon sink radiculopathy", where neck extension (often sustained) caused by having your hair washed can be painful. Single axon recordings during cervical extension/lateral flexion in humans have been correlated with associated pain and paraesthesia (Ochoa et al. 1987). Pinching pains can be nasty and often lead to postural changes. Some of these root pains are shooting and severe and lead to postural changes such as a forward head posture. Fear of what can be a shooting, stabbing, unremitting and electrical pain dictates movement behaviours as much as the pain itself.

Cervical nerve root problems are frequently at C6 or C7, so the lower cervical spine should be examined. As part of the routine evaluation, include lower cervical extension (Fig. 15.11A) and also (if required) a quadrant (Maitland 1986) or Spurling's (1944) test (Fig. 15.11B). I suggest cervical extension and then lateral flexion towards the test side. You can perhaps explore with small ranges of rotation in either direction, while in this position. Be careful though and guide the movement backwards. There is often some distal spread of pain or ache in the nerve root situations. More subtle cases may just show differences between the test on the left and on the right. In this case, other clinical data will be helpful to support a hypothesis of nerve root disorder.

The tissues of the shoulder girdle are also "containers". Elevation of the arm sometimes provides significant relief of low cervical nerve root disorders. This has been noted and referred to as the "shoulder abduction relief sign" (Davidson et al. 1981; Fast et al. 1989). The relief it provides is probably due to shoulder elevation. A pure abduction movement without shoulder elevation as in the ULNT1 will place more load on neural tissues. Gentle axial traction will also frequently ease symptoms. Axial traction, the shoulder abduction relief sign and Spurling's test are highly specific (though not sensitive) for nerve root disorders related to cervical disc disease (Viikari-Juntura et al. 1989).

It is difficult to be specific with neurodynamic tests and individual nerve roots (Kleinrensink et al. 2000), but clinically, you may find ULNT 3 with its bias on lower roots will be more sensitive than the ULNT1. It may also be worthwhile testing from the shoulder first (chapter 12, Fig. 12.17) and positioning the neck first. The neurodynamic tests may not be very sensitive in some cervical nerve root disorders, probably due to neural/connective tissue arrangements such as connections which allow nerve roots to be protected from tensile forces (chapter 5, Fig. 5.4). However, these patients may have pinch sensitive nerve root disorders.

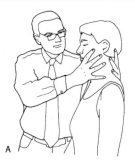
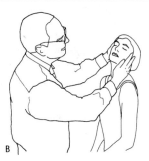

15.11A,B Lower cervical nerve root examination. Testing for pinching forces on nerve roots. A. Low cervical extension. B. Low cervical extension plus ipsilateral lateral flexion.

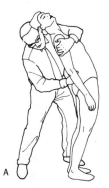
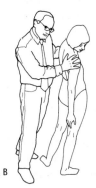

15.12A,B Lower lumbar nerve root examination. Testing for pinching forces on nerve roots. A. Lumbar extension. With my right hand I can focus extension to particular levels. B. Extension plus ipsilateral lateral flexion.

LUMBAR ROOTS

The pattern of acute lumbar nerve root injury is often very clear. Patients may stand with a flat lumbar spine, their knee flexed, listing (often, but not necessarily towards the injured side) and there may be neurological signs. Sometimes they are sensitive enough, or the container tissues are degenerated enough, for both pinching (lumbar extension) and elongation (lumbar flexion) to be sensitive. You need skilled and practised handling here for pinching tests. Pay attention to lumbar extension (Fig. 15.12A and lumbar extension combined with ipsilateral lumbar flexion (Fig. 15.12B). Routine neurodynamic testing will include straight leg raise, passive neck flexion and perhaps a slump test. You will need to break the tests down depending on the severity of the injury.

In container dependent neuropathies, it would be nice to do something for the container as part of the conservative decompression. Dependent on individual presentations, this may be mobilising tissues, strengthening muscles, postural and ergonomic adjustments, gentle traction. It could be rest also, including monitored collar use. In acute nerve root disorders it may not cause any harm to let your patient rest in the antalgic posture while the AIGS settles. Let her rest, with faith in your and her ability to restore tissue health and sensitivity when the appropriate time comes. Most nerve root disorders are likely to have a container component. For the more acute neural dependent presentation, some gentle movements could also be encouraged. This could involve movements from the other side, teasing out neck movements while the arm and body is placed in an antalgic and pain relieving position. Patients with nerve root disorders also require a lot of neurobiologically based education.

NEUROBIOLOGY AND THE NERVE ROOT COMPLEX

If the source is nerve root, then pain and symptoms probably involve a high proportion of peripheral neurogenic mechanisms and the pattern will reflect it (chapter 3). Nerve roots will overlay their own particular variation on the pattern, dependent on spinal level, part of the root complex injured and kind of injury. Dermatomal and myotomal presentations (chapter 9, Figs. 9.2-9.4) may occur although not always. Pain rarely goes to the extremities, although numbness and tingling will (Murphey et al. 1973). In addition to pain, a variety of symptoms emerge, including coldness, shooting and tiredness. It is the horrible and often persistent nature of some nerve root pains, and the persistence and the potential for nerve root disorders to set up chronic pain states including perturbed homeostatic systems which needs consideration.

Traditional manual therapies include collars, traction and mobilisation. Results are variable. On the basis of current neurobiology, we should be able to define the structural and molecular targets of manual therapy better. These patients need education and understanding first. This is a biologically active technique in itself, and in addition it will enhance the effectiveness of any manual therapy technique.

In general, an explanation aims to take away the need for enhanced peripheral and central sensitivity. As far as the injured site is concerned, it is likely that appropriate education will lessen the amount of noradrenaline and other stress chemicals available, and presumably signal cell nuclei that production of receptors for excitatory neurotransmitters such as noradrenaline is no longer required (it really is talking to molecules!). So in general, and adapted where appropriate, try and explain to them what is wrong, provide a prognosis, and provide and discuss options for management by therapists and by patient. Review the evidence based management list at the start of chapter 14. Some key educational points will relate to decreasing fear and catastrophising. Patients need to be told that it will get better, yet have an up and down course to improvement, that fears and anxiety may make it worse, and that others have the same problem. When they have pain and have been told that there is a "disc collapse" tell them that we all have disc degeneration, but the body eventually adapts well. Some short term goals may need to be made and you can make them comfortable about ringing your practice to discuss problems.

Your educational input should take away some of the need for them to be sensitive. Understanding provides control. You may have to wean some patients from biologically incompatible techniques such as repeated manipulation and local treatments to referred pain areas or sites of secondary hyperalgesia.

MINOR NERVE ROOT DISORDERS

A wide spectrum of nerve root disorders exists. We should all be able to pick the hot and acute nerve root disorder very quickly. Sometimes, not only the mechanism (peripheral neurogenic) is obvious but so is the source (nerve root at a particular level). However at the other end of the spectrum is the more minor nerve root injury. Sunderland (personal communication 1989) commented a number of times that there was need for a profession to manage the more minor, yet sometimes debilitating nerve injuries.

There are occasional research reports of minor cervical nerve root injuries attracting convenient diagnoses such as tennis elbow (Gunn and Milbrandt 1976) and shoulder complaints (Mimori et al. 1999). Diagnostic difficulties occur due to the minor nature of the injury, but probably also because there may be associated secondary hyperalgesia and neurogenic inflammation at the ends of the neurones all making a very convincing clinical picture that a tissue dominant problem is in existence. For example, a patient may have a minor but ongoing cervical nerve root problem associated with a tender point on the lateral elbow and a tender spot lateral to the T4 level. Palpation of the spot in the thorax evokes the elbow pain. If the T4 area is treated by manual means, neck and elbow symptoms and signs may ease but only to return some hours later or the next day. You have probably treated tissues underlying secondary hyperalgesia. Skilled fingers may well have identified tissue changes around the T4 area. However these may be due to centrally generated antidromic impulses, or local motor responses or perhaps (being speculative) the value that CNS processing has placed on the T4 area has resulted in allocation of pro-inflammatory immune based molecules to the area. If you were to return to this patient and perform a skilled neurological examination (chapter 9) and use tests which both pinch and elongate neural tissues, you may find that cervical nerve root is the culprit.

Perhaps some of the recalcitrant hamstring injuries could also be minor nerve root disorders.

THE RECALCITRANT "HAMSTRING" PAIN

Neural contributions in patients with hamstring pain, those with especially repetitive hamstring problems and dysfunction have often been suspected and have been demonstrated via slump tests (eg. Kornberg and Lew 1989; Turl and George 1998). But what does "neural contribution" mean in these often problematic patients? We can hypothesise about the nervous system's possible contributions in a number of ways.

A neural injury may have occurred at the same time as the injury which caused the tear (eg. blood around nerve or nerve root) and during healing, scar tissue has developed in the mesoneurium or epineurium. Perhaps an abnormal impulse generating site has been set up somewhere along the nerve tract and is maintaining a low grade inflammation via neurogenic inflammation (chapter 3). Or maybe the nerve injury, (more likely if nerve root) has set up a central sensitivity so that the residual hamstring pain to testing and palpation is actually secondary hyperalgesia. It will still show positive on a slump test. Maybe some of these processes were there before the injury. As all clinicians know, there are many situations where the patient has not "done enough" to actually tear the muscle.

In table 15.1 I have listed possible evaluation techniques, based on neurodynamics theory and the particular anatomy of the lumbar spine. The suggested evaluation will involve all lower limb nerve trunks, positioning the spine "from above" the root level as well as below and be carried out as an evaluation of sensitivity rather than just a pure tissue chase. An evaluation of sensitivity means consideration of both peripheral and central mechanisms.

Neurodynamic tests could show positive for both primary and secondary hyperalgesia. The sensitive movement could be mobilised. I am sure we have treated primary and secondary hyperalgesia in the past without knowing the difference. It may have been the "finding it", which helped. Mobilisation in the case of primary hyperalgesia may well have helped a stiff area of nerve whereas the mobilisation in the case of more secondary hyperalgesia may have comprised signals to that person's CNS, that it was not a threat to experience that pain. In

NEURODYNAMIC TEST EVALUATION	REASONING
Use SLR combinations	
SLR	Base test
Ankle DF/Ev + SLR	Test tibial based fascicles and roots
Ankle PF/In + SLR	Test peroneal based fascicles and roots
Ankle + SLR (as above) + hip MR/Ad	Adding further sensitivity + change relationship to piriformis
Use order of movement	
SLR + ankle positions as above	Neurodynamics are different to above
Hip flex/Adduction + knee extension	Different neurodynamics, loads closer to spine first
Spine positioned (eg. LF) + SLR	As above plus access to intracanal roots and fixation
Spine positioned + Hip flex/Adduction + knee extension	Access to intracanal roots and fixation
Use pinching movements	
Lumbar extension, ipsilateral lateral flexion, combined	Place a pinching force on the nerve roots, evaluate "container dependent" roots
Use pinching movements + tension	
As above plus SLR	Make a pinch sensitive pathology more sensitive
Slump and other combinations	
Sitting slump and slump long sit Plus sensitising additions	More tension forces, added intracanal components
Consider also muscle contraction in test positions, piriformis and strain	Tests nerve/canal relationship dynamically

Table 15.1   Examples of neurodynamic test evaluations for a patient with persistent hamstring pain and suspected peripheral neurogenic contribution.

particular, the experience of having the pain in a helpful clinical environment may have dampened down the meaning of the pain when evoked in the future.

The principles of conservative decompression apply here. In minor neuropathies, use the position that "finds it" as a mobilisation technique. Bio-psycho-social considerations are necessary here. Fear of reinjury, awareness of the younger and faster athlete coming though, the lack of diagnosis and a thorough evaluation could contribute via a number of nervous system processes. An example of a useful mobilisation for a settling nerve root problem is shown in figure 15.13A and 15.13B.

DOUBLE CRUSH – REVIEW OF AN OLD FRIEND

The double crush concept is discussed and updated. Double crush encourages a more global look at peripheral neurogenic pain and the need for multi-tissue evaluation skills. It may also provide explanations for some common pain states.

The double crush hypothesis was originally proposed by Upton and McComas (1973). The basis of the hypothesis was a study of 115 patients with either carpal tunnel syndrome or lesions of the ulnar nerve at the elbow. They found that 81 patients had electrophysiological and clinical evidence of neural lesions at the neck. The proposal was that minor serial impingements along a peripheral nerve could have an additive effect and cause a distal neuropathy. Reversed double crush, ie. nerve lesions at the wrist predisposing proximal neural tissue to injury have been proposed (Lundborg 1988), as have multiple crush syndromes (Mackinnon and Dellon 1988). Upton and McComas (1973) also reported that one of the constraints could be metabolic, for example diabetes. For reviews of double crush see Mackinnon (1992), Simpson and Fern (1996), Wilbourn and Gilliatt (1997) and Osterman (1988).

SOME HISTORY

When I first began to read about double crush and the work of Upton and McComas (1973) and others, and integrate their evidence and concepts into my clinical setting, it was something of a relief. It was at a time when my entire patient clientelle were suffering whiplash or upper limb repetitive strain injury. The neurodynamics concepts were new in the 1980s and I was trying to clinically test their relevance. Positive tests in both patient groups

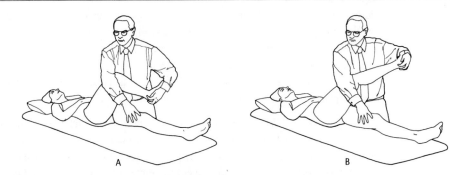

5.13A,B Example of a passive mobilisation technique for a settling nerve root injury.
A. Her knee is well supported on my chest and her foot can be placed in either dorsiflexion or plantarflexion. Her spine can be placed in some rotation or lateral flexion.
B. The mobilisation is through the knee. This movement can be easily converted into a home exercise.

were extremely common and a test such as the ULNT would often reproduce more than one symptom in those with the clinical diagnosis of repetitive strain injury. The double crush concept provided an explanatory model. In particular, it provided an explanation for the spread of symptoms and the coexistence of symptoms. It initiated a concept of dynamic neuropathy and it provided a freedom from the clinically stifling manual therapy rules of the day, which was to examine no further than the site of pain and the nerve root which was capable of referring to that anatomical site. The concept helped to formulate "Mobilisation of the Nervous System" (Butler 1991).

The clinically reasoned impression was that many people were helped by the explanation, active and passive movement strategies and attention to the health of the whole body, which the concept encouraged. I have no doubt that my own youthful exuberance was a major contributor also. However, there was also a group within the repetitive strain injury who did not get better and who were sometimes made sore by physical examinations and who were non-responsive to treatment, or responsive only for a day or so. In retrospect, these may have been patients with significant maladaptive components of central sensitivity or particularly sensitive AIGS sites.

CURRENT THOUGHTS ON DOUBLE CRUSH

The literature on double crush can be confusing. Some electrodiagnostic studies deny the existence of the disorder (eg. Bednarik et al. 1999) and others are are supportive (eg. Golovchinsky 1998). Numerous clinicians and clinical based researchers (eg. Sunderland 1978; Hurst et al. 1985; Osterman 1988; Mackinnon 1992; Goldner and Hall 1997) support the notion. There are also case studies which use the concept to explain findings (eg. Raps and Rubin 1994).

Clinical use of the double crush concept requires some quite judicious clinical reasoning. The failure of electrodiagnostic studies to identify a statistically relevant second lesion is not surprising. The pathological changes behind a second "crush" symptom may be minor and not be picked up electrodiagnostically. Biologically, second crush symptoms may be due to receptor upregulation in the dorsal root ganglion (chapter 3), and increased expression of the proinflammatory cytokine IL-1 and nerve growth factor in the dorsal root ganglia (Yamamoto et al. 1988). Dahlin et al (1987) showed that compression similar to that recorded in the carpal tunnels of patients with carpal tunnel syndrome, will block the retrograde axonal flow and induce changes in the cell bodies in the dorsal root ganglia. In addition the compression will alter the transport of tubulin, an important part of the axonal cytoskeleton (Dahlin et al. 1993). Dellon and Mackinnon (1991) also provided experimental support for the double crush notion in a rat model of nerve compression. They demonstrated that placing a band around a nerve would affect the electrophysiological responses to proximal or distal banding, if the band was placed on simultaneously or at a later time.

I consider double crush to be a useful concept if it can be used in relation to the "big picture" evidence list presented in the previous chapter and integrated into the pain mechanisms reasoning model proposed. It should not be a reason for clinicians to continually find sources of symptoms elsewhere to treat. But it does inspire the linking of symptoms. The explanation that a second pain is "not a new problem but just the old one showing itself" may be gratefully received. There is some experimental support (Nemoto et al. 1987) for the notion that in double neuropathies, all sites of nerve compression should be managed. The concept is useful if it encourages an understanding of whole body health, fitness and understanding. For example, it may help make sense of how a shoulder instability may be a contributing factor to a wrist problem and it may encourage therapeutic movement of the entire limb and body.

Conceptually, double crush could help predict or explain patients who have a poor result after a surgical release of a neuropathy (Osterman 1988; Idler 1996). Generally, the cervical spine could be excluded if cervical extension with lateral flexion to the affected side was clear (see cervical nerve roots above). Although the original concept was based on cervical nerve root and the median nerve at the wrist, the concept can be used elsewhere, for example, thoracic outlet syndrome, associated radial tunnel syndrome (Putters et al. 1992) and sciatic nerve lesions linked with tarsal tunnel syndrome (Augustijn and Vanneste 1992; Sammarco et al. 1993).

Double crush is a very peripheralistic concept. But multiple nerve compression, especially involving nerve roots and unexplained pain will not go unnoticed by the CNS. Or perhaps some sites of sensitivity may only exist because of CNS upregulation (chapter 4) or are maintained by antidromic CNS originated reflexes (chapter 3). Science has yet to confront these issues, but the clinicians need to consider it and reason with it in their daily patient management.

THE FOOT AND NEURODYNAMICS – THE PLACE TO START

When concepts of neurodynamics are new to you, foot disorders are a good place to start. Neurogenic contributions to foot disorders are quite common and are fast and easy to evaluate. It is also a place to challenge some long held diagnostic entities such as heel spur pain.

SPRAINED ANKLES AND THE PERONEAL NERVES

Peroneal nerve involvement, as suggested by positive neurodynamic tests for the nerve is a very common clinical finding in patients with acute and chronic ankle sprains. This has also been shown experimentally via the SLR (Mauhart 1990) and slump tests (Pahor and Toppenberg 1996). Injury to the superficial peroneal nerve during ankle inversion sprains has also been reported by Nobel (1966), Nitz et al. (1985) and Kleinrensink et al. (1994). A recent surgical study by Johnson and Howell (1999) involving eight patients with superficial peroneal neuralgia after ankle sprains, found anatomical abnormalities such as tethering fascial bands which caused radiating pain during ankle plantar flexion.

With a sprained ankle, all nerves of the foot should be assessed. In Pahor and Toppenburg's ankle sprain study (1996), slump tests biased to the tibial nerve (ankle dorsiflexion) and also the test in the neutral foot position were more sensitive on the injured side. This may suggest some degree of central sensitivity to the injury and your slump test input. I suggest performing an SLR first, then perform tests biased to the individual nerves (chapter 11). Then do a slump test with biases to the individual nerves if required. You can palpate these nerves at the feet also (chapter 8) and don't forget to perform a sensory examination as well (chapter 9). The sural nerve (chapter 8, Fig. 8.27) is often forgotten. It could easily be irritated or compressed in post sprain exudate pooling posterior to the malleollus. It is not only ankle sprains, but also Achilles tendon injury and fractures where the sural nerve is worth considering. This little nerve can be easily compressed (Reisin et al. 1994).

Clinically, a patient at, say 2 months post sprain, still with a resistant ankle pain with positive neurodynamic tests can be helped quite rapidly. An appropriate technique could be to place the patient in 90 degrees of hip flexion, add ankle plantarflexion/inversion to the point of pain and then mobilise knee extension. The ankle could also be mobilised in the slump position. It doesn't need to be done vigorously, just teasing into symptoms. Review the guidelines in chapter 14. An initial treatment may involve 2-3 minutes of mobilising. There could be a slight increase in pain for a few days along with better movement, but you have probably disturbed the CNS which was just getting used to a new movement/sensitivity relationship. It may well be therapeutic to perform slump manoeuvres challenging the tibial and sural divisions as well, given the research of Pahor and Toppenburg (1996).

HEEL SPURS

"Heel spur" is an ominous sounding diagnosis with the overtones of "how can a spur of bone be helped". There is increasing evidence of a peripheral neurogenic contribution to some heel spurs, either of the lateral plantar nerve or the medial calcaneal nerve (chapter 8, Fig. 8.28, 8.30) (Rask 1978; Baxter and Thigpen 1984; Henricson and Westlin 1984; Schon et al. 1993). These nerves could also contribute to a diagnosis of plantar fasciitis.

Nonspecific heel pain usually goes with a standard non-operative approach including heel cushions, Achilles stretching and anti-inflammatory medication (Davis et al. 1994). Heel cushions may ease pain by taking off some of the mechanical stretch forces on the tibial nerve. The interest here in a neurodynamics evaluation is in the examination needs to focus on the lateral plantar or the medial calcaneal nerve. It is also a reminder of the importance of ankle eversion to place load on the tibial pathway. Thus ankle eversion is critical and this clinical observation is supported experimentally by cadaver studies (Daniels et al. 1998; Trepman et al. 1999). If only dorsiflexion is added there is a tendency for the ankle to fall into inversion and thus take load off the tibial based nerves. The handling described and illustrated earlier (chapter 11 and figure 11.4) should accommodate the eversion component.

Heel spurs are also one pain state where the exact pain may not be replicated on physical evaluation, but on neurodynamic testing there are clues that something is not quite right. This could be minimal restrictions in range of motion, or symptoms evoked on the problem side but not the "good" side. In some cases, to assist with a clinical diagnosis, it is worthwhile getting your patient to exercise and sensitise the nerve prior to testing.

The suggestion is to assess SLR and also assess ankle dorsiflexion/eversion plus the SLR (chapter 11, Fig. 11.4). Also consider that pronation of the forefoot will place more load on the plantar nerves, especially the lateral plantar nerve. In some patients I have reproduced heel spur pains by starting with the leg off load (ie. approximately 40 degrees of hip and knee flexion), then I have taken up the ankle dorsiflexion/eversion and forefoot pronation, then extended the knee, then flexed the hip. If the position replicates the pain it may be worth mobilising in this position.

The importance of palpating over the proximal aspect of the abductor hallucis muscle and origin of the plantar fascia from the medial tubercle of the calcaneus is mentioned by Schon et al. (1993). Shacklock (1995) encourages palpating the tibial nerve in the posterior tibial tunnel (chapter 8, Fig. 8.29). This could be a useful adjunct to diagnosis and a way of showing the patient that the problem is not a calcaneal spur.

NEURODYNAMICS AND THE THORAX

The slump test in longsitting offers refined assessment and techniques which are not possible with other neurodynamic tests. It is also a gentle way to initiate active mobilisation techniques. Clinical creativity and adaptation to individual patients is possible. The thorax houses a variety of neural structures. The same mobilisation techniques can be used for different sources.

TECHNIQUES AND THE SLUMP LONG SITTING (SLUMP LS)

Like any manual technique, slump LS (chapter 11, Figs. 11.25 -11.28) will place loading forces upon a number of tissues. It will also load a variety of neural tissues including thoracic cord, dura mater, thoracic nerve roots, intercostal nerves, cutaneous branches of the thoracic dorsal rami and the sympathetic trunk. Some judgements about the actual source may be made from history and areas of symptoms. If required, you can review your thoracic neuroanatomy in chapter 5, figure 5.8.

ACTIVE AND PASSIVE SLUMP LS MOBILISATION

Slump LS is a useful position because patients can perform the mobilisations themselves. Even when sensitive, the starting position (Fig. 15.13) takes a lot of pressure off the nervous system and it can be used to encourage movement even when straight leg raise or passive neck flexion are particularly sensitive. In figure 15.14 some thoughts on the variety of techniques available are listed.

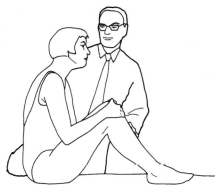

SLIDERS

Cx flexion + knee flexion
Cx flexion + ankle plantar flexion
Cx extension + knee extension
Cx extension + ankle dorsiflexion
Shoulder girdle elevation + knee extension

TENSIONERS

Cx flexion + knee extension
Cx flexion + ankle dorsiflexion (for tibial)
Shoulder girdle depression plus knee extension
As above plus ankle dorsiflexion

IN SLUMP LS

+ lateral flexion
+ rotation
+ rib mobilisation
+ costovertebral joint mobilisation
+ breathing exercises

Any of the above could be combined

15.14 Slump long sitting: examples of active and passive mobilisation techniques.

For stronger mobilisation in the slump long sitting position, passive movements could be added. This could just be an extension of the examination procedures, for example, adding thoracic lateral flexion or rotation or it could be a local focus on a particular level (chapter 11, Fig. 11.27B,C) via a spinous process or a rib. Your working hypothesis in this case would include local tissue dysfunction and a positive relevant slump, SLR or PNF for that patient. Patients will happily accept your techniques if you explain the treatment rationale. Most say it "feels right". Try to convert this to an active mobilisation as soon as possible

A useful technique for local thoracic dysfunction that includes the nervous system, is to perform a flexion mobilisation during the slump LS (Fig. 15.15). This can be performed with the slump LS position adjusted, for example with pillows under your patient's knees as in the figure, or even sitting her over the side of the bed in more sensitive and restricted cases. Some patients with flat thoraces or those with a slight thoracic lordosis may benefit. My right hand, just distal to my carpal tunnel "hooks" onto the spinous process of the joints above the level(s) you want to mobilise. My left hand is on the patient's sternum. Both hands work together during the technique to encourage flexion. The arrows in figure 15.15 exaggerate the directions. If you were trying to get some active input into the exercise you could ask her to extend both her knees at the same time while you were performing the mobilisation.

EXTENSION MANOEUVRES AND THE THORAX

Some upper thoracic pain states can be hard to alleviate. If your clinical diagnosis is that there is some local pathology worth mobilising, then a wedge could be used to provide an antero-posterior (AP) mobilisation for local joints and associated neural tissues. With an AP glide a remarkable amount of intervertebral movement can be appreciated, much more so than with a PA glide. Note figure 15.16. A wedge has been placed at a predetermined thoracic level, in this case at T5. I have cradled my patient's head on my arm (with a little bit of help from my stomach), but the index and ring fingers from my cradling hand are palpating for movement at the edge of the wedge. With my right hand spread wide I now place a downward pressure on the sternum, at the same time allowing her head, neck and upper thorax to go with the movement. Perhaps place a towel or pillow on the patient's chest for a bit more support and patient comfort. Try performing the mobilisation during expiration. If you wish to avoid sternal pressure, have her place her hands on her opposite shoulders and then perform the

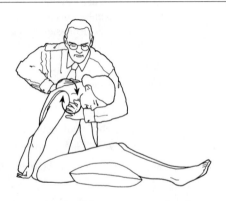

15.15   Thoracic mobilisation in slump longsitting.
See text for details.

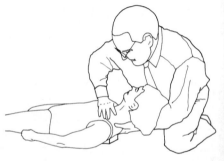

15.16   Antero-posterior pressures to the thoracic
spine via the sternum, using a wedge. See
text for details.

technique via her elbows, with pressures down through the humeri. It's a gentle technique and gentle pressures will elicit a significant amount of easily palpated movement at the intervertebral levels.

In figure 15.17, a wedge based technique on the upper thorax is demonstrated. Note that my left arm is in a similar position to the previously described technique. The ulnar border of my right hand is on her clavicles and I am gently resting the web space of my right hand on her chin. The head and neck move backwards as one and a localised movement at the lip of the wedge should be palpated. There is no need to take any pressures through the jaw. Patients can take wedges home, but it should assist accurate compliance if the techniques can be performed passively first.

These wedge based mobilisations can be combined with nervous system mobilisation if your examination reveals a relevant nervous system dysfunction. In figure 15.18, the thoracic wedge technique has been performed with the legs in a bilateral straight leg raise position. You could also alter the spinal position, by placing the patient in some lateral flexion. In figure 15.19, the upper thoracic wedge technique has been performed, but this time the patient has his arm in some degree of neural loading. Of course, this neural loading could be adjusted to place load on the median, ulnar or the radial nerve.

When positions such as the SLR and the ULNT are added to these wedge techniques, the amount of movement palpable at the edge of the wedge decreases very quickly. Try adding just a small amount of neural loading to your AP wedge technique at first. While there may be an increase in the tension in the tissues there may be motor responses as well to this novel technique. Remember, the central nervous system processing behind these responses is also being treated with your technique.

THOUGHTS ON THE SYMPATHETIC CHAINS

Proposals have been made (Butler 1991; Butler and Slater 1994; Slater et al. 1994) that a physically unhealthy thorax may also involve the sympathetic trunk, rami and ganglia. Since these are continuous tissues, inhibitory and excitatory effects may arise just like in a peripheral nerve. Pain may arise from the trunk itself or be related to tissues that the trunk supplies. This is of course speculative, but attractive for clinicians who continually ask the

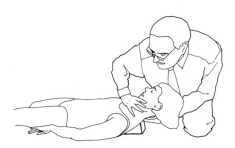

15.17 *Antero-posterior pressures to the upper thoracic spine and the cervicothoracic junction, using a wedge. See text for details.*

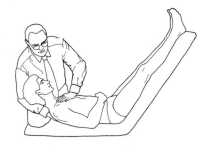

15.18 *Antero-posterior pressures to the thoracic spine via the sternum, using a wedge. Technique performed in some neural loading via bilateral straight leg raises. See text for details.*

question "why?" in regard to symptom presentation, in particular, responses to thoracic manual therapy.

The sympathetic trunk and the axes of movement in relation to the spine have been described in chapter 5 and illustrated in figures 5.8 and 5.9. Lipschitz et al. (1988) and Nathan (1987) documented widespread pathoanatomical changes in and around the sympathetic ganglia and trunk in 1000 cadavers. In particular, it was found that costovertebral osteophytic encroachment upon the trunk occurred in over 60% of cadavers. Nathan also proposed that that excitation/deficits could occur if the system lost its normal mechanics. In this regard it is no different to any other part of the nervous system.

In earlier publications (Butler 1991; Butler and Slater 1994; Slater et al. 1994) proposals were put forward for postures such as ipsilateral thoracic lateral flexion in slump long sitting and cervical flexion (see figure 11.27C) to load the contralateral sympathetic chain, more so if rib mobilisations were performed. Slater et al. (1994) demonstrated that this "sympathetic slump" plus mobilisation of T6 could produce an increase in skin conductance of 200% above baseline values and 50% above placebo measures, thus supporting an increase in peripheral sympathetic activity. Similar results were found when the test was performed on patients with frozen shoulder (Slater and Wright 1995), although there was only a tenuous link to clinical correlates.

The term sympathetic slump is no longer used as it is unrealistic to place such a focus on one tissue. Sympathetic contributions to pain states are more likely to be central nervous system generated. However, arthritic encroachment, open heart surgery, forward head postures, and blunt trauma to the side of the neck may injure the trunk and ganglia. In the big picture, there should be a place for the sympathetic chain.

Neural injury in the thorax has been reviewed in depth in Butler and Slater (1994). In figure15.20 A,B,C, some thoracic based techniques are demonstrated which could be useful for meninges, roots, intercostal nerves and sympathetic trunks. They are also processes to encourage movement, lessen fear of movement and can be quickly converted to an active mobilisation.

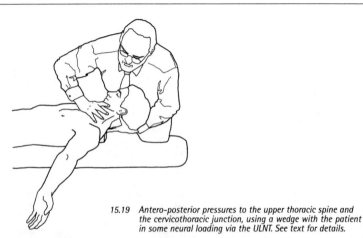

15.19   *Antero-posterior pressures to the upper thoracic spine and the cervicothoracic junction, using a wedge with the patient in some neural loading via the ULNT. See text for details.*

NOTALGIA PARAESTHETICA

Notalgia paraesthetica is used as a reminder that small nerves can hurt and also that some "trigger points" may actually be abnormal impulse generating sites in peripheral nerves.

Notalgia paraesthetica is regarded as a rare compression lesion of the posterior rami of the dorsal roots, usually from the second to the sixth thoracic nerve (chapter 8 figure 8.7) (Pleet and Massey 1978). There may be sensory symptoms in the innervation field, often itchiness, and an association with pigment disorders in the skin. Some suggest the nerve may by irritated by friction from the deposition of amyloid materials (Goulden et al. 1994). A recent report of twelve cases by Raison-Peyron et al. (1999) demonstrated the condition in older people and especially in the second to the sixth dermatomes. Most were associated with spinal disorders and reportedly benefited from electrotherapy. Raison-Peyron et al. (1999) also comment that the syndrome is common. This is certainly the clinical indication. A more minor manifestation of the syndrome may be in the form of an itchy spot or nodule.

Various therapies have been suggested and reported successful, such as hydrocortisone injection and exercises (Narakas 1989), topical application of local anaesthetic cream (EMLA) (Layton and Cotterill 1991) and capsaicin (Wallengren and Klinker 1995). Note that hydrocortisone also acts as membrane stabiliser and will thus suppress the activity in an AIGS as well as being as having an anti-inflammatory effect (Travell and Simons 1984; Devor and Seltzer 1999). This disorder is also a reminder that some trigger points may well be abnormal impulse generating sites in peripheral nerves (Maigne and Maigne 1991).

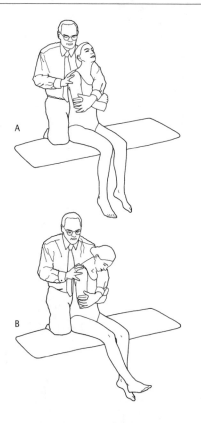

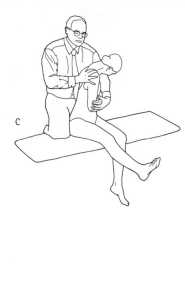

15.20A,B,C *Examples of mobilisation techniques for the thorax using the slump. The patient is guided from a relatively unloaded position in A. through to a neurally loaded position in C. Rotation of the thorax is included.*

The principles of conservative decompression of the nerve can be applied here. These nerves can be examined in the slump longsitting position (chapter 11, Figs. 11.25-11.27). Consider performing the slump LS as the base test and also in ipsilateral thoracic lateral flexion (Fig. 11.27B). If you place your patient in this position and then palpate the emergence of the nerve, you may feel a thickened nodule and perhaps evoke some local or referred pain. The sensitivity to palpation often eases if the neck is put in a little extension or the knee is flexed. If this spot is tender, massage laterally along the nerve, which will probably pull the nerve a little out of the container. This massage may well be therapeutic in patients with a defined and settling or stable local peripheral neurogenic disorder. Treatment of underlying joint and particularly soft tissue stretch and release techniques for the interscapular tissues appears helpful and biologically sound. An example of a self mobilisation technique, useful for the office is shown in figure 15.21A and 15.21B. Try it now. Hold your right knee in your hands. Keep your head relatively neutral. Let your hip relax and the knee sink down taking the upper limb and shoulder girdle with it. Imagine the weight slowly pulling your arms out of their sockets and the flat scapulae parting and sliding around your rib cage. Use breathing. Take a breath and then let the process occur again and again. You can then add cervical flexion to further move and glide the fascia (Fig. 15. 20B). And of course, cervical and thoracic lateral flexion away from the painful side further loads all the tissues, including nerves.

CHAPTER SUMMARY: WHAT'S IN A TECHNIQUE?

Manual therapists have sought a golden click, a magic technique for many years, it's part of the allure of going to a continuing education course. There will always be magic moments in manual therapy, but the reality is that the rapid changes we may see have probably occurred because your patient has rapidly altered the way they think and feel about their problem. Your manual technique and the way you delivered it and timed it, may have been the key to that change. Tissue health recovery is just one important part of it.

I haven 't covered manual techniques for all areas. If I had to, then the book's clinical decision making theme and the push to understand the basic science behind patient's presentations would all be in vain. Once you have techniques, either taught, self constructed or wrested from a research paper, the timing of application, the patient selection, the progression, the allied management strategies are all up to you. Modern and uncorrupted clinical reasoning should be as empowering to clinicians as the results will be to patients.

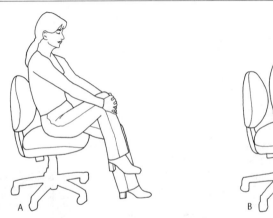

15.21A,B. Mobilisation of the interscapular tissues. See text for details.

REFERENCES CHAPTER 15

Augustijn P & Vanneste J (1992) The tarsal tunnel syndrome after a proximal lesion. Journal of Neurology, Neurosurgery and Psychiatry 55: 65-67.

Baxter D & Thigpen CM (1984) Heel pain-operative results. Foot and Ankle International 5: 16-25.

Bednarik J, Kadanka Z & Vohanka S (1999) Median nerve neuropathy in spondylotic cervical myelopathy: double crush syndrome. Journal of Neurology 246: 541-545.

Butler DS (1991) Mobilisation of the Nervous System, Churchill Livingstone, Melbourne.

Butler DS & Slater H (1994) Neural injury in the thoracic spine: a conceptual basis for manual therapy. In: Grant R (ed.) Physical Therapy of the Cervical and Thoracic Spine, 2nd edn. Churchill Livingstone, New York.

Coveney B, Trott P, Grimmer KA, et al. (1997) The upper limb tension test in a group of subjects with a clinical presentation of carpal tunnel syndrome. In Proceedings: Tenth Biennial Conference: Manipulative Physiotherapists Association of Australia , Melbourne.

Dahlin LB, Archer DR & McLean WG (1993) Axonal transport and morphological changes following nerve compression. An experimental study in the rabbit vagus nerve. Journal of Hand Surgery 18B: 106-110.

Dahlin LB, Nordborg C & Lundborg G (1987) Morphological changes in nerve cell bodies induced by experimental graded compression. Experimental Neurology 95: 611-617.

Daniels TR, Lau JT & Hearn TC (1998) The effects of foot position and load on tibial nerve tension. Foot & Ankle International 19: 73-78.

Davidson RI, Dunn EJ & Metzmaker JN (1981) The shoulder abduction test in the diagnosis of radicular pain in cervical extradural compressive monoradiculopathies. Spine 6: 441-445.

Davis PF, Severud E & Baxter DE (1994) Painful heel syndrome: results of nonoperative treatment. Foot and Ankle International 15: 531-535.

Dellon AL & Mackinnon SE (1991) Chronic nerve compression model for the double crush hypothesis. Annals of Plastic Surgery 26: 259-264.

Devor M & Seltzer Z (1999) Pathophysiology of damaged nerves in relation to chronic pain. In: Wall PD & Melzack R (eds.) Textbook of Pain, 4th edn. Churchill Livingstone, Edinburgh.

Durkan JA (1991) A new diagnostic test for carpal tunnel syndrome. Journal of Bone and Joint Surgery 73A: 536-538.

Fast A, Parikh S & Marin E (1989) The shoulder abduction relief sign in cervical radiculopathy. Archives of Physical Medicine and Rehabilitation 70: 402-403.

Garfinkel MS, Singhal A, Katz WA, et al. (1998) Yoga-based intervention for carpal tunnel syndrome: a randomized trail. Journal of the American Medical Association 280: 1601-1603.

Goldner JL & Hall RL (1997) Nerve entrapment syndromes of the lower back and lower extremities. In: Omer GE, Spinner M & Van Beek AL (eds.) Management of Peripheral Nerve Problems, 2nd edn. WB Saunders, Philadelphia.

Golovchinsky V (1998) Double crush syndrome in lower extremities. Electromyography and Clinical Neurophysiology 38: 115-120.

Goulden V, Highett AS & Shamy HK (1994) Notalgia paresthetica - report of an association with macular amyloidosis. Clinical and Experimental Dermatology 19: 346-349.

Gunn CC & Milbrandt WE (1976) Tennis elbow and the cervical spine. Canadian Medical Journal 8: 803-809.

Gunnarsson LG, Amilon A, Hellstrand P, et al. (1997) The diagnosis of carpal tunnel syndrome. Journal of Hand Surgery 22B: 34-37.

Henricson AS & Westlin NE (1984) Chronic calcaneal pain in athletes: Entrapment of the calcaneal nerve? American Journal of Sports Medicine 12: 152.

Hurst LC, Weissberg D & Carroll RE (1985) The relationship of the double crush to carpal tunnel syndrome: (an analysis of 1,000 cases of carpal tunnel syndrome). Journal of Hand Surgery 10B: 202-205.

Idler RS (1996) Persistence of symptoms after surgical release of compressive neuropathies and subsequent management. Orthopedic Clinics of North America 27: 409-416.

Johnston EC & Howell SJ (1999) Tension neuropathy of the superficial peroneal nerve: associated conditions and results of release. Foot & Ankle International 20: 576-580.

Kleinrensink GJ, Stoeckart R, Meulstee J, et al. (1994) Lowered motor conduction velocity of the peroneal nerve after inversion trauma. Medicine and Science in Sport 26: 877-883.

Kleinrensink GJ, Stoeckart R, Mulder PGH, et al. (2000) Upper limb tension tests as tools in the diagnosis of nerve and plexus lesions. Clinical Biomechanics 15: 9-14.

Kornberg C & Lew P (1989) The effect of stretching neural structures on grade one hamstring injuries. Journal of Orthopedic and Sports Physical Therapy June: 481-487.

LaBan MM, MacKenzie JR & Zemenick GA (1989) Anatomic observations in carpal tunnel syndrome as they relate to the tethered median nerve stress test. Archives of Physical Medicine and Rehabilitation 70: 44-46.

Layton AM & Cotterill JA (1991) Notalgia paraesthetica - report of three cases and their treatment. Clinical and Experimental Dermatology 16: 197-198.

Lipschitz M, Bernstein-Lipschitz L & Nathan H (1988) Thoracic sympathetic trunk compression by osteophytes associated with arthritis of the costovertebral joint. Anatomical and clinical considerations. Acta Anatomica 132: 48-54.

Lundborg G (1988) Nerve Injury and Repair, Churchill Livingstone, Edinburgh.

Mackinnon SE (1992) Double and multiple "crush" syndromes. Hand Clinics 8: 369-390.

Mackinnon SE & Dellon AL (1988) Surgery of the Peripheral Nerve, Thieme, New York.

Maigne JY & Maigne R (1991) Trigger point of the posterior iliac crest: painful iliolumbar ligament insertion or cutaneous dorsal ramus pain? An anatomic study. Archives of Physical Medicine and Rehabilitation 72: 734-737.

Maitland GD (1986) Vertebral Manipulation, 6th edn. Butterworths, London.

Mauhart D (1990) The effect of chronic ankle inversion sprains on the plantarflexion/inversion straight leg raise test (abstract). Australian Journal of Physiotherapy 36: 277.

Millesi H, Zoch G & Riehsner R (1995) Mechanical properties of peripheral nerves. Clinical Orthopedics and Related Research 314: 76-83.

Mimori K, Muneta T, Komori H, et al. (1999) Relation between the painful shoulder and the cervical spine with narrow canal in patients without obvious radiculopathy. Journal of Shoulder and Elbow Surgery 8: 303-306.

Murphey F, Simmons JC & Brunson B (1973) Ruptured cervical discs, 1939-1972. Clinical Neurosurgery 20: 9-17.

Narakas A (1989) Compression syndromes about the shoulder including brachial plexus. In: Szabo RM (ed.) Nerve Compression Syndromes, Slack, Thorofare.

Nathan H (1987) Osteophytes of the spine compressing the sympathetic trunk and splanchnic nerves in the thorax. Spine 12: 527-532.

Nathan PA, Meadows KD & Keniston RC (1993) Rehabilitation of carpal tunnel surgery patients using a short surgical incision and an early program of physical therapy. Journal of Hand Surgery 18A: 1044-1050.

Nemoto K, Matsumoto N, Tagaki K, et al. (1987) An experimental study on the "double crush" hypothesis. Journal of Hand Surgery 12: 552-559.

Nitz AJ, Dobner JJ & Kersey D (1985) Nerve injury and grades II and III ankle sprains. The American Journal of Sports Medicine 13(3): 177-182.

Nobel W (1966) Peroneal palsy due to hematoma in the common peroneal nerve sheath after distal torsional fractures and inversion ankle sprains: report of two cases. Journal of Bone and Joint Surgery 48A: 1184-1195.

Ochoa JL, Cline M, Dotson R, et al. (1987) Pain and paresthesias provoked mechanically in human cervical root entrapment (sign of Spurling). Single sensory unit antidromic recording of ectopic, bursting, propagated nerve activity. In: Pubols LM & Sessle BJ (eds.) Effects of Injury on Trigeminal and Spinal Somatosensory Systems, Liss, New York.

Olmarker K, Rydevik B & Nordborg C (1993) Autologous nucleus pulposus induces neurophysiologic and histologic changes in porcine cauda equina nerve roots. Spine 18: 1425-1432.

Osterman AL (1988) The double crush syndrome. Orthopedic Clinics of North America 19: 147-155.

Pahor S & Toppenberg R (1996) An investigation of neural tissue involvement in ankle inversion sprains. Manual Therapy 1: 192-197.

Panjabi MM, Takata K & Goel VK (1983) Kinematics of lumbar intervertebral foramen. Spine 8: 348-357.

Penning L (1992) Functional pathology of lumbar spinal stenosis. Clinical Biomechanics 7: 3-17.

Phalen GS (1966) The carpal-tunnel syndrome. Seventeen years experience in diagnosis and treatment of six hundred fifty four hands. Journal of Bone and Joint Surgery 48A: 211-228.

Phalen GS (1972) The carpal-tunnel syndrome. Clinical evaluation of 598 hands. Clinical Orthopedics and Related Research 83: 29-39.

Pleet AB & Massey EW (1978) Notalgia paresthetica. Neurology 28: 1310-1313.

Putters JL, Kaulesar Sukul DM & Johannes EJ (1992) Bilateral thoracic outlet syndrome with bilateral radial tunnel syndrome: a double-crush phenomenon. Case report. Archives of Orthopedic Trauma and Surgery 111: 242-243.

Raison-Peyron N, Meunier L, Acevedo M, et al. (1999) Notalgia paraesthetica: clinical, physiopathological and therapeutic aspects. Journal of the European Academy of Dermatology and Venereology 12: 215-21.

Raps SP & Rubin M (1994) Proximal median neuropathy and cervical radiculopathy: double crush revisited. Electromyography and Clinical Neurophysiology 34: 195-196.

Rask MR (1978) Medial plantar neurapraxia (jogger's foot): Report of three cases. Clinical Orthopedics and Related Research 134: 163-168.

Reisin R, Pardal A, Ruggieri V, et al. (1994) Sural neuropathy due to external pressure: report of three cases. Neurology 44: 2408-2409.

Rosenbaum R (1999) Carpal tunnel syndrome and the myth of El Dorado. Muscle & Nerve 22: 1165-1167.

Rozmaryn LM, Dovelle S, Rothman ER, et al. (1998) Nerve and tendon gliding exercises and the conservative management of carpal tunnel syndrome. Journal of Hand Therapy 11: 171-179.

Saal JS, Franson RC, Dobrow R, et al. (1990) High levels of inflammatory phospholipase A2 activity in lumbar disc herniation. Spine 15: 674-678.

Sammarco GJ, Chalk DE & Feibel JH (1993) Tarsal tunnel syndrome and additional nerve lesions in the same limb. Foot Ankle 14: 71-77.

Schon LC, Glennon TP & Baxter DE (1993) Heel pain syndrome: electrodiagnostic support for nerve entrapment. Foot and Ankle 14(3): 129-135.

Schonstrom N, Lindahl S, Willen J, et al. (1989) Dynamic changes in the dimension of the lumbar spinal canal: An experimental study in vitro. Journal of Orthopedic Research 7: 115-121.

Shacklock MO (1995) Clinical Application of Neurodynamics. In: Shacklock MO (ed.) Moving in on Pain, Butterworth-Heinemann, Sydney.

Simpson RL & Fern SA (1996) Multiple compression neuropathies and the double-crush syndrome. Orthopedic Clinics of North America 27: 381-388.

Slater H, Vincenzino B & Wright A (1994) "Sympathetic Slump". The effect of a novel manual therapy technique on peripheral sympathetic nervous system function. The Journal of Manual and Manipulative Therapy 2: 156-162.

Slater HA & Wright AW (1995) An investigation of the physiological effects of the sympathetic slump on peripheral sympathetic nervous system function in patients with frozen shoulder. In: Shacklock MO (ed.) Moving in on Pain, Butterworth-Heinemann, Sydney.

Spurling RG & Scoville WB (1944) Lateral rupture of the cervical intervertebral disc. Surgery, Gynaecology and Obstetrics 78: 350-358.

Stitik TP, Nadler SF & Foye PM (1999) Salon sink radiculopathy. American Journal of Physical Medicine and Rehabilitation 78: 381-383.

Sunderland S (1978) Nerves and Nerve Injuries, 3rd edn. Churchill Livingstone, Melbourne.

Travell JG & Simons DG (1984) Myofascial pain and dysfunction: the trigger point manual, Williams & Wilkins,

Baltimore.

Trepman E, Kadel NJ, Chislolm K, et al. (1999) Effect of foot and ankle position on tarsal tunnel compartment pressure. Foot and Ankle International 20: 721-726.

Turl SE & George KP (1998) Adverse neural tension: a factor in repetitive hamstring strain? Journal of Orthopedic and Sports Physical Therapy 27: 16-21.

Upton ARM & McComas AJ (1973) The double crush in nerve entrapment syndromes. Lancet August 18: 359-361.

Viikari-Juntura E, Porras M & Laasonen E (1989) Validity of clinical tests in the diagnosis of root compression in cervical disc disease. Spine 14: 253-257.

Wallengren J & Klinker M (1995) Successful treatment of notalgia paraesthetica with topical capsaicin, vehicle controlled, double-blind crossover study. Journal of the American Academy of Dermatology 32: 287-289.

Wilbourn AJ & Gilliatt RW (1997) Double-crush syndrome: a critical analysis. Neurology 49: 21-29.

Yamamoto S, Ochi M, Shu N, et al. (1988) Expression of cytokines in the dorsal root ganglion cell body in an experimental entrapment neuropathy. Hand Surgery 3: 175-183.

Yoo JU, Zou D, Edwards WT, et al. (1992) Effect of cervical spine motion on the neuroforaminal dimensions of human cervical spine. Spine 17: 1131-1136.

CHAPTER 16

EPILOGUE

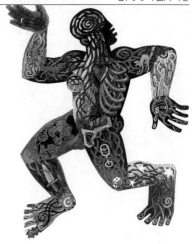

EPILOGUE

EPILOGUE

There is an intriguing and demanding future ahead for the movement based professions, I believe and I hope that intra and extraprofessional forces will lead to a search for greater commonality and a merging of the various manual therapy systems. I have expressed this in figure 1.1.

Awareness of what is common between groups and professions must facilitate mutual growth. Pain and disability come instantly to mind and placebo could also be considered a common central feature in manual therapy as it is in all areas of medicine and anywhere humans interrelate. Definition of the critical manual therapy product is also needed. I believe that the essential tenet common to all fields of manual therapy must be "pathological movement" (chapter 6). This should be the starting point, since it is faulty movement and sensitivity which we manage, not necessarily tissues or structures.

We now know some of the management strategies which can help people in acute and chronic pain. These features must be common to all approaches and concepts. In this book, a system of engaging neurobiology with manual therapy and ultimately altering manual therapy is proposed. It needs overall validation of course, but it is based on the widest possible basic sciences foundations.

There is a theme in this book which I hope has emerged for readers. That is for the movement based professions to maintain the skills of precise examination and management, but to also place their particular movement enhancement skills in a framework which includes evidence based medicine both from basic sciences and clinical trials.

The science of neurodynamics represents only a percentage of the overall message in this book. There is a conceptual approach proposed which could embrace problems in any tissue including nervous system. There is a difficulty introducing and encouraging attention to what may be a new tissue to contemplate in a physical sense. Yet the basic sciences, repeated clinical interpretations and emerging clinical research show that this mobile, sensitive, plastic and often injured structure is worthwhile introducing into clinical strategies. The strategy is no more than a search for the nature and mechanisms of the pain states and the disabilities which may follow. The words "big picture" and "broad perspective" have been used throughout. Neurodynamics must fit within that big picture of overall sensitivity and evidence.

The word "evidence" has been used throughout. We are far from the stage where we can say with certainty that a certain treatment protocol can be followed for a certain diagnosis. But as Matheson comments in chapter 13, being an evidence based clinician is not just blind adherence to the randomised controlled trials. It is becoming a critical user of and contributor to the literature as it relates to our interventions. A blend of reasoning skills and experience is all part of this. Randomised controlled trials have shown that traction does not work for non-specific low back pain. But what are we to do with the woman seeking help who has some nerve root irritation, gets better when lying down, has a feeling the back needs "pulling apart" to make it better, and then says her late husband found traction the best thing for his back? It's the overall outcome not the immediate solution which is important. And traction is a tool to the outcome. Of course I would dust off my traction machine and give her some traction. She may be in the subgroup which exists at a level which randomised controlled trials will never embrace. The traction may be a tool to use alongside other management strategies such as stabilisation and mobilisation exercises and movement enhancing explanations. I may even make the traction more dynamic and get her to perform some neural mobilising while in traction. This clinical creativity would still be defensible in terms of neurobiology and clinical experience.

In my view, the ultimate skill in manual therapy involves harnessing the central nervous system power (call it placebo if you wish) to allow the best possible safe and effective delivery of appropriate manual and educational skills. Those skills will be attuned to all tissues, pathobiological processes and all movements and consequences of injury, and will be a combination of hands on, education, guidance and patient empowerment.

Noigroup.com

Neuro Orthopaedic Institute Australasia have set up a web site with the main aim of creating an active network for discussion and exchange of ideas. Material includes:

• Reviews, case studies, relevant research data, reference lists

• Course schedules world wide

• Discussion forum and feedback page

• Book list with links to booksellers

• Resources

• Product sales

• More things to come

We regularly update the material at noigroup.com, and each time we do this we email a brief summary to all our members. This is like having a bite-sized injection of up to date information to digest each month!

If you would like to be a part of this network please visit noigroup.com and become a member by filling out the membership form or email info@noigroup.com with your details. It is free.